PUBLIC HEALTH LIBRARY

MORPHOGENESIS AND MALFORMATION OF THE EAR

BOOKS PUBLISHED BY ALAN R. LISS, INC.
FOR THE MARCH OF DIMES BIRTH DEFECTS FOUNDATION

Birth Defects Compendium, Second Edition, Daniel Bergsma, *Editor*

BIRTH DEFECTS: ORIGINAL ARTICLE SERIES

1980 – Volume XVI

No. 1 **Enzyme Therapy in Genetic Diseases: 2,** Robert J. Desnick, *Editor*
No. 2 **In Vitro Epithelia and Birth Defects,** B. Shannon Danes, *Editor*
No. 3 **Diet in Pregnancy: A Randomized Controlled Trial of Nutritional Supplements,** by David Rush, Zena Stein, and Mervyn Susser
No. 4 **Morphogenesis and Malformation of the Ear,** Robert J. Gorlin, *Editor*
No. 5 **Dentistry in the Treatment of Genetic Diseases,** Carlos F. Salinas and Ronald J. Jorgenson, *Editors*

See pages 355–356 for other volumes in this series published by Alan R. Liss, Inc.

March of Dimes Birth Defects Foundation
Birth Defects: Original Article Series, Volume XVI, Number 4, 1980

MORPHOGENESIS AND MALFORMATION OF THE EAR

Fifth International Workshop on Morphogenesis
and Malformation
held at Gulf State Park Resort, Gulf Shores, Alabama
Sponsored by
March of Dimes Birth Defects Foundation

Editor: **Robert J. Gorlin, DDS, MS,** Regents' Professor and Chairman, Department of Oral Pathology and Genetics, University of Minnesota, Minneapolis

Associate Editors: **Robert J. Ruben, MD,** Professor and Chairman, Department of Otorhinolaryngology, Albert Einstein College of Medicine of Yeshiva University, Bronx, New York

Harold F. Schuknecht, MD, Professor of Otology and Laryngology, Harvard Medical School, Boston, Massachusetts, and Chief, Department of Otolaryngology, Massachusetts Eye and Ear Infirmary, Boston, Massachusetts

Natalie W. Paul, March of Dimes Birth Defects Foundation

Assistant Editor: **Florence Dickman,** March of Dimes Birth Defects Foundation

ALAN R. LISS, INC., NEW YORK

To enhance medical communication in the birth defects field,
the March of Dimes Birth Defects Foundation publishes the
Birth Defects Compendium (Second Edition), an *Original
Article Series, Syndrome Identification*, a *Reprint Series*,
and provides a series of films and related brochures.

Further information can be obtained from:

March of Dimes Birth Defects Foundation
Medical Education Division
1275 Mamaroneck Avenue
White Plains, New York 10605

Published by:

Alan R. Liss, Inc.
150 Fifth Avenue
New York, New York 10011

Copyright © 1980 by March of Dimes Birth Defects Foundation

All rights reserved. No part of this publication may be reproduced or transmitted
in any form or by any means, electronic or mechanical, including photocopying
and recording, or by any information storage and retrieval system, without permission in writing from the copyright holder.

Views expressed in articles published are the authors', and are not to be attributed to
the March of Dimes Birth Defects Foundation or its editors unless expressly so stated.

Library of Congress Cataloging in Publication Data

International Workshop on Morphogenesis and Malformation,
    5th, Gulf Shores State Park, Alabama, 1978.
    Morphogenesis and malformation of the ear.

    (Birth defects original article series; v. 16, no. 4)

    Sponsored by the March of Dimes Birth Defects Foundation
    Includes index.
    1. Ear – Abnormalities – Congresses. 2. Morphogenesis – Congresses. 3. Deafness – Genetic aspects – Congresses.
I. Gorlin, Robert J. II. Birth Defects Foundation. III. Title. IV.
Series. [DNLM: 1. Ear – Abnormalities – Congresses. W1
BI966 v. 16, no. 4 / WV201 I61m 1978]
RG626.B63 vol. 16, no 4 [RF187] 616'.043s [617.8'043]
ISBN 0-8451-1038-1   80-18892

Printed in the United States of America

The **March of Dimes Birth Defects Foundation** is dedicated to the goal of preventing birth defects and ameliorating their consequences for patients, families, and society.

As part of our efforts to achieve these goals, we sponsor or participate in a variety of scientific meetings where all questions relating to birth defects are freely discussed. Through our medical education program we speed the dissemination of information by publishing the proceedings of these and other meetings. From time to time, we also reprint pertinent journal articles to help achieve our goal. Now and then, in the course of these articles or discussions, individual viewpoints may be expressed which go beyond the purely scientific and into controversial matters. It should be noted, therefore, that personal viewpoints about such matters will not be censored but this does not constitute an endorsement of them by the **March of Dimes Birth Defects Foundation**.

Contents

Participants ix

Preface
   Robert J. Gorlin xi

Morphogenesis and Malformation of the Ear:
An Overview
   Robert J. Ruben 1

Ontogenic Aspects of Mammalian Inner Ear
Development
   Thomas R. Van De Water, Cheuk W. Li,
   Robert J. Ruben, and Cathy A. Shea 5

Dysmorphogenesis of the Inner Ear
   Harold F. Schuknecht 47

Discussion of Inner Ear Anomalies — Reply to
Dr. Schuknecht
   Isamu Sando 73

Biochemistry of the Inner Ear
   Ruediger Thalmann, Daniel C. Marcus, and
   Isolde Thalmann 83

Glutamate Mimics the Afferent Transmitter in the
Xenopus laevis Lateral Line
   Richard P. Bobbin and Dorothy N. Morgan 107

Morphogenesis and Malformation of Otoconia: A Review
   David J. Lim 111

The Morphogenesis of the Middle and External Ear
   Thomas R. Van De Water, Paul F. Maderson, and
   Tina F. Jaskoll 147

Pathoembryology of the Middle Ear
   Joseph B. Nadol, Jr. 181

Discussion of Middle Ear Anomalies—Reply to Dr. Nadol
   Isamu Sando 211

Assessment and Consequence of Malformation
of the Middle Ear
   LaVonne Bergstrom 217

Genetic Malformations of the Inner Ear in the Mouse
and in Man
  Malkiat S. Deol 243

The Genetic Analysis of Profound Prelingual Deafness
  Walter E. Nance 263

Neurophysiology of Auditory Deprivation
  Ben M. Clopton 271

Microtia–Clinical Observations
  Jon M. Aase 289

Ear Muscles and Ear Form
  David W. Smith and Hirotada Takashima 299

The Etiology of External Ear Malformations and Its
Relation to Abnormalities of the Middle Ear, Inner Ear,
and other Organ Systems
  Michael Melnick 303

Intervention in Mild-to-Moderate Conductive and
Sensorineural Hearing Losses
  Charles I. Berlin 333

Concluding Remarks of Chairman Ruben,
Schuknecht, and Gorlin 347

Index 349

Participants

Jon M. Aase, MD, Associate Professor, Department of Pediatrics, University of New Mexico School of Medicine, Albuquerque, New Mexico 87131 [289]

LaVonne Bergstrom, MD, FACS, Associate Professor of Surgery, Division of Head and Neck, UCLA School of Medicine, Los Angeles, California 90024 [217]

Charles I. Berlin, PhD, Kresge Hearing Research Laboratory of the South, Department of Otorhinolaryngology and Biocommunication, Louisiana State University Medical Center, New Orleans, Louisiana 70119 [333]

Richard P. Bobbin, PhD, Kresge Hearing Research Laboratory of the South, Department of Otorhinolaryngology and Biocommunication, Louisiana State University Medical Center, New Orleans, Louisiana 70119 [107]

Ben M. Clopton, PhD, Associate Professor, Department of Otolaryngology, University of Washington School of Medicine, Seattle, Washington 98195 [271]

Malkiat S. Deol, PhD, DSc, Department of Genetics and Biometry University College London, Wolfson House, London NW1 2 HE, England [243]

Robert J. Gorlin, DDS, MS, Regents' Professor and Chairman, Department of Oral Pathology and Genetics, University of Minnesota, Minneapolis, Minnesota 55455 [xi, 347]

David J. Lim, MD, Professor and Director, Otological Research Laboratories, The Ohio State University Hospitals, Columbus, Ohio 43210 [111]

Michael Melnick, DDS, MS, Laboratory for Developmental Biology, Andrus Gerontology Center, University of Southern California, Los Angeles, California 90007 [303]

Joseph B. Nadol, Jr., MD, Assistant Professor of Otolaryngology, Massachusetts Eye and Ear Infirmary, Boston, Massachusetts 02114 [181]

Walter E. Nance, MD, PhD, Professor and Chairman, Department of Human Genetics, Medical College of Virginia, Virginia Commonwealth University, Richmond, Virginia 23298 [263]

Isabelle Rapin, MD, Professor of Neurology and Pediatrics, Albert Einstein College of Medicine of Yeshiva University, Bronx, New York 10461

Robert J. Ruben, MD, Professor and Chairman, Department of Otorhinolaryngology Albert Einstein College of Medicine of Yeshiva University, Bronx, New York 10461 [1, 347]

Isamu Sando, MD, DMS, Director, Division of Otopathology, Department of Otolaryngology, Eye and Ear Hospital, Pittsburgh, Pennsylvania 15213 [211]

The number in brackets following each participant's name is the opening page number of that author's paper.

x / Participants

Harold F. Schuknecht, MD, Professor of Otology and Laryngology, Harvard Medical School, Boston Massachusetts 02114, and Chief, Department of Otolaryngology, Massachusetts Eye and Ear Infirmary, Boston, Massachusetts 02114 [47, 347]

David W. Smith, MD, Professor of Pediatrics, University of Washington School of Medicine, Seattle, Washington 98195 [299]

Prof. Dr. Heinrich Spoendlin, Universitätsklinik für Hals-, Nasen- und Ohrenkrankheiten, Anichstrasse 35, A-6020 Innsbruck, Austria

Isolde Thalmann, MA, Department of Otolaryngology, Washington University School of Medicine, St. Louis, Missouri 63110 [83]

Ruediger Thalmann, MD, Professor of Otolaryngology, Washington University School of Medicine, St. Louis, Missouri 63110 [83]

Thomas R. Van De Water, PhD, Director, Developmental Otobiology Laboratory, Rose F. Kennedy Center, Albert Einstein College of Medicine of Yeshiva University, Bronx, New York 10461 [5, 147]

Ralph J. Wedgwood, MD, Professor and Head, Division of Arthritis/Immunology, Department of Pediatrics, University of Washington School of Medicine, Seattle, Washington 98195

Preface

Each year about 3,000 infants with profound hearing loss are born in the United States. Between 35 and 50% have a single gene etiology and probably over one-third of these cases are syndromal, ie associated in a pattern with other anomalies. Hereditary deafness is thus not rare. The development and functions of the ear are dependent upon hundreds or even thousands of genes interacting with each other and with the intra- and extrauterine environment. The form of the pinna, for example, is dependent upon many genes, but it may be grossly altered by single-gene mutation. The same applies to the external auditory canal, the ossicles, the oval window, the eustachian tube, the bony and membranous labyrinth, the semicircular canals, the utricle and saccule, and the auditory nerve. It is likely that the perilymph-endolymph balance and cochlear antigens are also under genetic control. It is thus surprising that as of this writing I know of but a single school that employs a full-time human geneticist for study of genetic hearing disorders. The encasement of the ear in one of the most dense bones has inhibited study of its biochemistry, both embryonal and postnatal. Growth of otocysts in tissue culture is one step in the right direction, but the milieu, being artificial, in no way guarantees that findings are necessarily valid for normal development.

The purpose of the Fifth International Workshop on Morphogenesis and Malformation: the Ear, sponsored by The National Foundation and held at Gulf Shores State Park, Alabama, was to forge a synthesis of our knowledge concerning ear morphogenesis and dysmorphology. What is not known – the obvious and not so evident lacunae – was also emphasized by the participants.

We are indebted for the success of the meeting to many individuals: Dr. Daniel Bergsma of the National Foundation, who together with Dr. Jan Langman, Dr. Ralph Wedgwood, Dr. David Smith, and Dr. Sydney Gellis conceived of these conferences; Dr. Robert Ruben and Dr. Harold Schuknecht, who moderated and edited the first and second days of the conference, respectively; Virginia Hansen, who recorded, edited, hosted, chauffeured and worried lest the success of the conference not meet her high expectations; and Natalie Paul, who so conscientiously put it all together into this volume.

Robert J. Gorlin, DDS, MS

Morphogenesis and Malformation of the Ear : An Overview

Robert J. Ruben, MD

Knowledge is the most valuable and least tangible of man's wealth. During this conference we are going to add to our own knowledge and, consistent with laws which govern our minds, we will individually and collectively synthesize new knowledge, thus adding to the store of this essential resource. It is, in this context, a privilege and a responsibility to open the conference with these thoughts concerning the morphogenesis of the ear and its clinical import. Our purpose is really the symbiotic relationship between scientific endeavor and clinical medicine.

Scientific endeavor has as its rationale the creation of knowledge for knowlege's sake. Clinical medicine's rationale is that of prevention, cure, and care of disease. Both of these motivating constructs share this: they are limited by the existing concepts of causality. The scientists will choose their problems and will, as the questions are proposed, carry out investigations which are limited by their conceptualizations of causality. Thus, the psychoacoustician will ask what sounds are discerned by the entire organism: the neurophysiologist will ask how does a nerve react to sound; the anatomist will ask what portion of the organism is needed to react to the sound: and the molecular biologist will ask what are the molecular changes which come about in response to the sound.

The concept of causality is also operative in the elucidation of knowledge in clinical medicine. Causality in clinical medicine is emergent from the corpus of available scientific information and this is our constraint. Examination of development of the three constructs of clinical medicine — prevention, cure, and care — in the study of the ear over the last century, demonstrates this principle. For example, there was almost no prevention of congenital deafness 100 years ago. Today, prevention of congenital deafness is practiced in a number of different ways including vaccination for rubella, genetic counseling, prenatal treatment of kernicterus, etc.

The cure of deafness a century ago, also was nonexistent. Today, our level of cure has modestly improved in that there are various surgical and medical interventions which will correct an underlying defect. However, it can be argued that some of these cures, for example a stapedectomy for otosclerosis, are really sophisticated types of care, since the intervention only corrects the phenotypic expression of the disease and not the fundamental process. There are still no cures for deafness which is characterized as sensorineural. The area of care during the last century has progressed from the practices of using ear trumpets, incising and draining of abscesses, using tuning forks, and (for the most part) institutionalizing the congenitally deaf. Today was have a large number of medical and surgical interventions for care: hearing aids, psychophysical and physiologic measures of hearing in man, and an earnest (if somewhat unsuccessful) structure for the education and socialization of the deaf.

The deficiency for clinical medicine, the factor limiting effective intervention, is the absence of knowledge, in almost all areas, of causality of the processes that result in deafness. The only area in which there is a substantial amount of knowledge, and this is far from complete, is in the pathology of the temporal bone. In biochemistry, molecular biology, embryology, physiology, genetics, study of deprivation, psychoacoustics of the abnormal ear, and epidemiology, our conceptualization of causality is insufficient. But congenital deafness results in the most severe form of morbidity. The effects of congenital deafness on linguistic, cognitive, economic, social, and psychologic functions — effects detrimental to the individual, family, and society — are well known.

In addition, there is one way of looking at congenital deafness which is not generally appreciated. Currently, the term "congenitally deaf" is used to describe a person who has a significant hearing loss at the time of birth. A broader and truer definition of congenital deafness includes all those cases of patients who lose hearing later in life due to an abnormality which was present at birth. This broader definition includes all the genetic deafnesses and also many of the craniofacial malformations which result in hearing loss. The expansion of the definition of congenital deafness that recognizes problems in later life as the result of processes that began before birth serves to further define the importance of genetic deafness and underlines the need to develop a scientific foundation of knowledge upon which clinical medicine can build efficacious systems of interventions for prevention, cure, and care.

During this conference several fundamental concepts will be articulated which should enable clinical medicine to become more effective. There will be other information for which there may not be any direct clinical utilization at this time. One would expect, as other information is obtained by various scientific endeavors, that this information, too, will eventually be utilized by clinical medicine.

Fundamental to our scientific consideration are studies of the mechanisms which control the normal, orderly development of the ear. Up to this time most of our scientific effort has examined the development of the inner ear. Scientists working in this area have already sought knowledge concerning not only what is responsible for the development of the inner ear, but what it is that the developing inner ear controls in its turn. Through the work of many scientists, including a number of the participants present, it is now apparent that there is a dialogue between the developing inner ear and the developing central nervous system. The developing central nervous system has a profound effect on the normal development of the inner ear; if there is a defect in part of the developing CNS, then there will be a defect in the associated inner ear. Conversely, the development of the central nervous system, both pre- and postnatally, is affected by the presence of the inner ear, by the reception of sound, or both. If the inner ear is defective, or if there is a decrease in the auditory input to the developing CNS, anatomic changes within the CNS will result. These anatomic changes effect associated physiologic and behavioral deficiencies.

The evidence for the brain/ear dialogue can be found, in hindsight, from clinical pathologic studies of the human inner ear performed at the turn of the century, and probably in the persistent failure of the prelingually deaf to develop normal language since the beginning of history. The scientific evidence for the ear/brain dialogue is constantly demonstrated when studied from the point of view of several different definitions of causality. The evidence that the developing central nervous system influences the developing inner ear has been shown by genetic and anatomic studies, and studies on cultured inner ears. That the inner ear affects the developing CNS has been shown by means of embryologic, anatomic, physiologic and behavioral investigations. The ramifications of this knowledge are significant. The answer to any scientific question results in more questions being asked. Scientists are now further defining the anatomic, physiologic, and behavioral effects of this dialogue. Further elucidation of the controlling genetic, molecular, and chemical processes is needed.

Clinical medicine can use and is utilizing this new knowledge in effecting its ends. Understanding of the ear/brain dialogue offers the opportunity to define mechanisms that result in prevention of deafness. More pragmatically, the recognition of the dialogue is bringing about strategies of intervention that may prevent some of the sequelae of congenital deafness. In initiation of early intervention and in the design of habilitative strategies that can circumvent or prevent the abnormalities of the central nervous system that result from congenital hearing loss, knowledge of the ear/brain dialogue has significantly lessened the constraints of ignorance for clinical medicine, and has added a new dimension in the prevention, cure, and care of deafness.

The effect of these scientific investigations, done initially in an Italian farmhouse and further carried out in laboratories in London, Seattle, New Haven, Richmond, Bethesda, New Orleans, New York, and other places, will be, in the broadest sense, the enrichment of the lives of many people. This is just one example of the excitement, joy, and sense of purposefulness which are the results of the symbiotic relationship of science and clinical medicine. The study of morphogenesis, in all of its aspects, has its own intrinsic justification. Furthermore, it provides the essential resource for those in clinical medicine to fulfill their purpose.

Ontogenic Aspects of Mammalian Inner Ear Development*

Thomas R. Van De Water, PhD, Cheuk W. Li, PhD, Robert J. Ruben, MD, and Cathy A. Shea, MS

INTRODUCTION

The ontogeny of the vertebrate inner ear was first studied by classic anatomic descriptive techniques. These early anatomic reports, as well as later reports of experimental surgical manipulation of otic anlage in submammalian vertebrate embryos, have been reviewed by Van De Water and Ruben [1] in a chapter on organogenesis of the ear in "Scientific Foundations of Otolaryngology." The most comprehensive analysis delineating mechanisms of otic embryogenesis in amphibian larvae is the classic presentation of Yntema [2]. His report showed 2 overlapping waves of induction, a mesodermal followed by a neural, and it plotted the response of the competent otic ectoderm as measured by histodifferentiation. Perhaps the first application of organ culture to analysis of otic development was done in 1959 by Chuang [3] at the Institute of Experimental Biology in China, employing explants of amphibian rhombencephalon and adjacent epidermis to demonstrate the importance of neural induction. Friedmann and associates [4–6] used organ cultures of chick otocysts as a model ear to study ototoxicity. Benoit [7] demonstrated in organ cultures of isolated periotic mesenchyme of chick embryos that crude extracts of chick embryonic otocysts prepared in a normal saline solution could induce this mesenchyme to undergo chondrogenesis. Orr [8] performed experiments using dissociation/reaggregation techniques with chick otocysts and observed in the otic reaggregates differentiating in vitro an association between the presence of mesenchyme and ectoderm and the differentiation of ectodermal sensory structures.

The developmental biologic technique of organ culture of the inner ear was first reported by Fell [10] in 1928, using otocysts extirpated from an avian em-

---

*The investigations were supported in part by grants from the National Institute of Neurological, Communicative Disorders and Strokes (2-R01-NS-08365), the March of Dimes Birth Defects Foundation, the Deafness Research Foundation, and the Nebur Trust Fund.

bryo. Organ culture of a mammalian inner ear was first applied to analysis of the factors influencing ontogeny of the inner ear by Van De Water and Ruben [9]. At present this provides a model system with which the mechanisms that control normal development and congenital malformation of the inner ear may be investigated. The following presentation reports the current state of knowledge of mechanisms influencing ontogeny of the mammalian inner ear as derived from organ culture experiments and discusses experimental data on the subjects of a) neurotrophic interactions, b) experiments on endolymphatic duct and sac anlage, c) fate mapping, d) neural induction, and e) epithelial/mesenchymal interactions.

DISCUSSION OF EXPERIMENTAL DATA

Neurotrophic Interactions

Trophic interactions are best defined as interactions between nerves and other cells which initiate or control molecular modification in the other cells and/or the neuron. The earliest observations by Todd [11] of a trophic influence were made in regenerating amphibian limbs. Farbman [12] has demonstrated the trophic effect of gustatory nerve ganglia upon the development of the taste buds in organ cultured explants of fetal tongue. The relationship between the statoacoustic ganglion and the developing sensory structures of the labyrinth was an unresolved question. Aspects pro and con have been presented by Van De Water and Ruben [1], and more recently by Van De Water [13].

An experiment was designed to answer the question whether or not the neural elements of the statoacoustic ganglion complex exert a trophic effect upon the development of sensory structures within organ cultured explants of mouse embryonic otic anlage. A detailed report of this experiment has been reported [13]. Embryonic otic anlage with associated cephalic mesenchyme and statoacoustic ganglion complex were excised from CBA/C57 mouse embryos of 11, 12, and 13

Fig. 1. Ventromedial wall of an 11-day-old mouse embryo at the time of explantation in vitro. No nerve fibers are present. (×500) (Figs. 1–10 from Van De Water TR: Effects of removal of the statoacoustic ganglion complex upon the growing otocyst. Ann Otol Rhinol Laryngol 85 (Suppl 33):1–32, 1976, with permission.)

Fig. 2. Ventromedial wall of a 12-day-old mouse embryo inner ear anlage at the time of explantation in vitro. A few pioneering nerve fibers are present in the wall of the inner ear anlage. A portion of the statoacoustic ganglion is present. (×500)

Fig. 3. Ventromedial wall of a 13-day-old mouse embryo inner ear anlage at the time of explantation in vitro. Several fascicles of nerve fibers are penetrating into presumptive sensory areas of the inner ear anlage. A portion of the statoacoustic ganglion is present. (×500)

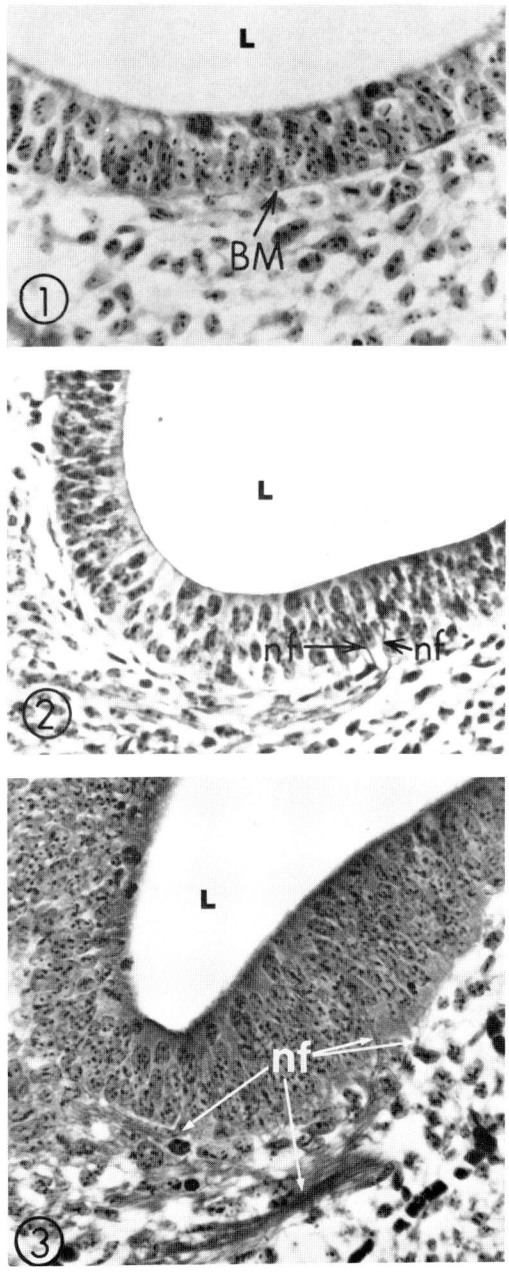

days' gestation. These explanted inner ears of each gestational age group were further divided into 2 groups: the first group, "A" (with statoacoustic ganglion), were explanted to the organ culture system [9] without further surgical intervention; the second group, "B" (without statoacoustic ganglion), underwent further microsurgical manipulation during which their statoacoustic ganglion complexes were dissected away prior to explantation in vitro.

The explanted otic anlage were grown in identical organ culture systems; the "A" (with) and "B" (without statoacoustic ganglion) cultures were organ-cultured in separate culture dishes to control for possible inductive factors that could be transmitted via the organ culture medium. The explanted inner ears were allowed to develop in the organ culture environment until the equivalent of gestational day 21 in vivo was reached for each gestational age group; all cultures were then fixed, histologically processed, and stained with a stain for nerve fibers (Bodian's protargol), in combination with a stain for glycoprotein membranes (Schiff's periodic acid). Specimens were code-labeled and then scored for light microscopic evidence of histodifferentiation of sensory structures and morphogenesis. Light micrographs of cross-sections of the ventromedial walls of otocysts of 11, 12, and 13 gestational days at the time of explantation in vitro are seen respectively in Figures 1–3.

These 3 gestational age groups represent 3 distinct stages of interaction between neural elements of the statoacoustic ganglion complex and the ectodermal cells which compose these otocysts. Photomicrographs of explanted 11-day-old otocysts of groups "A" (with) and "B" (without) are seen in Figure 4. The in vitro morphogenesis of the 11-day-old otocysts is somewhat variable, but given this variability, the morphogenesis of these explanted otocysts of Figure 4 after 10 days in vitro is similar in the 2 groups. Maculae of vestibular sensory hair cells that developed in the explanted 11-day-old otocysts of groups "A" and "B" are shown to be of similar character in the photomicrographs in Figure 5. Explanted 12-day-old otocysts from groups "A" and "B" are illustrated in Figure 6. The morphogenesis of these 12-day-old otocysts is of a more consistent character and, as can be seen in the photomicrographs of the explants after 9 days in vitro, the morphogenesis that occurred in the explants from groups "A" and "B" was very similar in character. Cristae that developed in the 12-day-old otocysts from groups "A" and "B" after 9 days in vitro are presented in Figure 7. These cristae are essentially similar in character and in level of cytodifferentiation of sensory hair cells.

The photomicrographs of Figure 8 illustrate the in vitro morphogenesis of the explanted 13-day-old otic anlage of specimens from groups "A" and "B." The morphogenesis of the explants of both groups is very similar in character, as was seen in the 12-day-old specimens of Figure 6. Formations of the organ of Corti in 13-day-old explants from groups "A" and "B" that developed for 8 days in vitro

Mammalian Inner Ear Development / 9

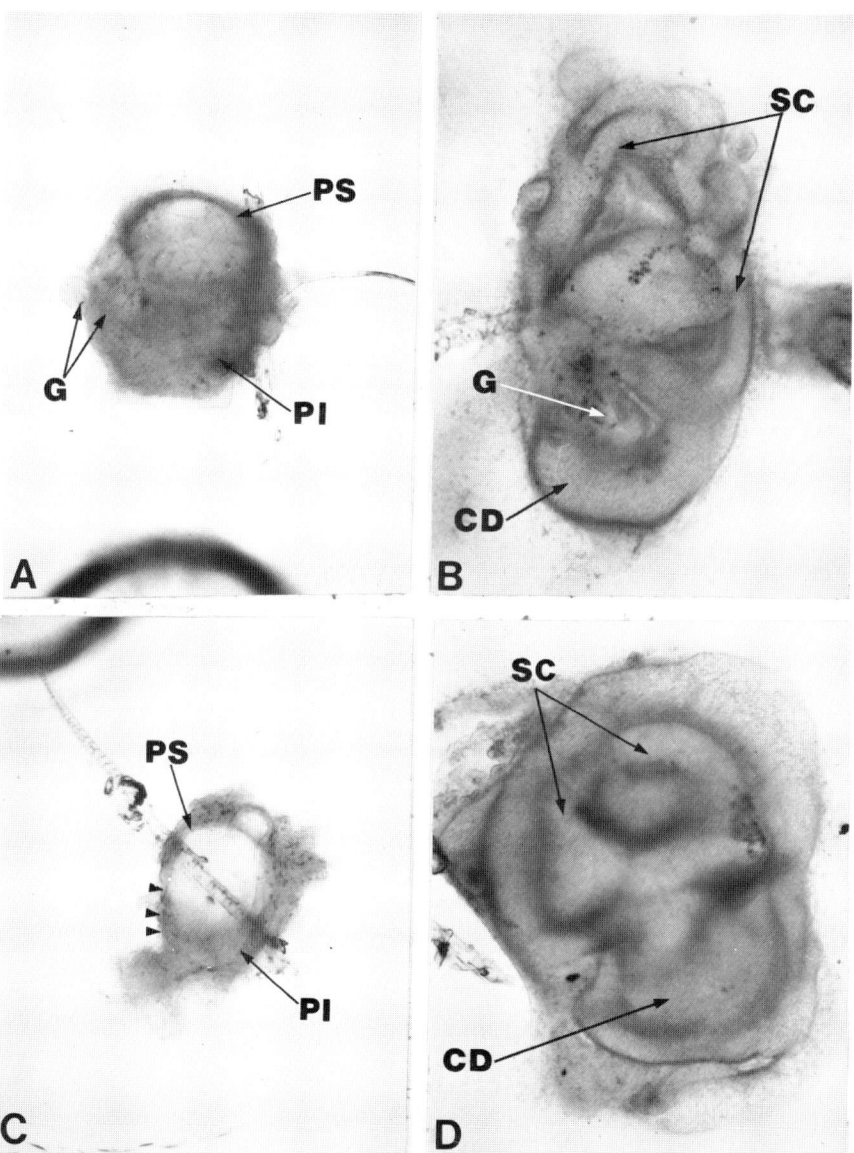

Fig. 4. Photomicrographs of living explants of 11-day-old mouse embryo otocysts after: A and C) 0 hours in vitro; B and D) 10 days in vitro. The culture in A and B has an intact statoacoustic ganglion complex. The culture in C and D has had its statoacoustic ganglion complex excised prior to explantation in vitro. Three arrowheads in B denote the site of excision of the ganglion complex. (×50)

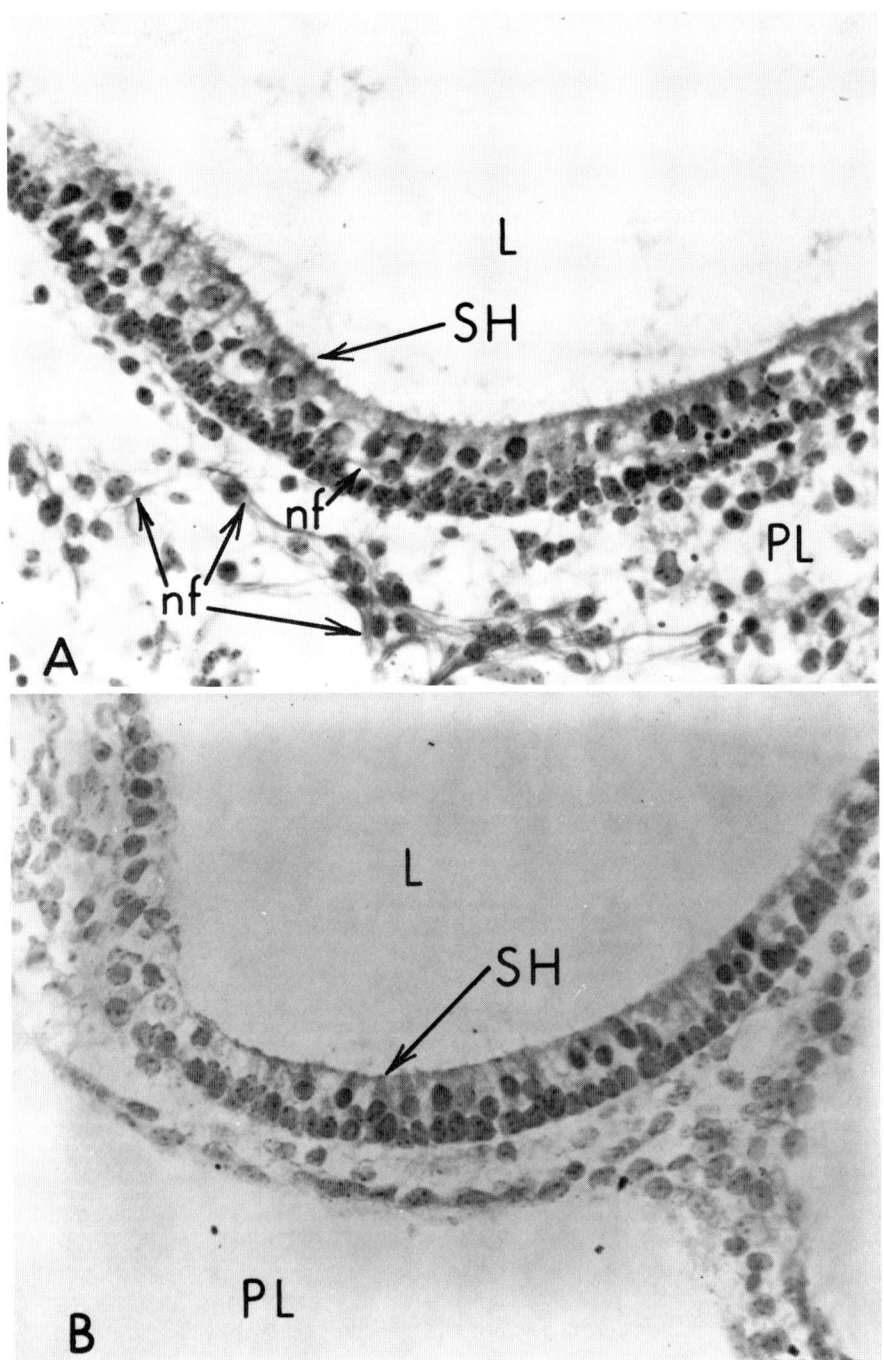

Fig. 5. Eleven-day-old otocyst, 10 days in vitro: A) with ganglion explanted – a macula with neural elements; B) without ganglion explanted – a macula without neural elements. (×500)

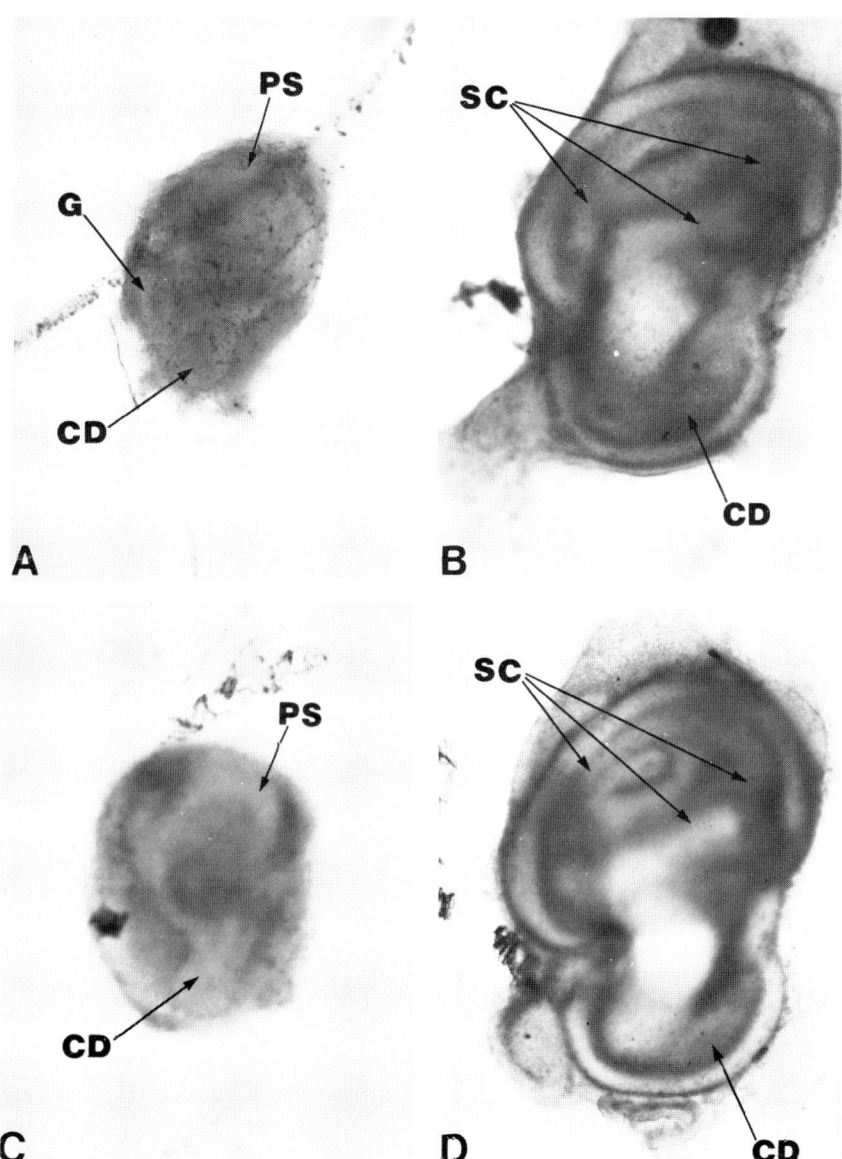

Fig. 6. Photomicrographs of living explants of 12-day-old mouse embryo inner ear anlage: A and C) after 0 hours in vitro; B and D) after 9 days in vitro. Cultures A and B have an intact statoacoustic ganglion complex. Cultures C and D have had their statoacoustic ganglion complex excised prior to explantation in vitro. (×50)

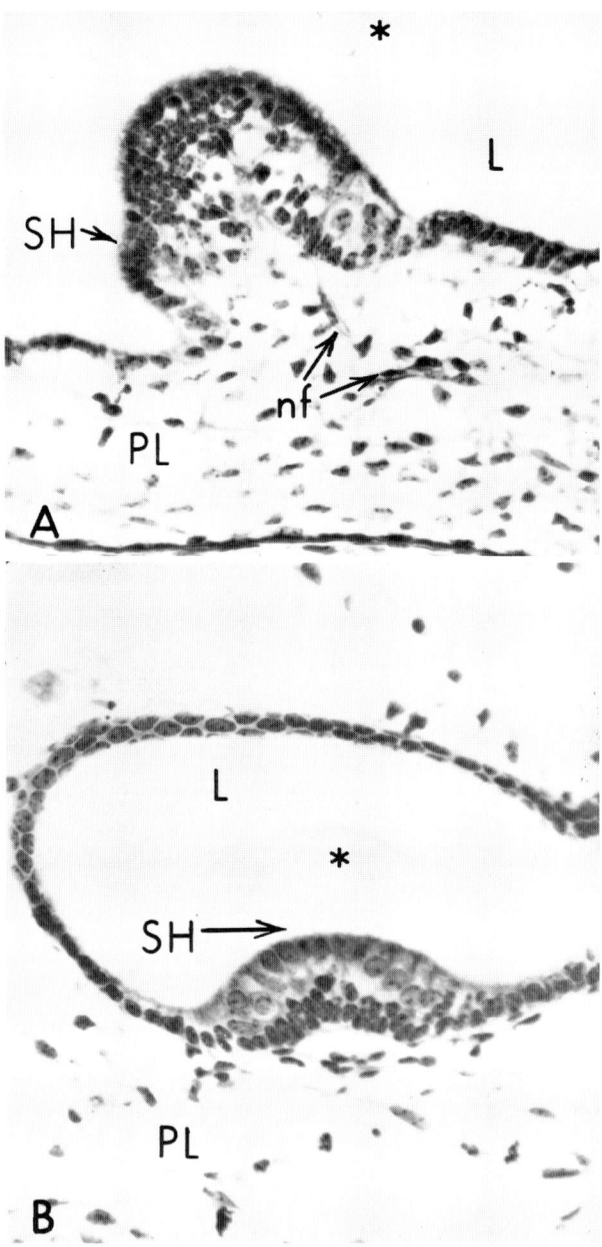

Fig. 7. Twelve-day-old inner ear anlage, 9 days in vitro: A) with ganglion explanted – a crista with neural elements; B) without ganglion explanted – a crista without neural elements. (×500)

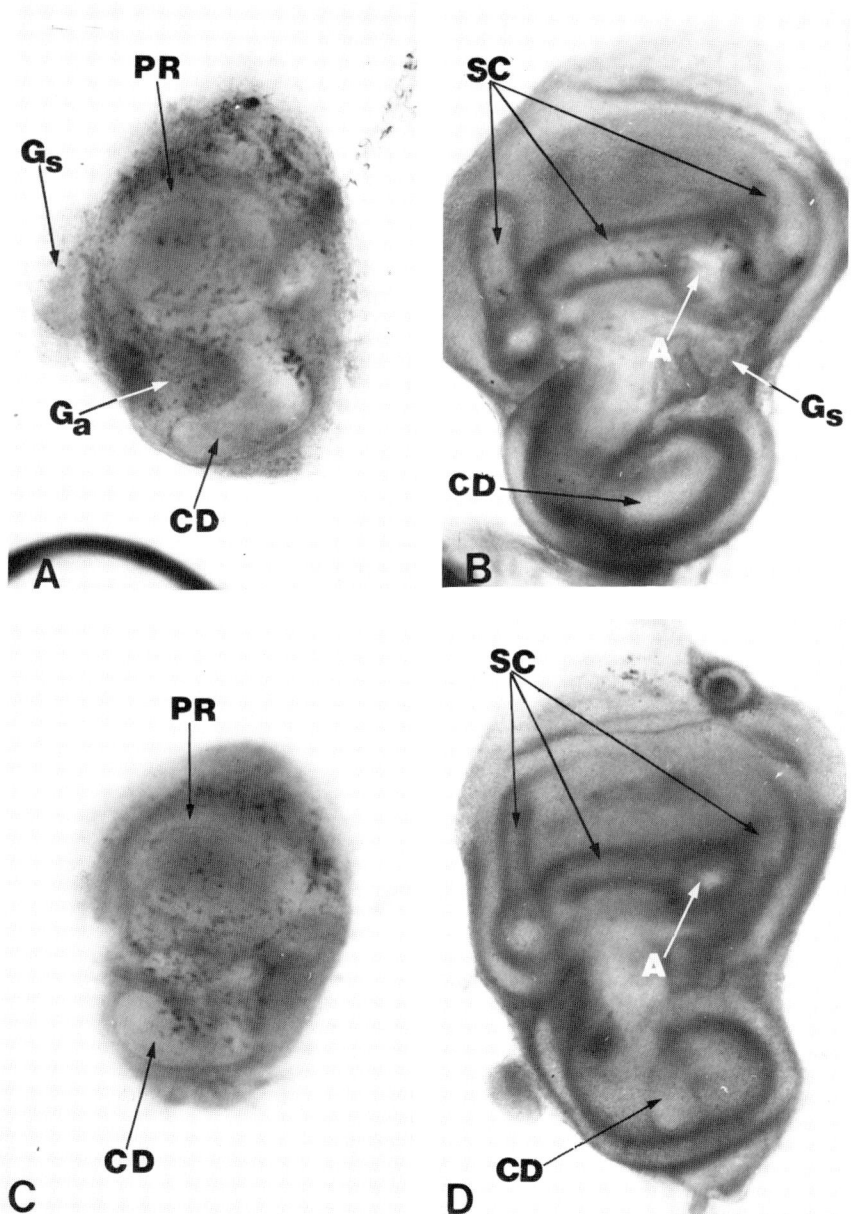

Fig. 8. Photomicrographs of living explants of 13-day-old mouse embryo inner ear anlage: A and C) after 0 hours in vitro; B and D) after 8 days. Cultures A and B have an intact statoacoustic ganglion complex. Cultures C and D have had their statoacoustic ganglion complex excised prior to explantation in vitro. (×50)

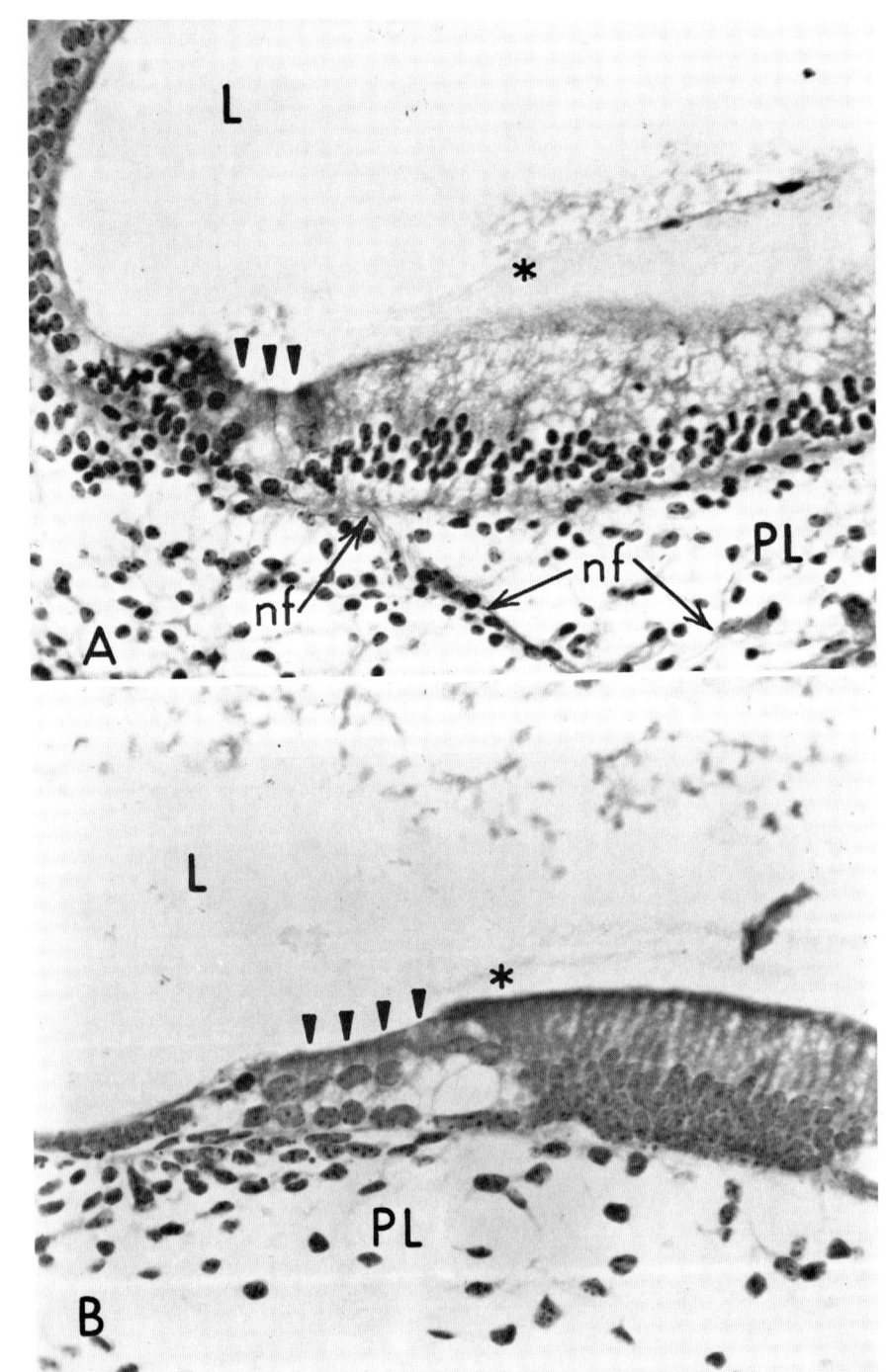

are seen in Figure 9. The level of cytodifferentiation in vitro attained by these 2 specimens is essentially similar in character. The organ of Corti was observed to histologically differentiate in a base-to-apex pattern in the explants in vitro in both group "A" and group "B" of all gestational ages. In the analysis of the histodifferentiation in vitro of the explanted embryonic inner ears from group "A" and group "B," the histologic sections were observed with oil immersion objectives for the structure of the hair cells. The following histologic qualities were observed: cell morphology, staining characteristics of the nucleus and cytoplasm, morphology of sensory hair tufts, and relationships of sensory membranes to the hair cells. In each gestational age group observed, these characteristics were found to be similar in the specimens from both groups "A" (with) and "B" (without).

Conclusions. The results of the histologic quantification of the specimens from the 11th, 12th, and 13th gestational days, groups "A" and "B," are presented in tabular form in Table 1. These data were then grouped into 2 general categories of explants, "A" (with) and "B" (without statoacoustic ganglion complex), and were presented in histographic form (Fig. 10) so that the significance of the data can be visualized better. (See ref. [13] for a detailed discussion of the results.) Light microscopic observations confirmed that in cultures of group "A," statoacoustic ganglion neurons and their nerve fibers were present in association with the developed sensory structures; neither ganglion cell neurons nor their nerve fibers were found to be present in the sensory structures that developed in the organ-cultured specimens of group "B." Quantification revealed no consistent trend toward greater occurrence of any sensory structure in any of the groups of explants analyzed.

The presence of such a trend would have signified the probable existence of a trophic effect of the statoacoustic ganglion neural elements upon development of the inner ear's sensory structures in the explants of group "A" of the 11-, 12-, and 13-day-old organ cultured specimens of embryonic inner ears when compared to the aganglionic cultured otocysts of group "B." Microscopic comparison of the sensory structures and their sensory hair cells that developed in the organ cultures revealed no differences in the quality of the histodifferentiation of sensory structures of either group "A" or group "B" explants. A base-to-apex pattern of histodifferentiation of the organ of Corti's sensory structures, which has been described to occur in vivo, was noted to occur in the cochlear ducts developed in vitro of all of the explanted inner ears without respect to whether neural elements were present ("A") or absent ("B") during development. It was concluded from

---

Fig. 9. Thirteen-day-old inner ear anlage, 8 days in vitro: A) with ganglion explanted — an organ of Corti formation with neural elements; B) without ganglion explanted — an organ of Corti formation without neural elements. (×500)

the quantification of the data on histodifferentiation and from the above observations on the differentiative pattern of Corti's organ that no trophic effect of the neural elements of the statoacoustic ganglion complex influenced the histodifferentiation of sensory structures of 11-, 12-, and 13-gestational-day-old embryonic mouse inner ear explants as they differentiated in vitro.

TABLE 1. Histologic Quantification With (A) and Without (B) Statoacoustic Ganglion

Histologic features	Gestation-day of explant					
	11th		12th		13th	
	A (%)	B (%)	A (%)	B (%)	A (%)	B (%)
Cartilaginous otic capsule	100	100	100	100	100	100
Perilymphatic spaces	100	100	100	100	100	100
Statoacoustic ganglion cells	100	0	100	0	100	0
Nerve fibers associated with sensory structures	100	0	100	0	100	0
Utriculosaccular space	100	100	100	100	100	100
Maculae						
1 only	0	7	9	12	3	15
2	97	93	91	84	93	85
Total	97	100	100	96	96	100
Semicircular canals						
1 only	33	30	0	12	0	11
2 only	50	70	58	52	14	27
3	10	0	42	36	86	62
Total	93	100	100	100	100	100
Cristae						
1 only	3	4	3	0	0	8
2 only	20	18	18	24	10	23
3	77	78	79	76	90	69
Total	100	100	100	100	100	100
Cochlear duct	97	100	94	96	100	100
Organ of Corti	93	93	94	96	100	96
Stria vascularis	90	93	94	92	100	96
Tectorial membrane	71	93	85	76	86	73
Endolymphatic duct	87	96	88	96	100	92
Endolymphatic sac	87	96	88	92	100	88
Total number of specimens analyzed	30	30	30	30	30	30

"A" – with statoacoustic ganglion complex.
"B" – without statoacoustic ganglion complex.

(From Van De Water TR: Effects of removal of the statoacoustic ganglion complex upon the growing otocyst. Ann Otol Rhinol Laryngol 85(Suppl 33):1–32, 1976, with permission.)

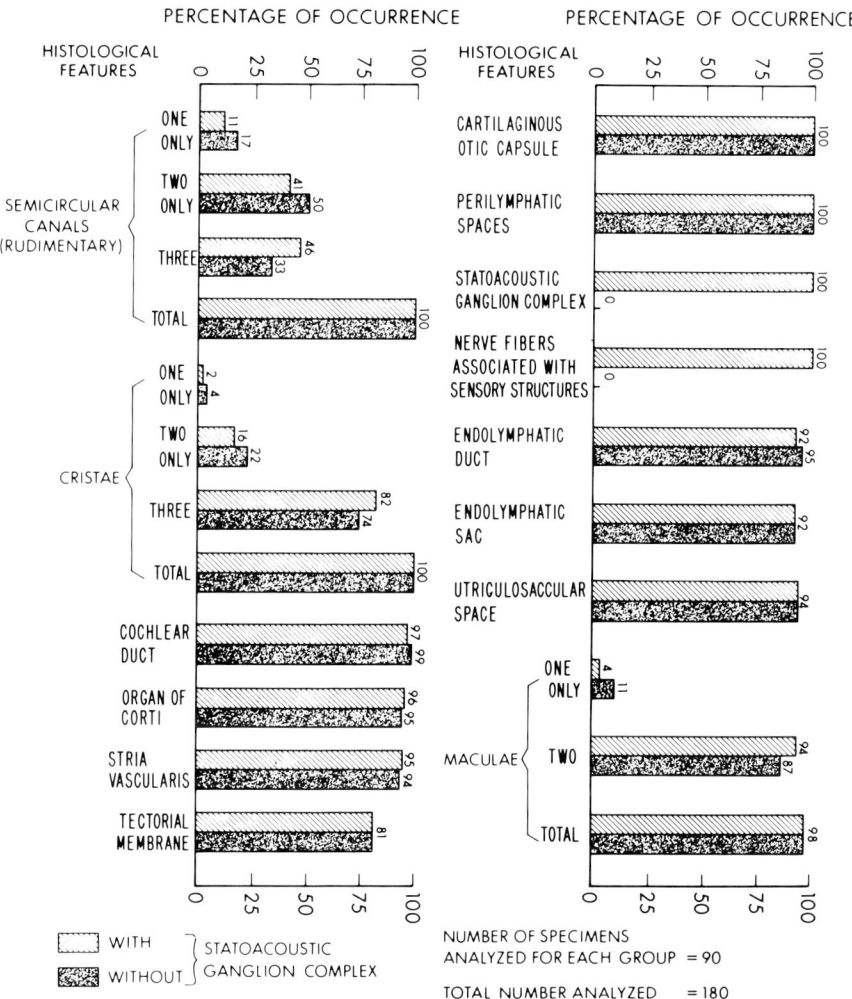

Fig. 10. Summary of histologic quantification with and without acoustic ganglion.

Experiments With Endolymphatic Duct and Sac

Harrison [14] suggested that the intactness of the endolymphatic appendage may be an essential factor in the orderly organogenesis of the amphibian inner ear. Bonnevie [15] and Hertwig [16], when studying the development of mutant mouse embryos (Shaker-short and Kreisler mice, respectively) that had congenitally malformed inner ears, noted that both homozygotic genotypes did not develop an endolymphatic duct and sac anlage in the early otocystic stage of development of the inner ear. Partsch [17], in a report on a histologic study of malformed human fetal material, drew the conclusion that the absence of an endolymphatic duct and sac system impairs regulation of labyrinthine pressure, and, in turn, impairs labyrinthine differentiation. Hendricks and Toerien [18] experimented with endolymphatic duct and sac anlage extirpation in developing chick embryos in ovo and reported that their results suggested that an intact endolymphatic duct and sac anlage was necessary for orderly organogenesis of the labyrinth. Van De Water and Ruben [19] reported on the organ culture of homozygotic and heterozygotic Kreisler otocysts. The homozygotic Kreisler otocyst was reported to reproduce phenotypically in vitro its pattern of malformation as observed to occur in vivo. These homozygotic Kreisler explants were observed to

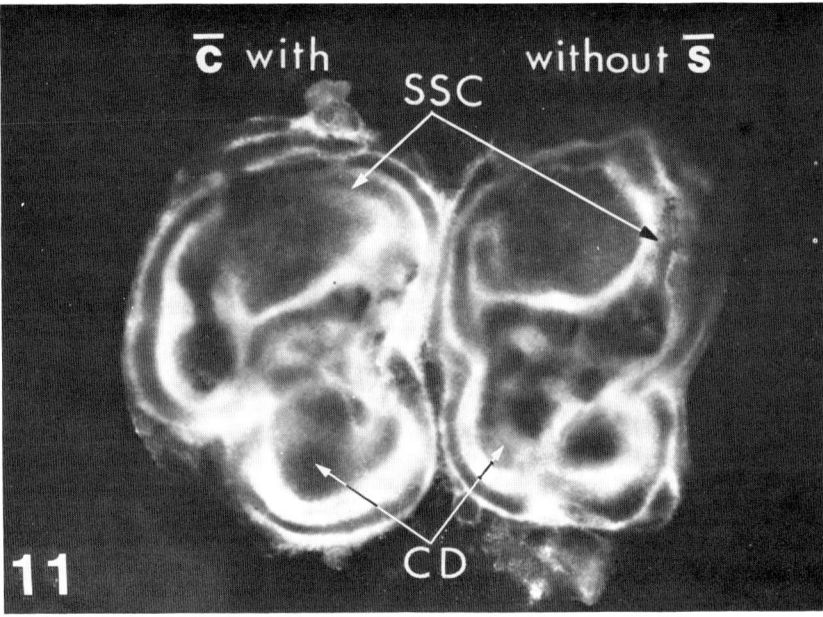

Fig. 11. A darkfield photomicrograph of 2 living mouse otocysts 13 gestational days old, that have developed for 8 days in vitro. The otocyst on the left ($\bar{c}$) was explanted with an intact endolymphatic duct and sac anlage, and the otocyst on the right ($\bar{s}$) had its endolymphatic duct and sac anlage excised prior to explantation in vitro. The areas of the semicircular canal (SSC) and cochlear duct (CD) are indicated. (×20) (Figs. 11–15 from Van De Water TR: The effect of the removal of the endolymphatic duct and sac anlage upon organogenesis of the mammalian inner ear "in vitro:" A preliminary report. Arch Otorhinolaryngol 217: 297–311, 1977, with permission.)

lack an endolymphatic appendage at the time of explantation to the organ culture system, when compared to otocysts explanted from comparably developed heterozygotic littermate embryos.

An experiment was designed to observe the effect of removal of the endolymphatic duct and sac anlage upon the organogenesis of a normal mouse's inner ear in vitro. Twelve and 13-gestational-day-old mouse embryonic inner ears were excised and each gestational age group of specimens was further divided into 2 groups. The first group did not undergo further surgical manipulation and were explanted directly into the organ culture dishes; the second group underwent further microsurgical dissection during which time the endolymphatic duct and sac anlage were removed at the point at which the anlage joined the dorsomedial aspect of the otocyst's pars superior. No other otocystic ectodermal tissue was excised. A piece of cephalic mesenchyme was placed at the operative site to effect wound closure, and the "without" explants were then placed into the organ culture dishes.

All specimens were allowed to develop in vitro to the equivalent of 21 days in vivo. The specimens were then fixed and processed histologically with a conventional hematoxylin and eosin staining technique. The specimens were code-labeled and histologically quantified [9] for development in vitro with the aid of a light microscope. A darkfield photomicrograph of two 13-day-old explants after 8 days of development in vitro, one with and the other without an endolymphatic appendage, were grown in the same organ culture dish for purposes of photographic demonstration, as seen in Figure 11.

The morphogenesis in vitro of these specimens is similar, with no gross distortion evident in either specimen. A low magnification of a histologic cross-section of cultured explants of inner ear, 13 gestational days old, 8 days in vitro "with" and "without" an endolymphatic duct and sac anlage, is seen in Figures 12 and 13, respectively. The histologic features of these organ-cultured specimens (Figs. 12 and 13) are similar. The histologic quantificational data of the explants of 12 and 13 gestational days' age is presented correspondingly in the histograms of Figures 14 and 15.

Conclusions. The resultant histologic quantification of the in vitro embryogenesis of the inner ear explants did not reveal any significant differences in morphogenesis, histodifferentiation of labyrinthine sensory structures, or presence of hydrops of the endolymphatic cavities in any of the organ-cultured specimens. It was concluded that, in the system studied, the absence of the endolymphatic duct and sac anlage did not have a significant effect on the organogenesis of the inner ear, with the exception of the resultant lack of development of an endolymphatic duct and sac. A more detailed presentation of the data and discussion of results is presented in Van De Water [20].

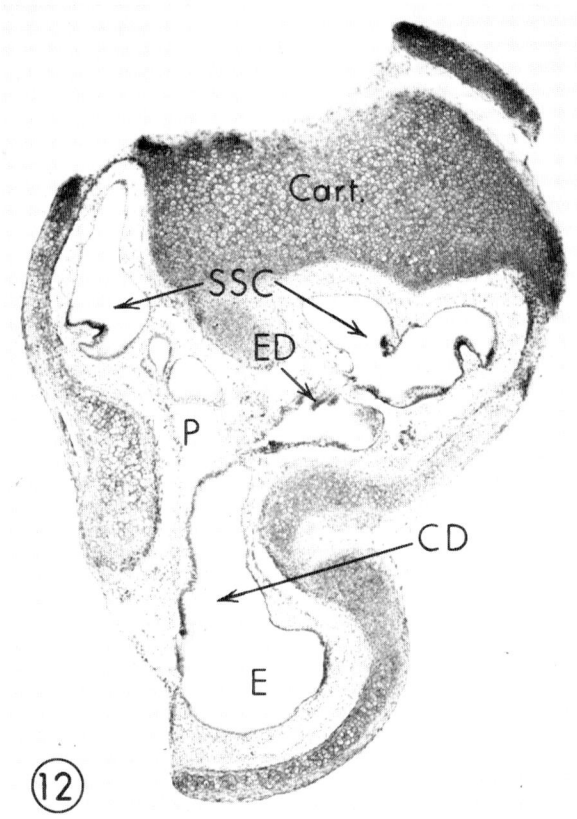

Fig. 12. An otocyst of the 13th gestational day, explanted "with" an intact endolymphatic duct and sac anlage, after 8 days in vitro. This photomicrograph is a cross-section showing the cartilaginous otic capsule (Cart.), perilymphatic (P), and endolymphatic (E) spaces. The semicircular canals (SSC) and cochlear duct (CD) are also indicated. (×55)

Fate-Mapping

Levy [21] observed that the cells of the amphibian otic cup developed independently of their environments, and the fates of the cells with regard to the membranous labyrinth were not determined. He postulated that any half of the otic cup would develop into a complete labyrinth half the size of a normal ear. Streeter [22] and Spemann [23] later arrived at a different conclusion from Levy's [21]. They felt that the open otic cup was not a harmonic equipotential system, and that considerable determination of cells had occurred by the time of formation of the otic cup.

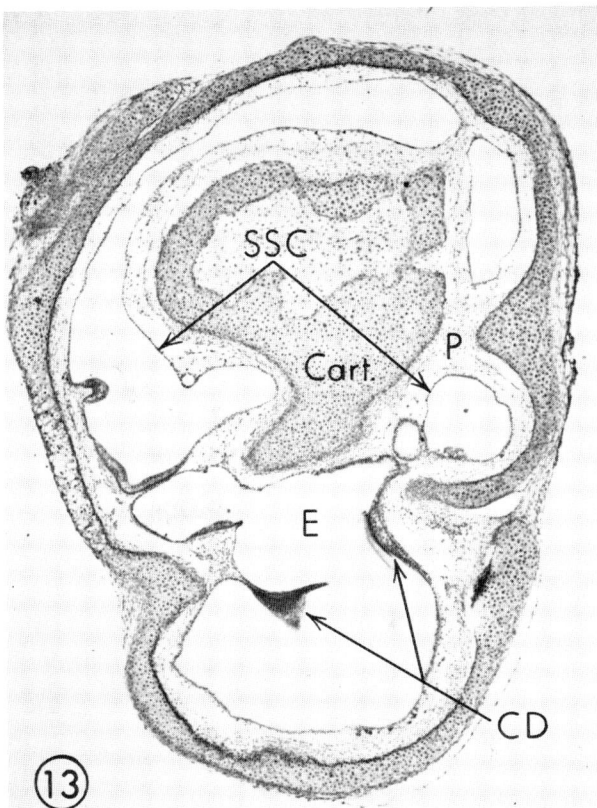

Fig. 13. An otocyst of the 13th gestational day, explanted "without" an endolymphatic duct and sac anlage, after 8 days in vitro. This photomicrograph is a cross-section of the explant showing the cartilaginous otic capsule (Cart.), perilymphatic (P), and endolymphatic (E) spaces. The semicircular canals (SSC) and cochlear duct (CD) are also indicated. (×55)

Harrison [24, 25] demonstrated that during the closure of the neural fold, the otic placode of *Amblystoma punctatum* was no longer isotropic, but was polarized in an anteroposterior axis. The polarization of cells determined the arrangement of sensory structures of the differentiating labyrinth along the anteroposterior axis. At this stage, cells along the dorsoventral axis of the placode were still subjected to the influence of the surrounding cells. Polarization along the dorsoventral axis appeared at a slightly later stage of development of the inner ear [26, 27]. Kaan [27] performed surgical ablation of otocysts in *Amblystoma punctatum* and concluded that after the developing inner ear passed the otic cup stage, regeneration of the inner ear became difficult. She showed that characteristic defects were

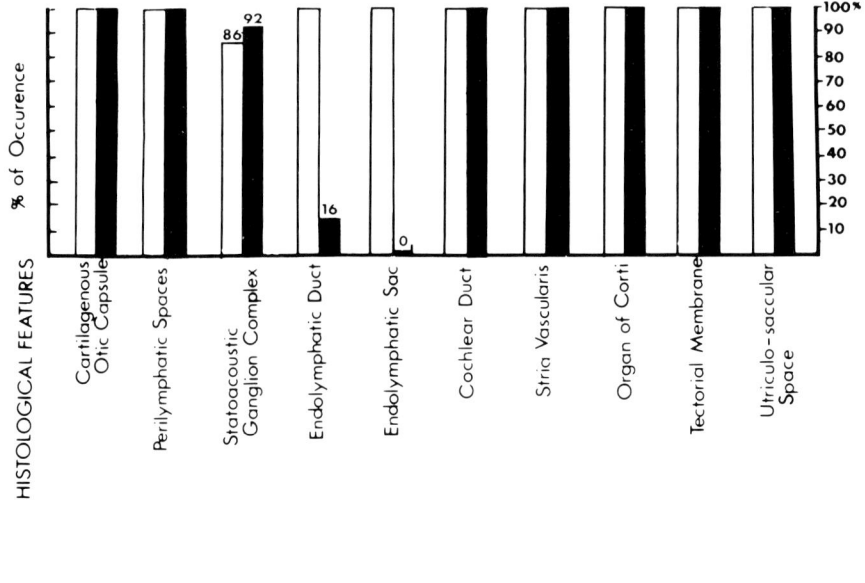
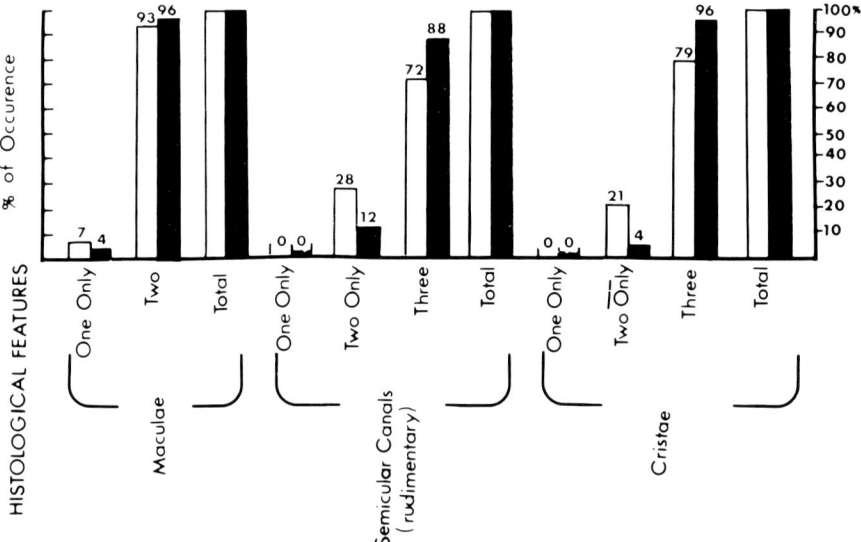

Fig. 14. A histogram depicting quantificational data for the histologic specimens 12 gestational days old.

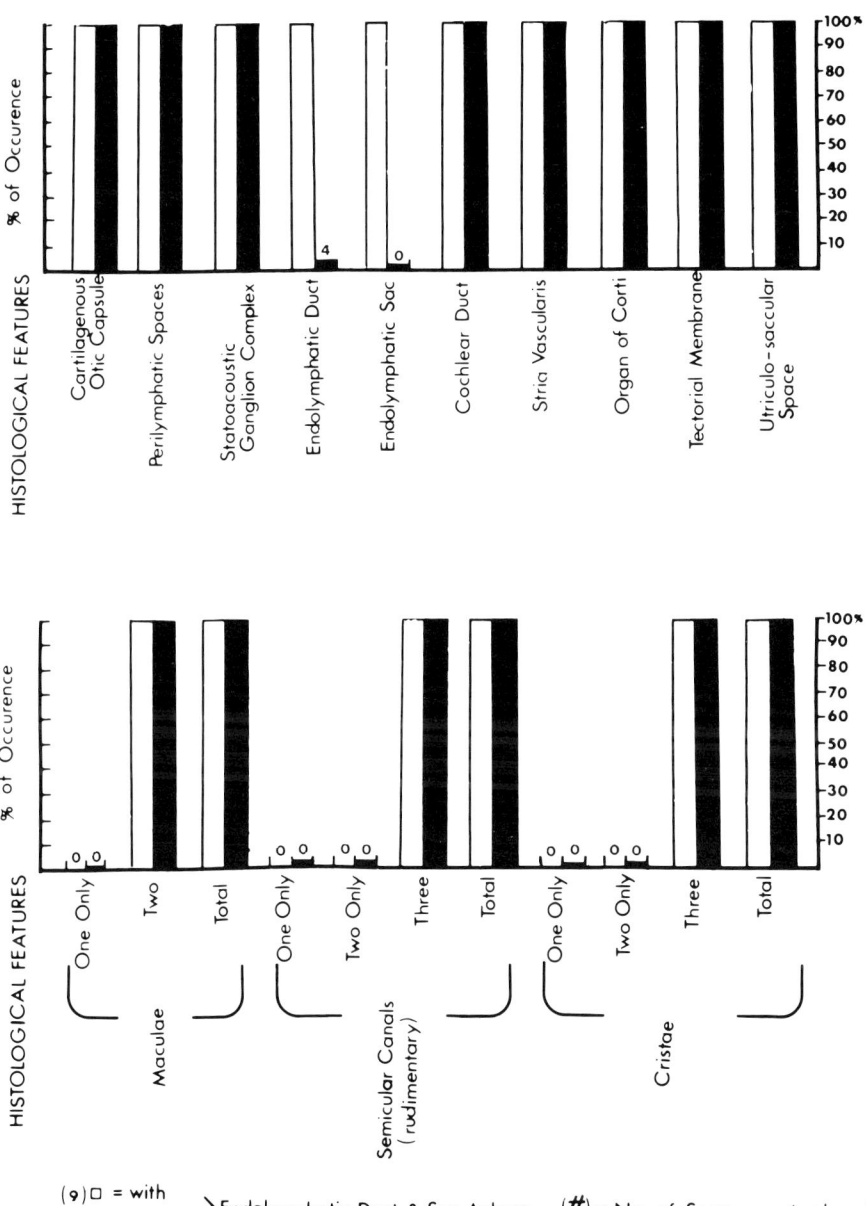

Fig. 15. A histogram depicting quantificational data for the histologic specimens 13 gestational days old.

reproducible depending on which portions of the otic cup were ablated and at which developmental stage the surgical operation was performed. Kaan's experiment [27] further demonstrated that cell determination has occurred by the time of formation of the otic cup.

In a study of the fate-mapping of the mouse otocyst, Li et al [28, 29] traced the mosaic for the development of the embryonic otic sensory structures. Otocysts of 11 and 12 days' gestation were dissected into 6 anatomic groups of dorsal, ventral, anterior, posterior, medial, and lateral halves. The dorsal and ventral halves were obtained by an anteroposterior incision midway through the 11- and 12-day-old otocysts. The anterior and posterior halves were obtained by a dorsoventral incision midway through the 11- and 12-day-old otocysts. The medial and lateral halves were obtained by mechanical ablation of either the respective lateral or medial wall of 12-day-old otocysts.

Because of surgical difficulty, the 11-day-old otocyst was not included in the medial/lateral anatomic group. Each anatomic group of otocysts was cultured separately in an incubator at 34.5°C for 10 days. Every 5th specimen was fixed as a histologic control for development. At the end of the experiment, the explants were histologically analyzed with light microscopy. The histologic control showed that the 11- and 12-gestational-day-old mouse otocysts were composed of histologically undifferentiated ectodermal cells, ranging from pseudostratified columnar cells composing the ventromedial wall to low cuboidal cells composing the dorso-

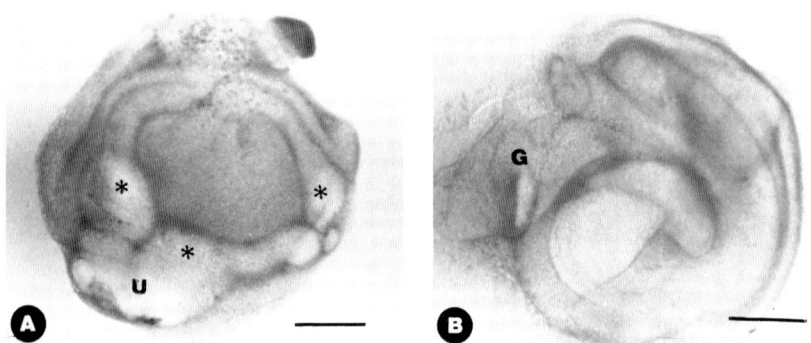

Fig. 16. A) Gross morphology of a dorsal half of a mouse otocyst, 13 gestational days old, 10 days in vitro. Note the development of the 3 semicircular ducts and their associated ampullae (*), and of the utricle (U). Line = 100 μm. B) Gross morphology of a ventral half of a mouse otocyst, 13 gestational days old, 10 days in vitro. Note the development of a coiling cochlea of one and a quarter turns. "G" denotes the VIIIth nerve's ganglion. Line = 100 μm. (Figs. 16 and 17 from Li CW, Van De Water TR, Ruben RJ: The fate mapping of the eleventh and twelfth day mouse otocyst: An "in vitro" study of the sites of origin of the embryonic inner ear sensory structures. J Morphol 157:249–268, 1978, with permission.)

lateral wall. Photomicrographs of dorsal and ventral explants of a 13-day-old mouse otocyst after 10 days of development in vitro are seen in Figure 16.

Data in Table 2 indicate that by the 11th day of gestation, the mouse otocyst has become a mosaic (Fig. 17) for the development of otic sensory structures with respect to the dorsoventral and anteroposterior axes. Data from the 12-day-old explants also reveal that mosaicism of otic sensory structures with respect to the mediolateral axis has occurred by at least the 12th day of gestation. The fate-map of the mouse otocyst is summarized by 8 anatomic sectors in Figure 17. The anterior duct and its associated crista-ampullaris developed from the dorsoanterior portion of the otocyst. The lateral duct originated from the dorsolateral wall of the otocyst and its associated crista-ampullaris from the dorsolateral anterior section of the otocyst. The posterior duct and its associated crista-ampullaris differentiated from the dorsoposterior portion of the otocyst. The utricle derived from the dorsal segment of the middle third of the otocyst and the utricular macula

TABLE 2. Fate-Mapping of the Mouse Otocyst: Combined Results of 11- and 12-Gestational-Day-Old Explants*

	Dorsal	Ventral	Anterior	Posterior	Medial	Lateral
Cartilaginous capsule	100%	100%	100%	100%	100%	100%
Statoacoustic ganglion	2	87	80	0	67	48
Utriculosaccular space	56	31	93	43	89	95
Maculae						
1 only	26	17	43	8	60	52
2	13	15	47	0	19	43
Semicircular canals						
1 only	2	2	16	34	26	2
2 only	34	0	80	60	52	14
3	64	0	0	0	2	81
Cristae						
1 only	31	2	27	84	31	7
2 only	35	0	69	0	21	23
3	24	0	0	0	4	67
Cochlear duct	0	98	77	89	88	88
Cochlear sensory epithelium	0	92	66	84	82	52
Tectorial membrane	0	83	58	60	29	33
Stria vascularis	0	52	24	16	6	4
Total number of specimens analyzed	62	48	70	61	57	42

*Data presented in this table are the combined data of the 11th and 12th gestational days for the dorsal and ventral explants, the 11th and 12th gestational days for the anterior and posterior explants, and the 12th gestational day for the medial and lateral explants. (From Li CW, Van De Water TR, Ruben RJ: The fate mapping of the eleventh and twelfth day mouse otocyst: An "in vitro" study of the sites of origin of the embryonic inner ear sensory structures. J Morphol 157:249–268, 1978, with permission.)

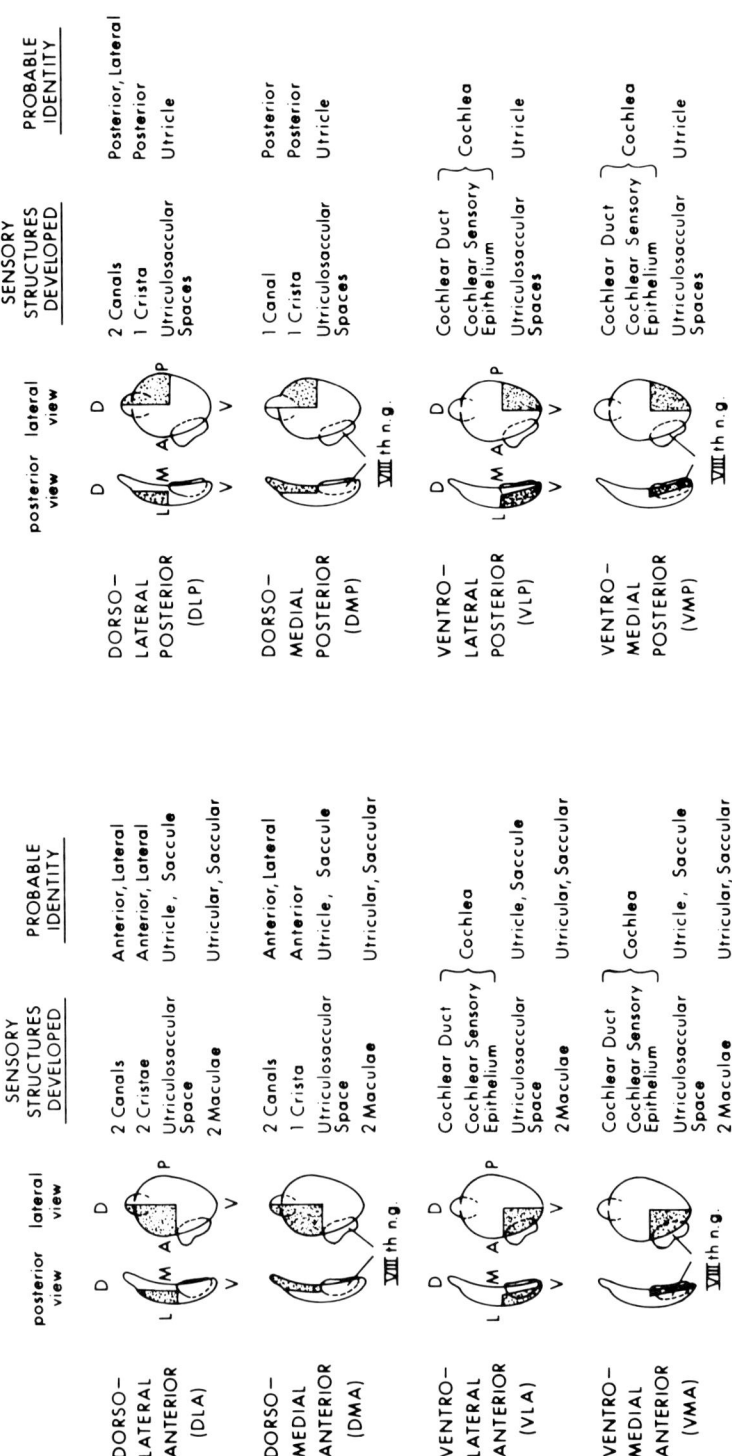

Fig. 17. Summary chart of the fate-mapping of the 8 anatomic sectors of the mouse otocyst.

from the anterior portion of the same segment. The saccule and its associated macula developed from the middle third of the anterior wall, ventral to the site of origin of the utricle. The cochlear duct and its sensory epithelium differentiated from the ventral portion of the otocyst.

The fate-mapping of the normal mouse otocyst provides 2 important pieces of information. First, it shows that cell determination has already occurred by the 11th day of gestation. It was shown in the same experiment [28, 29] that the otocyst of 10 days' gestation, grown in isolation, failed to show gross morphologic differentiation. It is evident that induction of some kind, whether neural or mesodermal or both [2], is essential during this embryonic period of early otic development. Second, the fate-map of the normal mouse otocyst will provide a model and an outline for structural development of normal inner ear such that it could be used to compare the pathologic morphogenesis of congenital mutants.

Van De Water and Ruben [19] reported that in vitro explants of homozygotic Kreisler otocysts reproduced the phenotypic expression of this congenital malformation as it occurs in vivo [16]. Li [30] examined the cell determination of the Kreisler mouse and found that the heterozygotic Kreisler (+/kr) otocyst differentiated according to the fate-map of the normal mouse otocyst [28, 29]. In contrast, the homozygotic Kreisler (kr/kr) otocyst followed a developmental course that was both variable and different from that of the heterozygotic Kreisler otocyst, and which resulted in the formation of an abnormal labyrinth. However, in spite of this variable pattern of development, the kr/kr otocyst appeared to follow, in a general pattern, the normal outline for dorsoventral development of otic sensory structures. Sensory structures, abnormal in size and shape, were often recognizable in histologic preparation of both dorsal and ventral explants of homozygotic Kreisler otocysts. Semicircular ducts and their cristae differentiated in the dorsal half of the kr/kr otocyst, and the middle portion of the kr/kr otocyst developed into utriculosaccular structures. Cochlear structures were derived from the ventral half of the kr/kr otocyst.

Neural Induction

Many experimental studies of avians and amphibians have demonstrated that the development of the embryonic inner ear is dependent upon the influence of the neural tube [2, 3, 14, 24, 31–35]. Waddington [31] further proposed that inducing factors other than the neural elements are active during differentiation of the chick otic ectoderm. One of these factors, he believed, was the mesoderm adjacent to the otic ectoderm. Yntema [2], in a study of the induction of salamander inner ear, demonstrated that induction of otic placode and formation of otic vesicle is dependent on mesodermal influences and that differentiation of the otic vesicle depends on inductive influences of the rhombencephalon. In studying the abnormalities of the inner ear in Kreisler mice, Deol [36] observed that the otic vesicle of homozygotic embryos formed in an abnormal position where close apposition with the rhombencephalon was not possible during early embryogenesis. Deol [36] suggested that it is unlikely that the Kreisler gene expresses itself directly within the cells of the otic anlage during otic development. On the contrary, development of the Kreisler inner ear appears to proceed along a course that one would expect from experimental work [2, 24, 33, 34]. It has been demonstrated experimentally in amphibians and avians that when the normal embryonic relationship between the otic vesicle and the rhombencephalon is disturbed, abnormal development of the otic vesicle may result, ranging from an undifferentiated cyst-like state to a malformed labyrinth with an imperfect otic capsule [33, 34, 37, 38].

In studying the fate-map of the mouse otocyst, Li et al [28, 29] demonstrated that isolated 10-gestational-day-old mouse otocysts fail to differentiate in vitro, while explants of 11-gestational-day-old otocysts differentiate into labyrinths with well-formed sensory structures. In both cases, sufficient amounts of adhering periotic mesenchyme were included in the explants, so mesodermal interaction cannot account for the differences in differentiation of these two embryonic age-group explants of otocysts. A preliminary transfilter study reported by Li et al [39] suggests that the rhombencephalon exerts an inductive influence on the in vitro differentiation of 10-gestational-day-old explants of mouse otocysts.

A transfilter-apparatus used to study tissue interactions in vitro was first introduced by Grobstein [40]. Since then, many investigators have employed such a system for the study of embryonic induction [41–43]. A modified transfilter-apparatus was used by Li et al [39] which consisted of a Falcon's plastic organ culture dish containing a grid of stainless steel wire with a 10 mm hole in its center. A sterile nuclepore filter membrane with pore size ranging from 1 μm–8μm was placed over the hole in the wire grid. A segment of rhombencephalic tissue excised from an embryo of the 12th gestational day was held onto the underside of the membrane by a clot of chick plasma. Culturing medium (Neumann Tytell serumless medium supplemented with 20% fetal calf serum) was maintained at the level of the filter membrane. The control group was prepared in the same manner, with the exception that the clot of chick plasma on the underside of the filter membrane contained no rhombencephalic tissue.

In the control group, an otocyst of a 10-day-old embryo, freed of adhering brain tissue, was placed lateral side up on the filter membrane directly above the plasma clot, while the other otocyst of the same 10-day-old embryo was used in the experimental group. It was freed of brain tissue and placed on the filter membrane directly above the plasma clot containing rhombencephalic tissue obtained from a 12-day-old embryo. Because of the variations in age found among embryos of the same litter, the exact embryonic age of the otocyst was determined by the number of somites in the mouse embryo (21–25 somites = 9.5 days' gestation; 26–28 somites = 10 days' gestation; 29–36 somites = 10.5 days' gestation [63, 64]. The specimens were allowed to grow for a period of 11 days.

Examination at the end of the experiment showed degeneration of cells in the plasma-clotted control group of otocyst explants of 9.5 and 10 days' gestation. Otocysts of 10.5 days' gestation and those under the influence of the rhombencephalic tissue, however, exhibited development of sensory epithelia and formation of a cartilaginous capsule around the membranous labyrinth. The sensory structures of the otocysts explanted from embryos of 9.5 and 10 days of gestation did not achieve the same degree of histodifferentiation and structural integrity as those of the 10.5-day otocyst explants, but compartmentalization and maturation of explants' sensory structures were often observed to have occurred within these younger inner ear explants. Furthermore, rhombencephalic tissue with well-differentiated glial cells and neurons often induced more mature cartilaginous cells in the capsule and a higher degree of otocyst compartmentalization and cytodifferentiation of sensory structures than otocyst explants interacted with rhombencephalic tissue that showed signs of degeneration.

Epithelio-Mesenchymal Interactions

Morphogenesis within an organ system requires the organization of specific cell populations of the forming organ into unique configurations which will ultimately result in the final structure of the organ. The question that arises is, "What causes and controls the organization of these specific cell populations during the process of morphogenesis?" Certain portions of the developmental process are under direct genomic control, but substantial evidence [44] suggests that tissue interactions are the primary mechanism for regulating the assembly of specific populations of cells into organs. The development of organs composed of epithelial and mesenchymal components is particularly convenient for study since the interaction involves only 2 tissues. The interaction occurring between epithelial and mesenchymal tissues appears not to be isolated events, but rather a continuous process.

Grobstein and Cohen [45] reported on the disruptive effect of collagenase on epithelio-mesenchymal tissue interactions that control morphogenesis of salivary gland rudiments in vitro. Grobstein [46] in a later publication addressing the mechanisms of organogenetic tissue interactions, stressed the importance of epithelio-mesenchymal tissue interactions in organs such as kidney, salivary gland, limbs, tooth, lung, liver, pancreas, thymus, mammary gland, and eye. The 18th Hahnemann Symposium in 1968 was devoted to epithelio-mesenchymal interactions and their role in inductive and morphogenetic processes. At this symposium, McLoughlin [47] reported that various foreign mesenchymal tissues can specifically affect the differentiation of the ectodermal tissue with which they interact in an in vitro environment. Grobstein [48] focused his comments upon the importance of substances that accumulate at the epithelio-mesenchymal interface, which extended his original collagenase experiment. He reported experiments that utilized transfilter interaction of epithelial and mesenchymal tissues in the presence of tritiated 1-proline. The results suggested a greater accumulation of the tritium label at the epithelio-mesenchymal interface when both tissues were present, compared to tritium label accumulation observed when either tissue was cultured alone. Coulombre and Coulombre [49] have reported on the action of 1-azetidine-2-carboxylic acid in interrupting the production and excretion of collagen into the primary stroma of the cornea of developing chick eyes in ovo.

Hay [50] has also examined the origin and role of collagen in organogenesis in the chick embryo. She described in chronologic order 4 embryonic systems in which substantial evidence suggests that collagen present in basal lamina plays a role in organogenesis. The embryologic tissue interactions reported by Hay [50] were divided into 3 classes: a) epithelial-epithelial (eye–primary stroma of the cornea); b) epithelial-mesenchymal (induction of chondrogenesis of somitic mesenchyme by the neural tube); c) mesenchymal-epithelial (morphogenesis of the submaxillary gland). Her work also supported the theory that glycosaminoglycans (GAG) are involved within the collagen matrix of the epithelial basal lamina.

Bernfield et al [44] presented additional indirect evidence for a role of GAG in the formation of epithelial organs and their patterns of association at the epithlio-mesenchymal interface during morphogenesis. Glycosaminoglycans were shown to be distributed in specific patterns within the extracellular matrix of the epithelial basal lamina during morphogenesis of the mouse embryonic submandibular salivary gland as it developed in organ culture. Hay and Meier [51] reported on the synthesis of GAG by embryonic inductor tissues, such as neural tube, notochord, and lens. With the use of tritiated precursors and histochemical studies, these investigators also noted the distribution of the GAG in the basal lamina and compartments of extracellular matrix that surround these inductor tissues. Newsome [52] demonstrated that pigmented retinal epithelial cells of the chick excrete an extracellular matrix onto filter membranes that can, after lysis of the original cell population, stimulate cephalic neural crest mesenchyme to form cartilage.

The series of reports presented here indicates that the extracellular, collagen-bearing, GAG-containing matrix, often present at the site of embryonic induction, may play an important role in morphogenesis and differentiation of organ systems that involve epithelio-mesenchymal tissue interactions. The role of epithelio-mesenchymal tissue interactions in the development of the mammalian inner ear has had but one isolated report, by Grobstein and Holtzer [53], demonstrating the role of inductor of a mammalian otocyst upon somitic mesenchyme in a transfilter-interaction experiment in vitro. Benoit [7, 54] demonstrated that crude saline extracts of 3- and 4-day-old chick embryo otocysts could induce in vitro cultivated cephalic mesenchyme to form cartilage, while cephalic mesenchyme of the saline controls did not undergo chondrogenesis in vitro. In the following paragraphs, preliminary results of in vitro experimental manipulations of epithelio-mesenchymal tissue relationships of the embryonic mammalian inner ear explants are presented.

Whole Mesenchyme

A series of experiments involving a total of 126 explants of inner ear were performed to investigate the nature of the interactions occurring between the otocyst and its surrounding mesenchyme. The first series of 42 explants were 12- and 13-day-old otocysts that were pretreated with a dilute solution of trypsin (1:300) in Ca^{++} and Mg^{++} free, phosphate-buffered, saline for 1 hr at room temperature to aid in the dissection of adhering cephalic mesenchyme from the ectodermal cells of the otocyst. Trypsin is a proteolytic enzyme which is commonly used to aid in the separation of mesenchymal cells from epithelial tissue. When the explanted organ cultures were examined with a dissecting microscope, during their period of in vitro development, the control cultures treated with trypsin were found to deviate from the normal pattern of labyrinthine morphogenesis as has been observed to occur in vitro [9, 13]. The trypsin-treated otocysts that had the adhering cephalic mesenchyme removed exhibited a complete lack of labyrinthine morphogenesis in the organ culture system. Histologic sections of these 2 groups of specimens showed that many of the inner ear's sensory structures had developed in the control explants treated with trypsin, and that chondrogenesis of the otic capsule had taken place, but was abnormal in appearance. The trypsin-treated otocysts that had their adhering mesenchyme dissected prior to explantation showed that some mesenchyme had remained and there were small islands of abnormal cartilage. The ectodermal cells, of these otocysts from which mesenchyme had been dissected, tended to form many small cyst-like structures with small patches of differentiated sensory hair cells, but that these sensory cell areas had not organized into any definable inner ear sensory structure.

Because of the abnormalities that were evident in the trypsin-treated control specimens, a second series of experiments with mesenchymal removal was undertaken in which 11-, 12-, and 12.5-day-old mouse embryonic otocysts were stripped of most of their enveloping cephalic mesenchyme without the aid of proteolytic enzymes or Ca^{++} and Mg^{++} free saline solutions. This second series of experiments with mesenchymal extirpation was composed of 84 specimens. At the time of surgical removal of the otocysts from the embryo, one otocyst was excised in the normal manner with its surrounding cephalic mesenchyme (M) intact, while the contralateral otocyst was dissected with as little adhering cephalic mesenchyme (m) as possible. Only matched pairs of otocysts derived from the same embryo were employed in this study, to provide exact control for the developmental stage at time of explantation. Photomicrographs of all of the specimens were taken, to record gross morphology, at the time of explantation and again at the end of the period of development in vitro.

The experiment was divided into 3 groups for each gestational age studied. The first group consisted of explanted otocysts with adequate amounts of adhering periotic mesenchyme (M), while a second group consisted of otocysts that were explanted with a minimal amount of adhering periotic mesenchyme (m). The third group was composed of pairs of otocysts explanted from the same embryo. These otocysts were co-cultured in the same culture dish in close proximity to one another, with one otocyst being grown with its mesenchyme intact (M) as in group 1, while the other had had its mesenchyme reduced (m) as in group 2. Group 3 was included in the study to explore the possibility that there may be some factor from the normal mesenchyme "M" specimens that could be transmitted through the culture media to the specimens with reduced mesenchyme, thus causing differences in morphogenesis when these reduced mesenchyme specimens are compared to those of Group 2 with reduced mesenchyme (m) that were not co-cultured with normal mesenchyme specimens.

The morphogenesis observed in the organ-cultured specimens with reduced mesenchyme (m) was comparable in both groups of explants. The co-culturing of "M" and "m" specimens in close proximity within the same organ culture dish did not appear to affect the course of morphogenesis of the specimen with reduced mesenchyme (m). A series of photomicrographs of a co-cultured pair of otocysts of 11 gestational days with intact mesenchyme (M) and reduced mesenchyme (m), extirpated from the same embryo, are seen in Figure 18. The most striking feature is the difference in size due primarily to the development of a cartilaginous otic capsule in the "M" specimen and the apparent lack of it in the "m" specimen. More detailed analysis of the specimens also revealed that the "M" specimens had undergone morphogenesis into areas of vestibule and cochlear duct, while the "m" specimens did not undergo an organized pattern of morphogenesis, but appeared to form many small vesicular structures. A histologic presentation of the preceding morphogenesis is illustrated in Figures 19A and C which are photomicrographs of cross-sections of the "M" and "m" specimens, respectively, seen in Figure 18.

The histogenesis of sensory structures of "M" specimens was normal (Fig. 19A), but the histogenesis of the "m" specimens (Fig. 19C) was affected in relation to

---

Fig. 18. A series of photomicrographs of developing explants at A) 0 hours, B) 3 days, and C) 9 days in vitro, of 11-day-old mouse embryo inner ears. The specimen with reduced mesenchyme is marked "m" and the specimen with normal mesenchyme "M". Pars superior (PS), pars inferior (PI), semicircular ducts (SSC), and cochlear duct (CD) are as indicated by labels. (×8)

Mammalian Inner Ear Development / 33

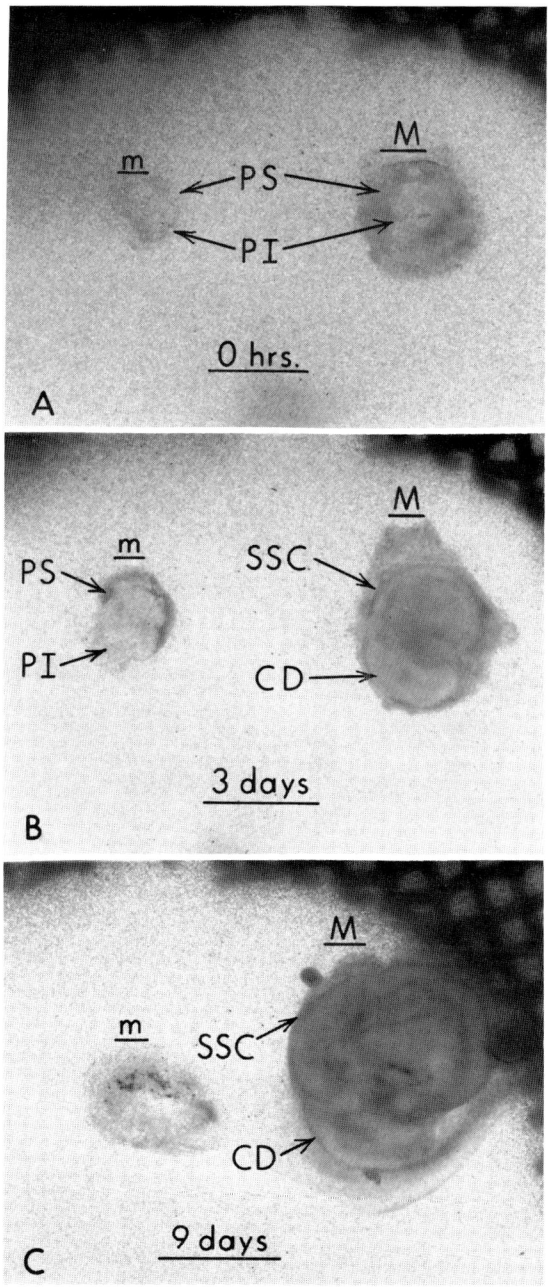

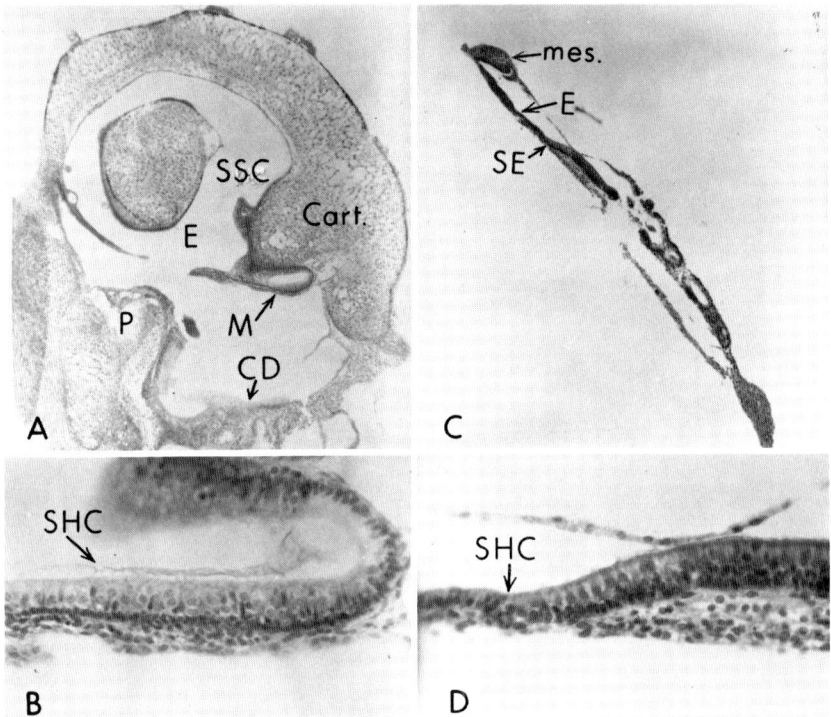

Fig. 19. Photomicrographs of histologic features of the specimens "M" and "m," 11 days old as in Fig. 18, after 10 days' development in vitro: A) a specimen with normal mesenchyme "M" in cross-section; B) a high-powered photomicrograph of the macula of sensory cells in 19A; C) a specimen with reduced mesenchyme "m" in cross-section; and D) a high-powered photomicrograph of the sensory cell area of Figure 19C. The following labels were employed in identification: (Cart.) cartilage, (CD) cochlear duct, (E) endolymphatic lumen, (M) macula, (Mes.) mesenchyme, (P) perilymphatic space, (SE) sensory epithelium, (SHC) sensory hair cell, and (SSC) semicircular canal. (A and C ×55; B and D ×300)

the formation of sensory structures. The cytodifferentiation of sensory hair cells in both specimens "M" and "m" was similar in nature (see Figs. 19B and D, respectively). These results were most dramatically evident in the 11-day-old specimens and tended to decrease in severity in proportion to increasing embryonic age. These preliminary observations, based on 126 specimens, suggest that there is a continuing influence of the mesenchyme upon the morphogenesis and histogenesis of sensory structures developing in the explants of mouse inner ear during the period of embryogenesis of the inner ear. This period of time in the fetal mouse extends from approximately the 8th to the 14th day of gestation.

Ventral Mesenchyme

Li and McPhee [55, 56] studied the effects of the removal of a piece of mesenchyme from the ventral portion of otic explants upon the development and coiling of the cochlear duct within these in vitro developing explants. Otocysts of the 11th, 12th, and 13th gestational day were excised and each gestational age group was treated as a unit. Each group was further subdivided into 2 groups: in the first, controls underwent no further microsurgical manipulation and were explanted directly to the system in vitro; the second (or reduced ventral-mesenchyme (VM) group), had adhering cephalic mesenchyme dissected away from the ventral half of the otocyst prior to their explantation in vitro. This ventral half of the otocyst represents the area from which the cochlear duct is fated to develop [28, 29].

All of the explanted otocysts were allowed to develop to the equivalent of the 21st day of gestation. All of the explanted inner ears showed normal development of vestibular sensory structures. The cochlear ducts of otocysts with ventral mesenchyme (VM) removed expanded in an unrestrained manner, forming a cyst-like extrusion (Fig. 20B). Cochlear ducts of the control specimens exhibited a normal pattern of morphogenesis in vitro and coiled inwards in a spiral pattern (Fig. 20A).

Additionally, the observation was made that a progressive amount of coiling was observed in specimens of the control groups, which correlated to the em-

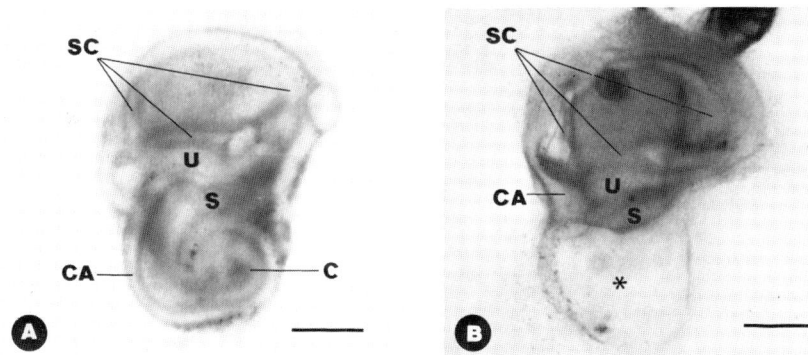

Fig. 20. A) Inner ear developed from a mouse otocyst 13 gestational days old in the control experiment, after 9 days in vitro. "SC" denotes the semicircular ducts, "U" the utricle, "S" the saccule, "C" the cochlea of one and one-half turns, and "CA" the cartilaginous capsule. Anterior side is on the right. Line = 200 μm. B) Inner ear developed from a mouse otocyst 13 gestational days old, with ventral mesenchyme removed, at the 9th day in vitro. "SC" denotes the semicircular ducts, "U" the utricle, "S" the saccule, "*" the defective cochlea in a cystic form, and "CA" shows a cartilaginous capsule with normal development in the dorsal area, and defective formation in the ventral area. Anterior side is on the right. Line = 200 μm. (From Li CW, McPhee J: Development of the cochlea and its coiling mechanism. Otolaryngology 86:292–296, 1978, with permission.)

bryonic age of the explanted otocyst. Thirteen-day-old otocysts exhibited coiling of the cochleae ranging from 1 to 1½ turns, while the 11-day-old otocysts merely produced cochleae in the form of a hook or ¼ turn. The 12-day-old otocysts showed varying degrees of coiling, from ¼ to one full turn. It is evident that the growth and shape of the cochlea are influenced by the formation of the cartilaginous capsule, which is in turn induced by the developing labyrinth. Coiling of the cochlea may be the result of epithelio-mesenchymal cell interactions or of a physical barrier and support provided by the cartilaginous cells differentiating from the surrounding ventral mesenchyme of the otocyst, or a combined effect of both factors.

Treatment with LACA

L-azetidine-2-carboxylic acid (LACA) is an analog of l-proline and has been shown to interfere with production of collagen [49]. Since collagen has been found to be one of the major constituents of basement membranes in developing systems [50], an experiment was designed to investigate the effect of this analog of l-proline, LACA, upon organogenesis of the inner ear as it occurs in vitro. Otocysts of 12, 12.5, and 13 gestational days were extirpated, surrounded by a gen-

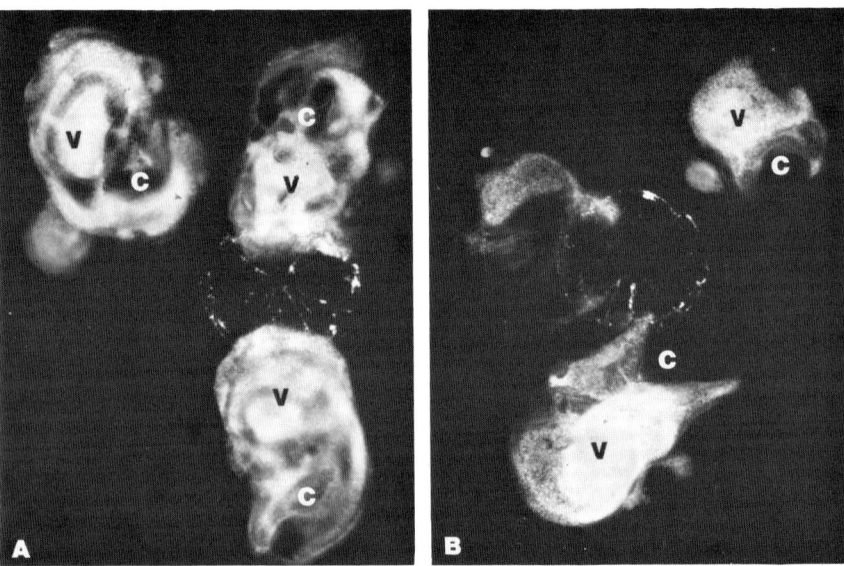

Fig. 21. Darkfield photomicrographs of living explants of inner ear 12 days old, that have developed for 9 days in vitro: A) control cultures exhibiting morphogenesis of vestibular (v) and cochlear ductal (c) cartilaginous capsules; B) cultures of inner ear that were grown in the presence of 100 μg/ml of LACA. The vestibular and cochlear capsular development is abnormal. (×12)

Mammalian Inner Ear Development / 37

erous amount of cephalic mesenchyme, and explanted to the organ culture system. Each gestational age was divided into 4 groups: the first were controls with normal media; in the next 3 groups, the nutrient media contained dosages of 25 µg/ml, 50 µg/ml and 100 µg/ml, respectively, of the 1-proline analog LACA. All media, both the normal and those containing dosages of LACA, were changed every 3rd day. All specimens were grown in vitro to the equivalent age of 21 days in vivo.

Specimens were observed every other day with the aid of a dissecting microscope, and photomicrographs were taken on the day of explantation and the day of fixation for histologic preparation. The entire cartilaginous capsule appeared abnormal in the 12-day-old specimens receiving either 50 or 100 µg/ml of LACA (Fig. 21B) when compared to the 12-day-old controls (Fig. 21A). The vestibular capsule of the 12.5-day-old specimens with 50 and 100 µg/ml of LACA appeared normal, but the area of the cochlear duct was abnormal (Fig. 22B) when compared to 12.5-day-old control specimens (Fig. 22A). Twelve- and 12.5-day-old otocysts receiving 25 µg/ml of LACA in the culture media showed no differences in morphogenesis of labyrinthine form when compared to their respective control specimens. The 13-day-old otocysts cultured in the presence of 100 µg/ml of

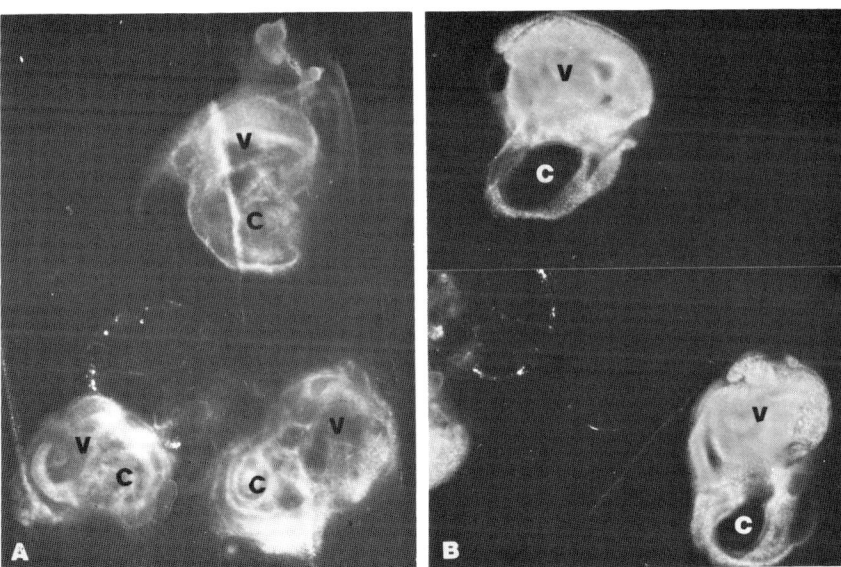

Fig. 22. Darkfield photomicrographs of living explants 12.5 days old, that have developed for 9 days in vitro: A) control cultures exhibiting morphogenesis of vestibular (v) and cochlea ductal (c) cartilaginous capsules; B) otocystic explants that were cultured in the presence of 100 µg/ml of LACA. The vestibular capsule appears normal in contrast to the abnormal development of the cartilaginous capsule of the cochlear duct. (×12)

LACA in the media did not differ in morphogenesis from that observed in the 13-day-old control otocysts.

Histologic details from a normal 12-day-old control after 9 days in vitro are seen in Figure 23A, and a high magnification of a normal crista is seen in Figure 23B. In contrast to this untreated control specimen, a photomicrograph of a 12-

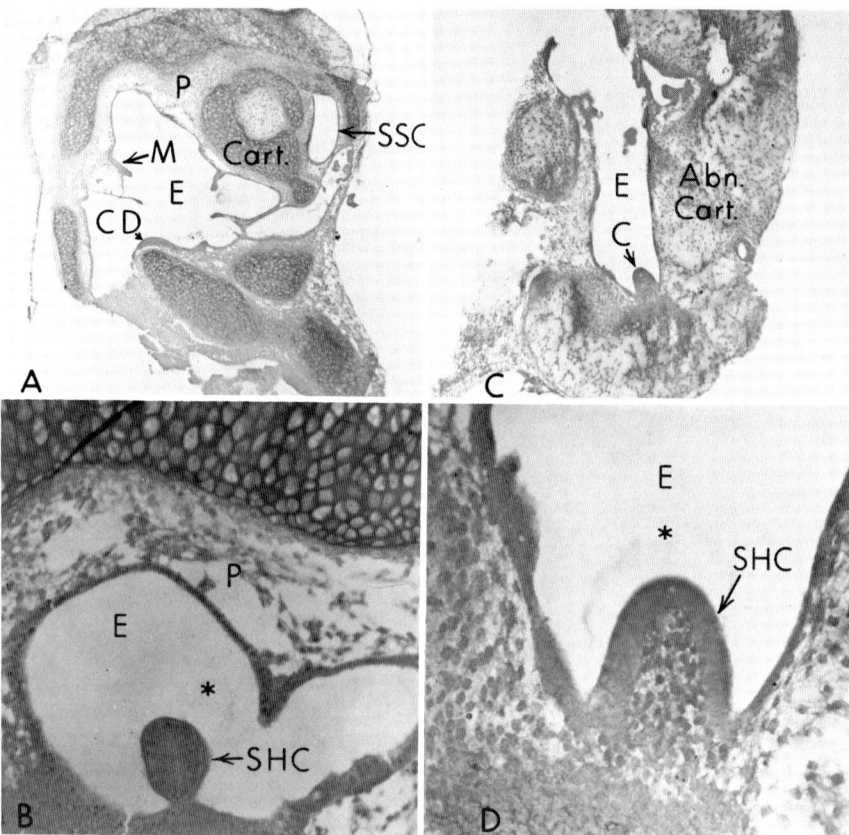

Fig. 23. Photomicrographs of the histologic features of otocysts 12 days old, that developed for 9 days in vitro: A) a normal culture showing well-differentiated sensory structures, endolymphatic and perilymphatic spaces, and a cartilaginous otic capsule; B) an ampulla with cristae from a normal culture; C) a culture grown in the presence of 100 μg/ml of LACA showing an abnormal capsule, poor development of perilymphatic spaces, and poor distribution of differentiated sensory epithelia; D) a crista that differentiated in the lumen of the otocyst of a culture with 100 μg/ml of LACA. The following symbols were used as labels: (Abn. Cart.) abnormal cartilage, (c) crista, (Cart.) cartilage, (CD) cochlear duct, (E) endolymphatic lumen, (M) macula, (P) perilymphatic spaces, (SHC) sensory hair cell and (*) to denote the cupula. (A and C × 55; B and D × 300)

day-old otocyst grown for 9 days in the presence of 100 µg/ml of LACA is presented in Figure 23C. A crista that developed in the specimen represented in Figure 23C is seen in greater detail in Figure 23D. The histogenesis of sensory structures in 12-day-old explants cultured in the presence of 100 µg/ml of LACA was impaired, but not totally prevented, as illustrated by the crista of Figure 23D. This crista, however, was the only defined sensory structure that formed in the specimen represented in Figure 23C; cytodifferentiation of hair cells occurred in other portions of the specimen, but without formation of specific sensory structures, as were observed to form in the 12-day-old controls (Fig. 23A). Thirteen-day-old inner ear anlage that developed for 8 days in vitro are seen in Figure 24, with 24A being a control culture and 24B a specimen that received 100 µg/ml of LACA in the culture media. No histologic differences were noted in the occurrence or distribution of sensory structures within these 13-day-old cultures.

The analog of 1-proline, LACA, appeared to affect both morphogenesis of labyrinthine form and histogenesis of sensory structures of 12- and 12.5-day-old explants. Cytodifferentiation of some sensory hair cells occurred in 12- and 12.5-day-old explanted otocysts treated with LACA. The 13-day-old specimens were

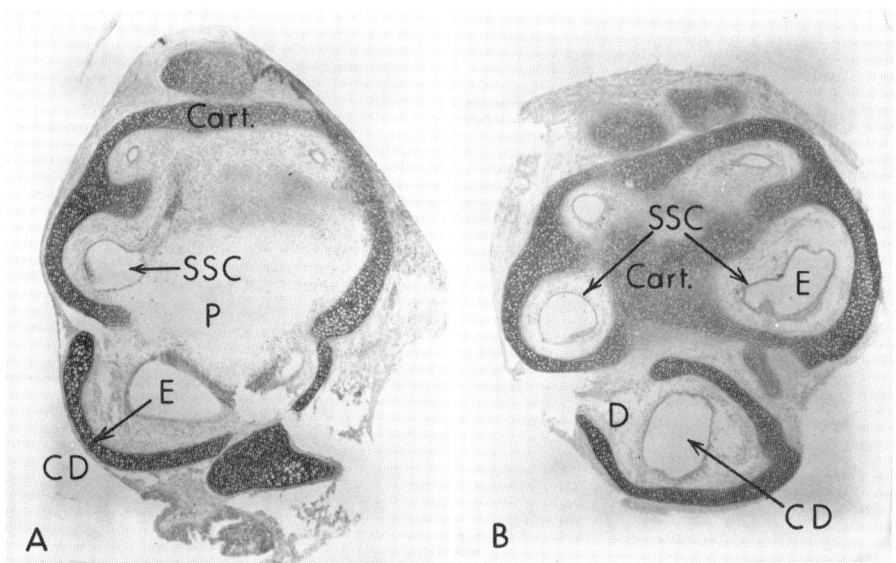

Fig. 24. Photomicrographs of explants of inner ear 13 days old, that developed for 8 days in vitro: A) an untreated explant showing normal development of sensory structures, endolymphatic and perilymphatic spaces, and a cartilaginous otic capsule; B) an explant treated with 100 µg/ml of LACA showing normal development as described in 24A. Symbols used as labels are: (Cart.) cartilage, (CD) cochlear duct, (E) endolymphatic spaces, (P) perilymphatic spaces and (SSC) semicircular ducts. (×55)

not affected by in vitro administration of LACA in the culture media. The work of Hay [50] and Coulombre [49] suggests that LACA may interrupt production of a basement membrane in the explants of otocysts and thereby affect the interactions taking place between the otocyst and its surrounding cephalic mesenchyme. This is only one of many mechanisms of action that could be responsible for the teratogenic effect of LACA upon development of the inner ear in vitro.

GENERAL OVERVIEW

The mechanisms involved in the development of the mammalian labyrinth in vitro have been experimentally explored in the preceding sections, and the resultant data condensed and presented. New data has also been presented in preliminary form. These findings of the in vitro model system of development of a mammalian inner ear have been combined with experimental embryologic data generated in other tetrapod species [1] to produce a generalized schema of tissue interactions that are important in the normal development of a tetrapod labyrinth. A flow-chart diagramming tissue interactions that occur during the period of embryologic development of a tetrapod labyrinth is presented in Figure 25.

In reports of embryologic investigations in avian [31] and amphibian [2, 32] species, it has been shown that determination of the cephalic ectoderm by the inductive action of chorda mesoderm results in the formation of an otic field. Recent ultrastructural studies in the chick [57, 58] present a temporal relationship which may suggest that migrating neural crest cells interact with ectodermal cells of the otic field to induce formation of an otic placode.

These ultrastructural findings are in contradiction to an earlier study [65] in chick embryos which reported that migrating avian cephalic neural crest cells did not appear to pass under the site of the auditory placode but instead split into 2 migrating columns of cells, one passing anterior and the other posterior to the site of the auditory anlage. Neurulation which is occurring during the otic cup stage of development causes this otic anlage to come into close apposition with the developing rhombencephalon. Experiments utilizing and examining amphibian [2, 3, 14, 24, 33, 34], avian [31, 59], and mammalian embryos [39] as well as analysis of the development of congenitally malformed labyrinths [15, 16, 30] provide evidence that the inductive interaction occurring between the otic anlage and the neural tube is essential for the continuation of orderly labyrinthine development. The occurrence of an endolymphatic projection at the otocyst stage of inner ear development was previously thought to be necessary for continuation of normal development of the labyrinth [14, 18]. Recent experiments in vitro [20] do not support this view, but rather suggest that the occurrence of the endolymphatic projection at the otocyst stage of inner ear development is an indicator that a normal neural inductive interaction has occurred during the otic cup stage.

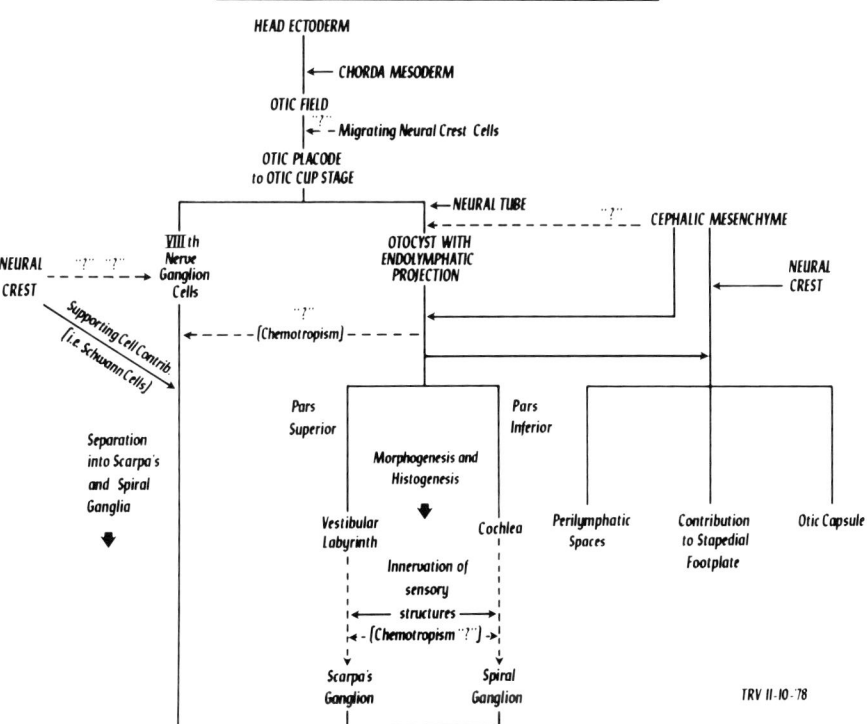

Fig. 25. Flow-diagram illustrating the tissue interactions which occur during the development of the labyrinth.

The lack of development of an endolymphatic projection at the otocyst stage of inner ear development may therefore be suggestive that a faulty neural inductive interaction has occurred between the rhombencephalon and the developing otic cup.

Direct trophic effects of neural elements upon histogenesis and differentiation of labyrinthine sensory structures have been suggested by anatomic studies of inner ear development within several species [1]. Experimentation in vitro involving reaggregates of dissociated avian otocysts [8] supports this view of a trophic action of neural elements upon labyrinthine development. Experimental surgical studies of explants of mammalian otocysts developing in vitro [20] do not demonstrate that the ingrowing neural components of the statoacoustic ganglion complex have any trophic effects on histogenesis of sensory structures of the inner ear or cytodifferentiation of sensory hair cells. As a possible interpretation of previous experimental observations [1, 8] it has been postulated [20] that trophic effects stemming from differentiating neuroblast cells (ie differentiating sensory hair cells) may result from the establishment of a chemotrophic gradient which causes the attraction of the growth cones of the ingrowing neural elements of the statoacoustic ganglion.

The contribution of the neural crest to the otic capsule and columella auris in birds has been documented in chick/quail embryo chimera experiments, but contribution of neural crest cells to the ganglion cell population of the VIII nerve ganglion of the avian inner ear was not observed during the course of these studies [60, 61]. Neural crest cells were observed [60, 61] to make extensive contributions to the supporting cell population of the VIII nerve ganglion. Deol [62] has suggested that there may actually be a dual origin of the VIII nerve ganglion in a mammalian species, based on his analysis of neural crest mutants, but, as yet, no definitive evidence has been presented to support this view. Documentation of the role of the otic vesicle during induction of its otic capsule and stapedial footplate has been reported in several species [2, 7, 27, 34, 37, 38, 53, 54], and more recently has been augmented by the experiments investigating the inductive role that a critical tissue mass of periotic mesenchyme plays in in vitro morphogenesis and cytodifferentiation of explanted otocysts.

The section on epithelio-mesenchymal tissue interaction demonstrates that reciprocal tissue interactions are taking place during early labyrinthine development. These experiments show that the otocyst not only acts as an inducer of chondrogenesis of its surrounding cephalic mesenchyme, but that tissue interactions occurring between the developing otocyst and this mesenchyme are also essential for orderly morphogenesis and histogenesis of sensory structures of the inner ear within the developing otocyst. The inductive events that are described in Figure 25 must not be viewed as single isolated events, but rather as a continuum of interrelated tissue interactions, each dependent upon some completed or still ongoing tissue interaction that allows for or directs the orderly organogenesis and cytodifferentiation of the tetrapod labyrinth.

ACKNOWLEDGMENTS

The authors thank Mr. M. Kurtz for his excellent photographic assistance, Mr. L. Montfries for the graphic arts, and Mrs. J. Cavalcante for the typing of this manuscript.

REFERENCES

1. Van De Water TR, Ruben RJ: Organogenesis of the ear. In Hinchcliffe R, Harrison D (eds): "Scientific Foundation of Otolaryngology." London: William Heinemann Medical Book, Ltd, 1976, pp 173–184.
2. Yntema CL: An analysis of induction of the ear from foreign ectoderm in the salamander embryo. J Exp Zool 113:211–243, 1950.

3. Chuang HH: Experiments concerning the induction and morphogenesis of the otic vesicle in urodelian amphibian. Acta Biol Exper Sinica. 6:352–363, 1959.
4. Friedmann I, Bird ES: The effect of ototoxic antibodies and of penicillin on the sensory areas of the isolated fowl embryo otocyst in organ cultures. J Pathol Bacteriol 81:81–90, 1961.
5. McAlpine JC, Friedmann I: A histochemical study of the effects of ototoxic antibiotics on the isolated embryonic otocyst of the fowl (*Gallus domesticus*). J Pathol Bacteriol 86:477–486, 1963.
6. Friedmann I: The chick embryo otocyst in tissue culture: A model ear. J Laryngol Otol 82:185–201, 1968.
7. Benoit JAA: Etude experimentale des facteurs de l'induction du cartilago otique chez les embryons de poulet et de truite. Ann Sci Naturelles Zool 12:327–385, 1960.
8. Orr MF: Histogenesis of sensory epithelium in reaggregate of dissociated embryonic chick otocysts. Dev Biol 17:39–54, 1968.
9. Van De Water TR, Ruben RJ: Quantification of the "in vitro" development of the mouse embryo inner ear. Ann Otol Rhinol Laryngol 82(Suppl 4):19–21, 1973.
10. Fell HB: Development "in vitro" of the isolated otocyst of the embryonic fowl. Arch Exp Zellforsch Besonders Gewebeznecht 7:69–81, 1928.
11. Todd JR: On the process of reproduction of the members of the aquatic salamander. QJ Sci Lit Arts 16:84–96, 1923.
12. Farbman AI: Taste bud regeneration in organ culture. Ann NY Acad Sci 228:350–354, 1974.
13. Van De Water TR: Effects of removal of the statoacoustic ganglion complex upon the growing otocyst. Ann Otol Rhinol Laryngol 85(Suppl 33):1–32, 1976.
14. Harrison RG: Relations of symmetry in the developing embryo. Trans Conn Acad Arts Sci 36:277–330, 1945.
15. Bonnevie K: Abortive differentiation of the ear vesicle following a hereditary brain-anomaly in the short-tailed-waltzing mice. Genetica 18:105–125, 1936.
16. Hertwig P: Die Genese der Hirn-und Gehörganmissibildungen bei röntgenmutierten Kreisler-Mäusen. Z Mensch Vereb Konst 28:327–354, 1944.
17. Partsch CJ: Entwicklungsstörungen des Ductus und Saccus endolymphaticus als Ursache der Innenohrmissbildung. Z Laryngol Rhinol Otol 45:529–538, 1966.
18. Hendricks DM, Toerien MJ: Experimental endolymphatic hydrops. S Afr Med J 47:2294–2300, 1973.
19. Van De Water TR, Ruben RJ: Symposium: New data for noise standards (III). Organ culture of the mammalian inner ear. A tool to study inner ear deafness. Laryngoscope 86:738–749, 1974.
20. Van De Water TR: The effect of the removal of the endolymphatic duct and sac anlage upon organogenesis of the mammalian inner ear "in vitro:" A preliminary report. Arch Otorhinolaryngol (NY) 217:297–311, 1977.
21. Levy O: Entwicklungsmechanische studien am Embryo von *Triton taeniatus*. (1) Orientierungsversuche. Roux' Arch Entw Mech 20:335–379, 1906.
22. Streeter GL: Experimental evidence concerning the determinations of posture of the membranous labyrinth in amphibian embryos. J Exp Zool 16:149–176, 1914.
23. Spemann H: Uber die Determination der ersten Organanlagen des Amphibienembryo, I–VI. Roux' Arch Entw-Mech 43:448–555, 1918.
24. Harrison RG: Experiments on the development of the internal ear. Science. 59:448, 1924.
25. Harrison RG: Relations of symmetry in the developing ear of *Amblystoma punctatum*. Proc Natl Acad Sci 22:238–247, 1936.

26. Hall EK: On the duration of the polarization process in the ear primordium of embryos of *Amblystoma punctatum* (Linn.). J Exp Zool 82:173–192, 1939.
27. Kaan HW: Experiments of the development of the ear of *Amblystoma punctatum*. J Exp Zool 46:13–61, 1926.
28. Li CW, Van De Water TR, Ruben RJ: "In vitro" study of fate mapping of the mouse otocyst. Trans Am Acad Ophthalmol Otolaryngol 82:ORL-273-280, 1976.
29. Li CW, Van De Water TR, Ruben RJ: The fate mapping of the eleventh and twelfth day mouse otocyst: An "in vitro" study of the sites of origin of the embryonic inner ear sensory structures. J Morphol 157:249–268, 1978.
30. Li CW: Congenital malformation of inner ear: 1. An "in vitro" study of cell determination of the homozygotic and heterozygotic Kreisler mouse otocysts. Dev Neurosci 2:7–18, 1979.
31. Waddington CH: The determination of the auditory placode in the chick. J Exp Biol 14:232–239, 1937.
32. Zwilling E: The determination of the otic vesicle in *Rana pipens*. J Exp Zool 86:333–342, 1941.
33. Detwiler SR: Further quantitative studies on locomotor capacity of larval *Amblystoma* following surgical procedures upon the embryonic brain. J Exp Zool 108:45–74, 1948.
34. Detwiler SR, Van Dyke RH: The role of the medulla in the differentiation of the otic vesicle. J Exp Zool 113:197–199, 1950.
35. Yntema CL: Experiments on determination of the ear ectoderm of *Amblystoma punctatum*. J Exp Zool 65:317–357, 1933.
36. Deol MS: Abnormalities of the inner ear in Kreisler mice. J Embryol Exp Morphol 12: 475–490, 1964.
37. Kaan HW: The relation of the developing auditory vesicle to the formation of the cartilage capsule in *Amblystoma punctatum*. J Exp Zool 55:263–291, 1930.
38. Kaan HW: Further studies on the auditory vesicle and cartilaginous capsule of *Amblystoma punctatum*. J Exp Zool 78:159–183, 1938.
39. Li CW, Van De Water TR, Ruben RJ, Shea CA: Rhombencephalic induction on the differentiation of the tenth gestation day mouse otocyst. (Abstract) Association of Research on Otolaryngology, Midwinter meeting, Clearwater, Florida, January, 1978.
40. Grobstein C: Morphogenic interaction between embryonic mouse tissues separated by a transmembrane filter. Nature 172:869–871, 1953.
41. Grobstein C: Some transmission characteristics of the tubule-inducing influence on mouse metanephrogenic mesenchyme. Exp Cell Res 13:575–587, 1957.
42. Saxen L: Transfilter neural induction of amphibian ectoderm. Dev Biol 3:140–152, 1961.
43. Gallera J: Quelle est la durée necessaire pour de clencher des inductions neurales chez le poulet? Experientia 21:218–219, 1967.
44. Bernfield MR, Cohen RH, Banerjee SD: Glycosaminoglycans and epithelial organ formation. Am Zool 13:1067–1083, 1973.
45. Grobstein C, Cohen J: Collagenase: Effect on the morphogenesis of embryonic salivary epithelium "in vitro." Science 150:626–628, 1965.
46. Grobstein C: Mechanisms of organogenetic tissue interaction. Natl Cancer Inst Monogr 26:279–299, 1967.
47. McLoughlin CB: Interaction of epidermis with various types of foreign mesenchyme. In Fleischmajer R, Billingham RE (eds): "Epithelial-Mesenchymal Interaction." Baltimore: Williams & Wilkins, 1968, pp 244–251.
48. Grobstein C: Developmental significance of interface materials in epitheliomesenchymal interaction. Ibid, pp 173–176.

49. Coulombre A, Coulombre J: Corneal development. IV. Interruption of collagen excretion into the primary stroma of the cornea with L-azetidine-2-carboxylic acid. Dev Biol 28: 183–190, 1972.
50. Hay ED: Origin and role of collagen in the embryo. Am Zool 13:1085–1107, 1973.
51. Hay ED, Meier S: Glycosaminoglycan synthesis by embryonic inductors: Neural tube notochord, and lens. J Cell Biol 62:889–898, 1974.
52. Newsome D: "In vitro" stimulation of cartilage in embryonic chick neural crest cells by products of retinal pigmented epithelium. Dev Biol 49:496–507, 1976.
53. Grobstein C, Holtzer H: "In vitro" studies of cartilage induction in mouse somite mesoderm. J Exp Zool 28:333–357, 1955.
54. Benoit JAA: Action inductrice de durée variable sur le mésenchyme otique de l'embryon de poulet en culture in vitro. CR Acad Sci (D) Paris 258:334–336, 1964.
55. Li CW, McPhee J: Development of the cochlea and its coiling mechanism. Otolaryngology 86:292–296, 1978.
56. Li CW, McPhee J: Influences on the coiling of the cochlea. Ann Otol Rhinol Laryngol 88:280–287, 1979.
57. Meier S: Development of the embryonic chick otic placode: I. Light microscopic analysis. Anat Rec 191:447–458, 1978.
58. Meier S: Development of the embryonic chick otic placode: II. Electron microscopic analysis. Anat Rec 191:459–478, 1978.
59. Muria Garcia F: Experimental contribution to the study of the neural influence in the development of the organ of hearing. Rev Esp Otoneuroatal 21:230–232, 1962.
60. Noden DW: The control of avian cephalic neural crest cytodifferentiation. I. Skeletal and connective tissues. Dev Biol 67:296–312, 1978.
61. Noden DW: The control of avian cephalic neural crest cytodifferentiation. II. Neural tissues. Dev Biol 67:313–329, 1978.
62. Deol MS: Deficiencies of the inner ear in the mouse and their origin. Colloques Internationaux CNRS. #266 Mechanisms of the Embryogenesis of the Organs of Vertebrate Embryos, 163–171, 1978.
63. Rugh R: "The Mouse: Its Reproduction and Development." Minneapolis: Burgess Publishing, 1968.
64. Theiler K: "The House Mouse: Development and Normal Stages From Fertilization to 4 Weeks of Age." Berlin, Heidelberg, New York: Springer-Verlag, 1972.
65. Noden DM: A radiographic analysis of the migration of avian cephalic neural crest cells. PhD Dissertation, Washington University, St. Louis, 1972.

Dysmorphogenesis of the Inner Ear

Harold F. Schuknecht, MD

Developmental defects of the inner ear may occur as anatomic variants, dysplasias associated with syndromes, or isolated dysplasias. They may be caused by genetic factors or noxious prenatal influences. The group of defects called anatomic variants by definition, consists of frequently occurring morphologic alterations which usually have no effect on function of the inner ear and should not be given undue significance. There are 5 common defects of the bony labyrinth, and 5 of the membranous labyrinth.

Microfissures of the bony labyrinth are small fissures found in all adult temporal bones and are presumed to result from stresses occurring during growth and remodeling of the bone. A constant fissure is found between the niche of the round window and the ampulla of the posterior semicircular canal (Fig. 1). The scala communis is a condition of the bony labyrinth consisting of a defect in the interscalar septum, and is most frequently seen between the middle and apical turns (Fig. 2) [1]. Defects of spiral lamina may allow the scala tympani and vestibuli to communicate, and nerve fibers may pass to the organ of Corti in bony canals (Fig. 3). Abnormal semicircular canals may be small, short, or missing (Fig. 3). The lateral canal is most frequently involved [2]. The principal significance of the variant of a large cochlear aqueduct is the role it plays in producing the copious flow of perilymph found occasionally during a stapedectomy (Fig. 1).

Defects of the membranous labyrinth include an absent utriculo-endolymphatic valve. This condition has no apparent effect on vestibular function. Or, there may be utriculosaccular confluence, which is associated with partial or total absence of utricular and saccular ducts (Fig. 4). Variations are found in the length of the cochlear duct. On 2-dimensional graphic reconstructions, the human cochlear duct varies from 27–35 mm with no apparent influence on cochlear function. Variations in length of the endolymphatic duct and size of the endolymphatic sac, however, do appear to have some correlation with Ménière disease, although the short duct and small sac can occur in normal inner ears [3]. Duplications, focal pro-

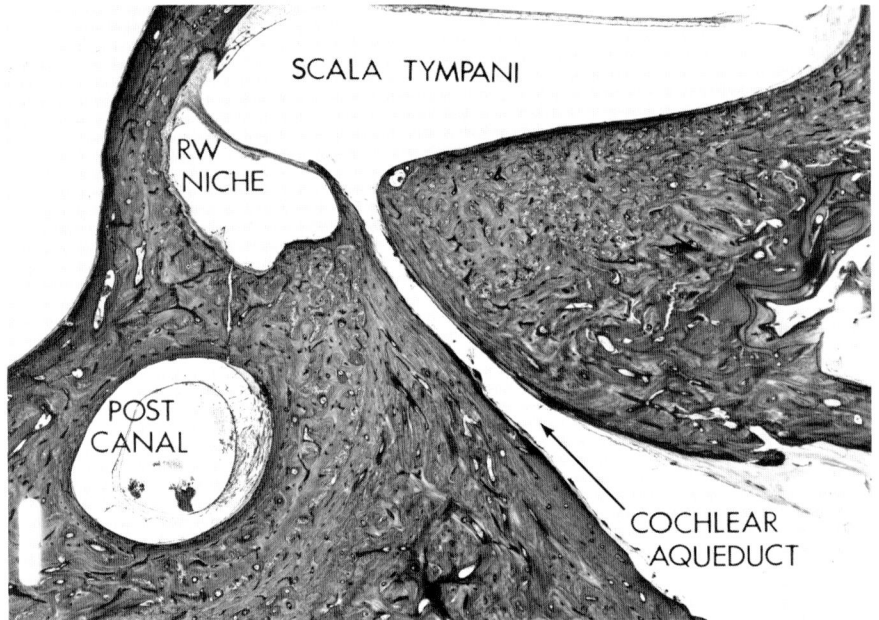

Fig. 1. A microfissure between the niche of the round window and crista of the posterior canal is a normal finding. This ear also has a large patent cochlear aqueduct.

liferations, and distortions of the membranous labyrinth are localized malformations causing no functional disturbance (Figs. 5 and 6).

Syndromes with associated dysplasia of the inner ear are caused principally by genetic factors. They are too numerous to be listed here. The reader is referred to the publication by Konigsmark and Gorlin [4] for a review of the subject. Suffice it to say that developmental defects of the inner ear may occur in association with defects of the external ear, eye, musculoskeletal system, skin, kidney, nervous system, endocrine glands, and in various chromosomal disorders. In general, our knowledge of morphology of the inner ear in these disorders is incomplete. Several examples will show the diverse dysplasias of the inner ear which accompany these syndromes.

ALPORT SYNDROME

Alport syndrome exhibits autosomal dominant inheritance principally affecting males and characterized by progressive nephritis and hearing loss [5].* Ocular manifestations are common and consist of cataracts, anterior lenticonus, spherophakia, and myopia. Histologic studies of temporal bones from individuals with

*It should be noted that there is a host of syndromes encompassing nephropathy and hearing loss (See ref. [4]).

Dysmorphogenesis of the Inner Ear / 49

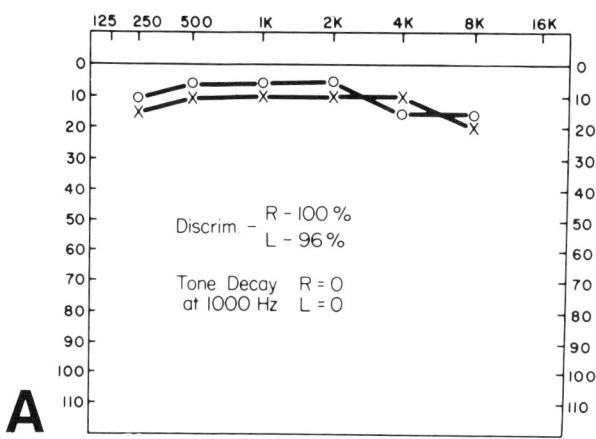

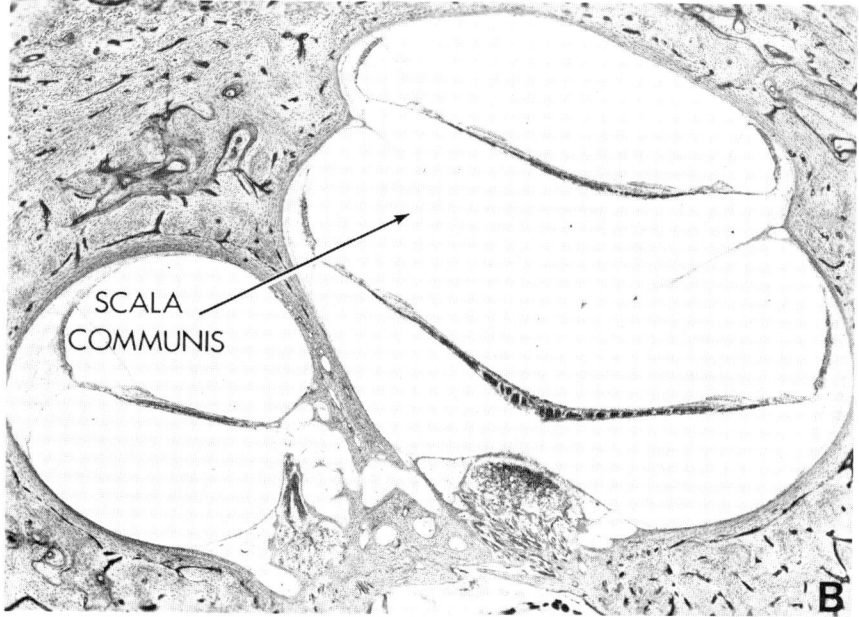

Fig. 2. Bilateral scala communis. A) This woman had normal hearing when tested at age 39. She died of multiple sclerosis one year later. B) Both ears show large defects of the cochlear partition between the 2nd and 3rd turns.

Alport syndrome have failed to reveal a consistent pathologic change [6]. Among the changes described in individual cases are loss of cochlear neurons, atrophy of the spiral ligament, loss of hair cells, endolymphatic hydrops, degeneration of the stria vascularis, and pigmentation of the substrial zone of the spiral ligament.

This subject first complained of hearing loss at age 15. He also had progressive nephritis. He was 1 of 6 sibs, 3 males and 3 females, 4 of whom showed evidence of nephritis. An older male sib died of renal failure at age 26. This individual died of renal failure at age 24. Histologic study shows similar findings in both ears of Case 1 (Alport Syndrome). The only abnormalities seen are a basophilic deposit in the substrial regions of the spiral ligaments and a moderate loss of cochlear neurons in the basal turns (Fig. 7).

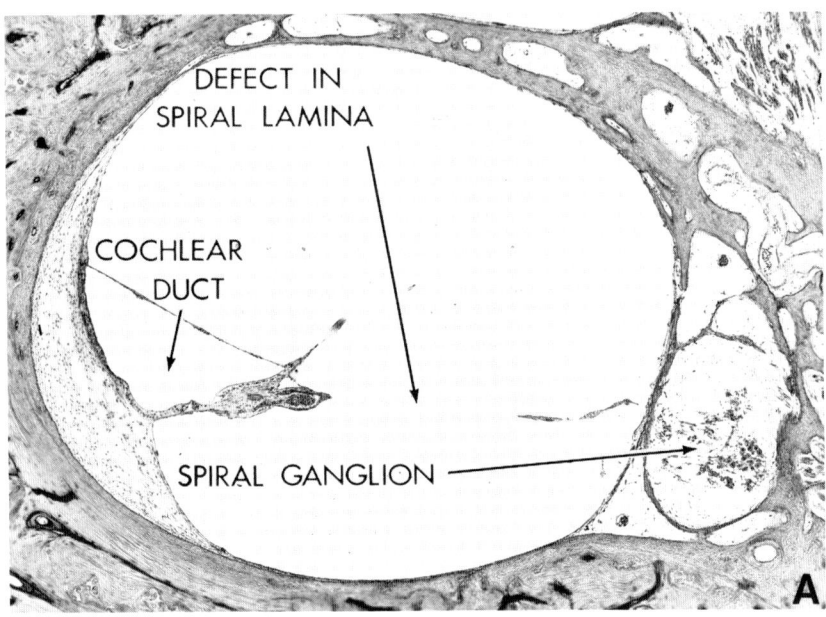

Fig. 3. This woman had multiple congenital malformations including bicornuate uterus, atresia of the left posterior communicating artery of the circle of Willis, spina bifida of the thoracic region, and fusion of the 2nd and 3rd cervical vertebrae. A) The inner ears show defects of the osseous spiral lamina in the right ear and B) absence of the posterior semicircular canal in the left ear. At the age of 41, she was found to have a moderately severe sensorineural hearing loss. She died at age 45 of nephrosclerosis. The hearing loss appears to be caused by atrophy of the hair cells and cochlear neurons.

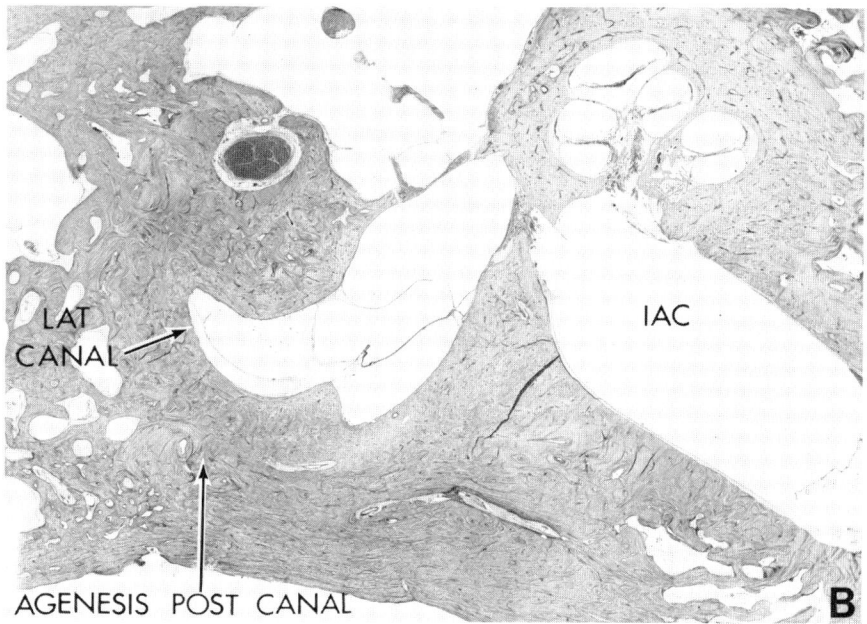

USHER SYNDROME

In 1914, Usher reported on 69 cases of retinitis pigmentosa of which 11 were profoundly deaf and 19 had some degree of hearing loss [7]. The subjects with severe hearing loss usually showed vestibulocerebellar ataxia. A recent study of temporal bones of a subject with moderately severe hearing loss showed loss of hair cells and neurons in the basal turn of the cochlea.

Case 2 (Usher Syndrome)

This person had a slowly progressive hearing loss beginning in early childhood.*
At age 11, audiometry showed a symmetric sensorineural loss varying from 20 dB for the low frequencies to 60 dB for the high frequencies (Fig. 8). At the age of 19, he complained of difficulty with night vision and was found to have retinitis

---

*Usher syndrome has recently been shown to have marked genetic heterogeneity. The more common types do not exhibit progressive hearing loss. This is probably Type III Usher syndrome. *R.J. Gorlin, Editor*

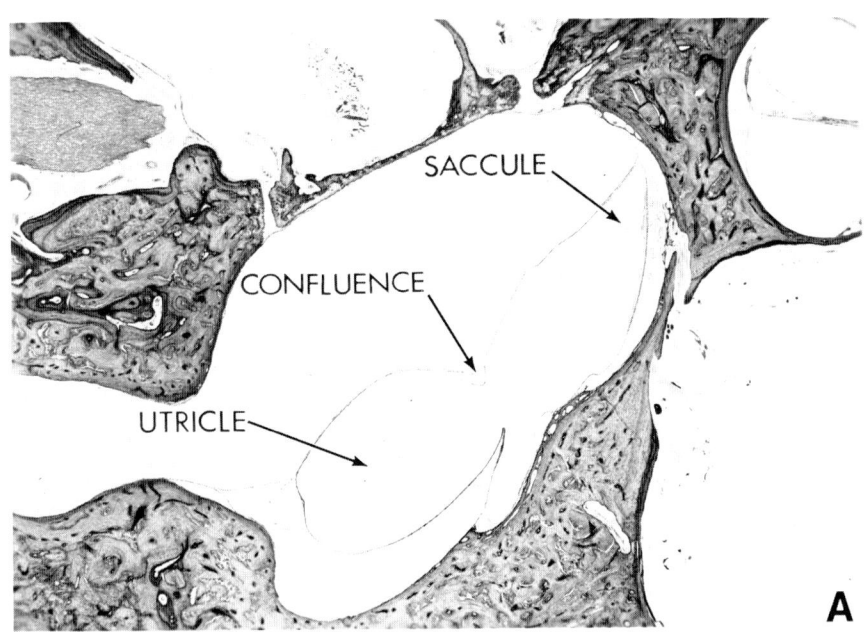

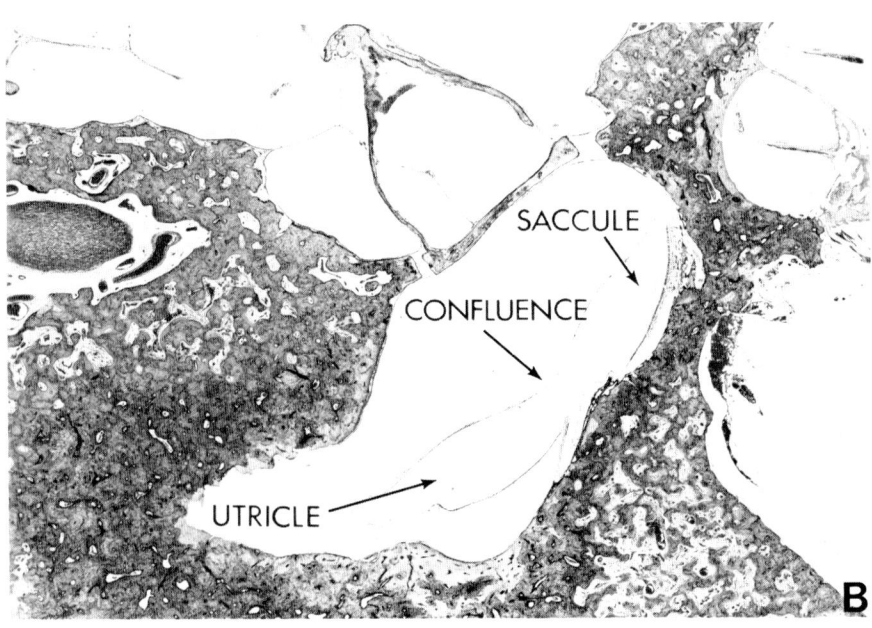

pigmentosa. At age 38, he died of hepatic cirrhosis. Histologic studies show similar findings in both ears. There is a partial loss of hair cells and cochlear neurons in the basal turns, and patchy areas of strial atrophy in the middle part of the basal turns. These changes do not adequately account for the severe hearing loss (Fig. 9).

In Klippel-Feil syndrome there is massive fusion of cervical vertebrae, with shortening of the neck, a low posterior hairline and restricted movement of the head and neck. Other anomalies which may occur are high scapulae, spina bifida, facial asymmetry, torticollis, cervical rib, cleft palate, vascular and pulmonary anomalies, and hearing loss [8]. The hearing loss may be unilateral or bilateral, sensorineural or conductive, or both, and of varying magnitude. Microtia and aural atresia may occur, and when present are often associated with fixation of ossicles and dysplasia of the inner ear of the Mondini type [9].

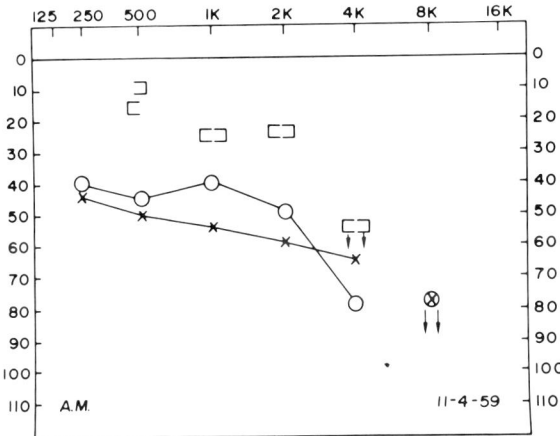

Fig. 5. Anomaly of cochlear duct apical turn. This woman had bilateral mild recurring otitis media. She died at age 84 of adenocarcinoma of the stomach. Audiogram at age 78 showed a predominantly conductive hearing loss. Bone conduction thresholds for the low frequencies were near normal for both ears.

Fig. 4. Utriculosaccular confluence. A) The utricle and saccule have a wide communication with each other and with the endolymphatic sinus. There were no vestibular symptoms attributable to this anomaly. B) The utricle and saccule have a wide communication with each other and with the lateral semicircular canal. There was severe Paget disease of the temporal bone but there were no symptoms attributable to the anomaly.

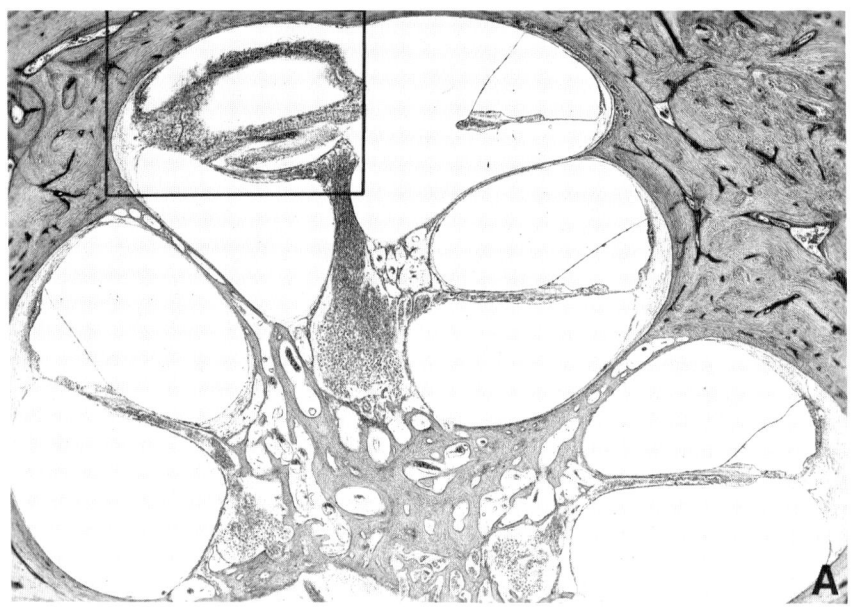

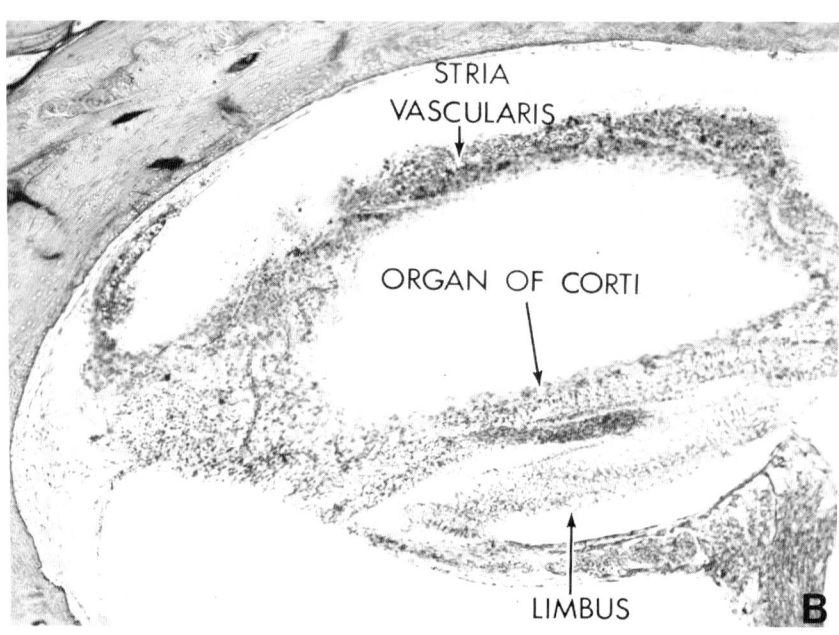

CHROMOSOMAL ANEUPLOIDY

Deviations from the normal number of autosomal chromosomes, in trisomic states, lead to serious alterations of the phenotype. Anomalies may also occur when the chromosomes are normal in number but exhibit partial trisomy by an unbalanced translocation or partial monosomy by deletion. The most familiar autosomal trisomy is that of chromosome 21 which causes Down syndrome, the incidence of which is 1 in 600 live births. Anomalies of the ear are rare in trisomy 21.

Trisomies of larger chromosomes such as 13 or 18 occur less frequently but are more disastrous. Infants afflicted with these aberrations fail to thrive, and die within a few days to a few months. Among the anomalies most frequently seen in these 2 syndromes are low-set ears, poorly differentiated pinnae, preauricular tags, aural atresia, absence of middle ear, cleft lip and/or cleft palate, micrognathia, microphthalmia, cataracts, retinal dysplasia, and aplasia of the optic nerve. Histologic studies have revealed a variety of anomalies of the inner ear including aplasia of the organ of Corti and stria vascularis, displacement and encapsulation of the tectorial membrane, collapsed cochlear duct with the Reissner membrane lying on the organ of Corti, aplasia of the saccule, scala communis, incomplete modiolus, large cochlear aqueduct, and aplasia of the cochlear nerve [10].

Case 3 (Trisomy 13)

This full-term white female, who has cochleosaccular dysgenesis, was born to a 41-year-old mother and a 42-year-old father. The infant presented multiple anomalies including microcephaly, cleft palate, cleft lip, microphthalmia, bilateral colobomata, low-set ears, polydactyly, seizures and failure to respond to sound. She died at the age of 25 days.

Both ears show cochleosaccular dysgenesis (Fig. 10). The external canals and middle ears are normal. In the basal turns the organs of Corti are either missing or replaced by a layer of fibrous tissue. In the middle and apical turns some of the supporting cells are present but hair cells are missing. The tectorial membranes have a spherical shape and are partly encapsulated by a thin layer of cells. The striae vascularis show patchy atrophy, and the Reissner membranes are collapsed to obliterate the endolymphatic spaces. The saccular walls are collapsed and the sensory epithelium of the saccules is disorganized, cystic, and missing in some areas. The cochlear neurons and saccular nerves are normal. The utricles and cristae are normal.

Fig. 6. In the left ear there is an anomalous organization of the cochlear duct in the apical turn. A) In this region the spiral ligament is rudimentary and the cochlear duct is displaced inward away from the cochlear wall. B) The abnormality appears to consist of hyperplasia and duplication of the stria vascularis, organ of Corti and limbus. There is moderate loss of hair cells and cochlear neurons in the basal turn.

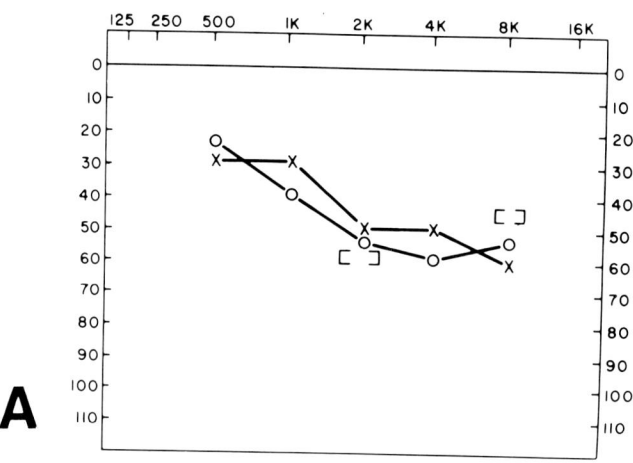

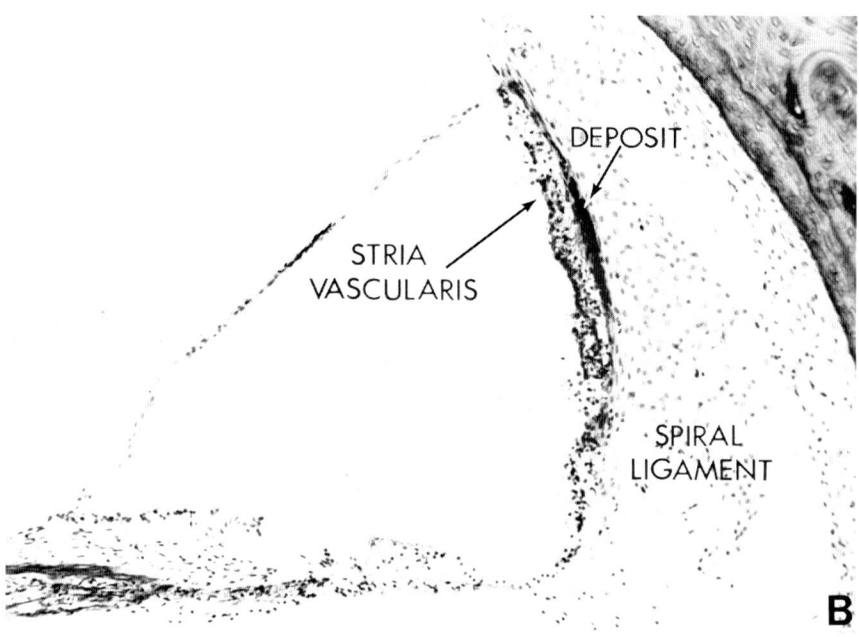

Fig. 7. Alport syndrome showing A) sensorineural hearing loss at age 15. B) There is a basophilic deposit in the substrial area. (Courtesy of Fujita and Hayden).

Case 4 (Trisomy 18)

This white male was the product of the 6th pregnancy of a 38-year-old mother and a 41-year-old father. Physical findings included bilateral inguinal hernias, prominent occiput, micrognathia, high-arched palate, low-set ears, rocker-bottom feet, and apparent deafness. He died at 10 weeks of age. Histologic study showed anomalies of the middle and inner ears (Fig. 11), which included aberrant courses of the facial nerves, large cochleariform processes and incudostapedial discontinuity. The cochleae showed flattening and scala communis. The modioli are incompletely developed and most of the cochlear neuronal cell bodies are missing. The few that remain are located in the internal auditory canals adjacent to the cribrose area. The hair cell populations of the organs of Corti appear normal as do the saccules, utricules, and semicircular canals.

TERATOGENIC AGENTS

Multiple anomalies of the organs may be caused by teratogenic drugs and maternal virus infections acting on the embryo during the 1st trimester. The best known examples are the tranquilizing drug, thalidomide [11], and rubella [12]. Thalidomide was found to produce ectromelia (hypoplasia of one or more limbs), as well as malformations of the intestinal tract, urinary tract, heart, and ears. There may be any degree of malformation of the auricles, external auditory canals and middle ears, and of the inner ears. Even total absence of the inner ear (Michel dysplasia) can occur [13]. Maternal rubella may cause numerous congenital defects including cataracts, patent ductus arteriosus, and other cardio-

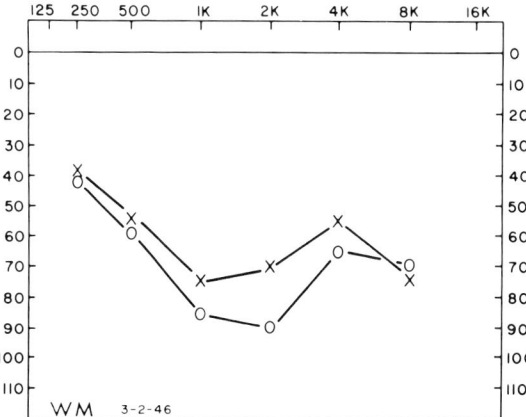

Fig. 8. Usher syndrome. Audiogram at age 11. See text and Figure 9. (This is probably is an example of Usher syndrome type III.)

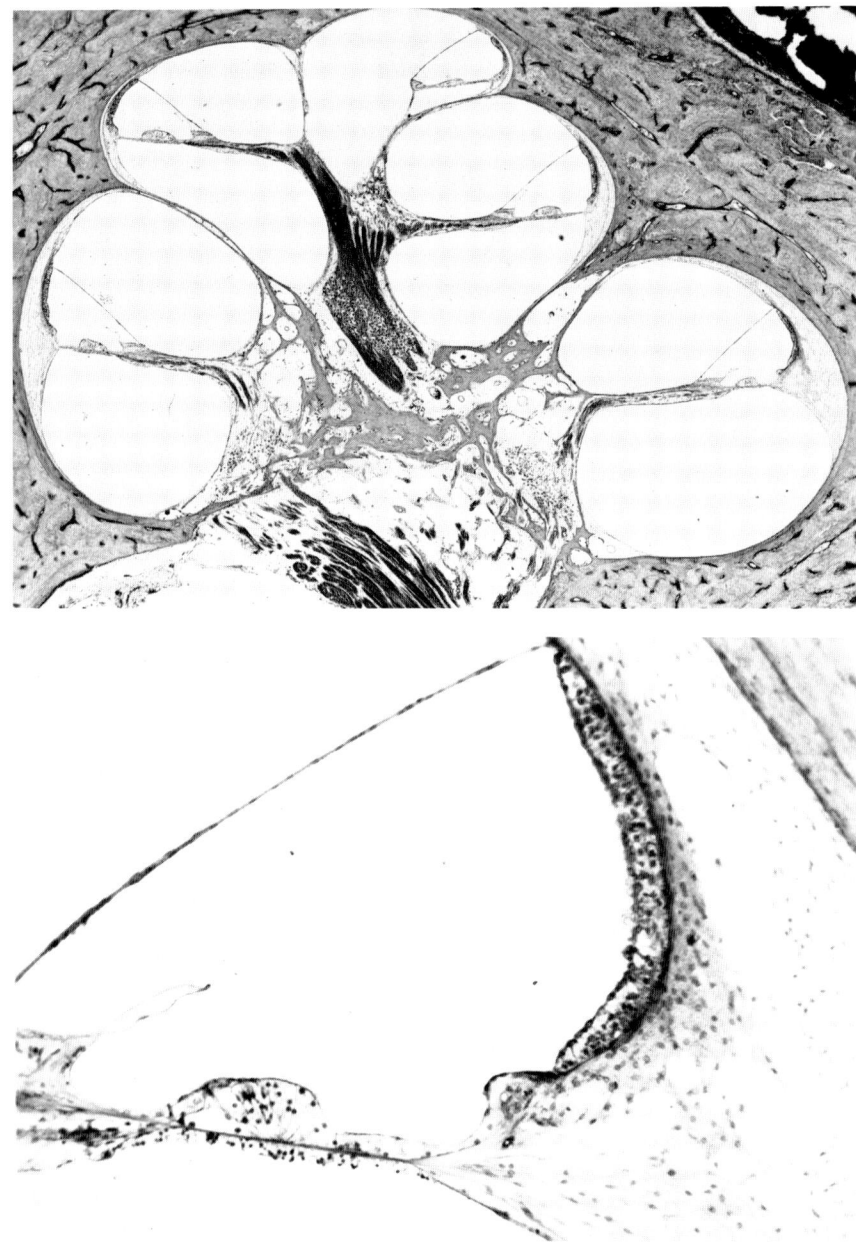

Fig. 9. Usher syndrome. There is a loss of hair cells and cochlear neurons in the basal turn but these changes do not appear to be of sufficient magnitude to explain the hearing loss. See Figure 8.

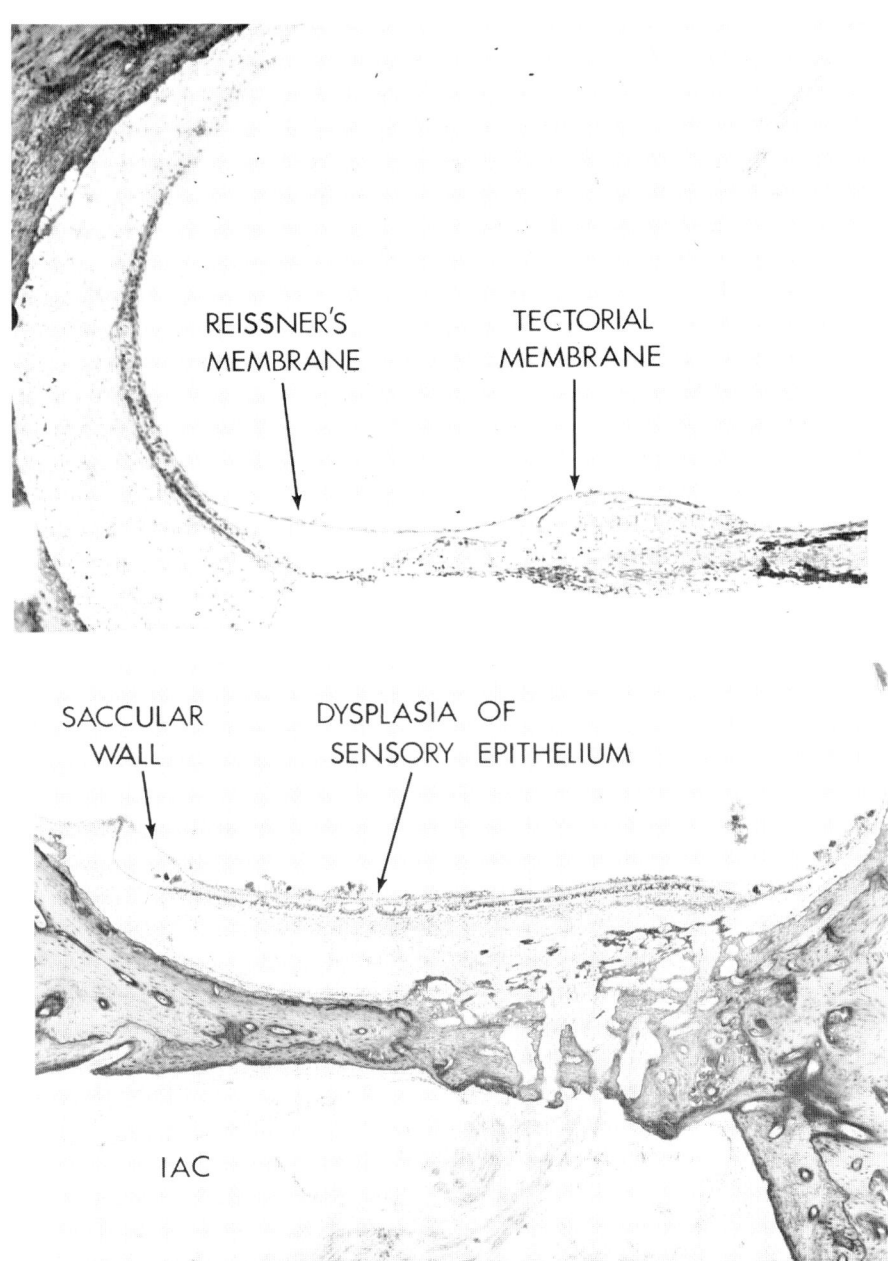

Fig. 10. Trisomy 13 showing cochleosaccular dysgenesis.

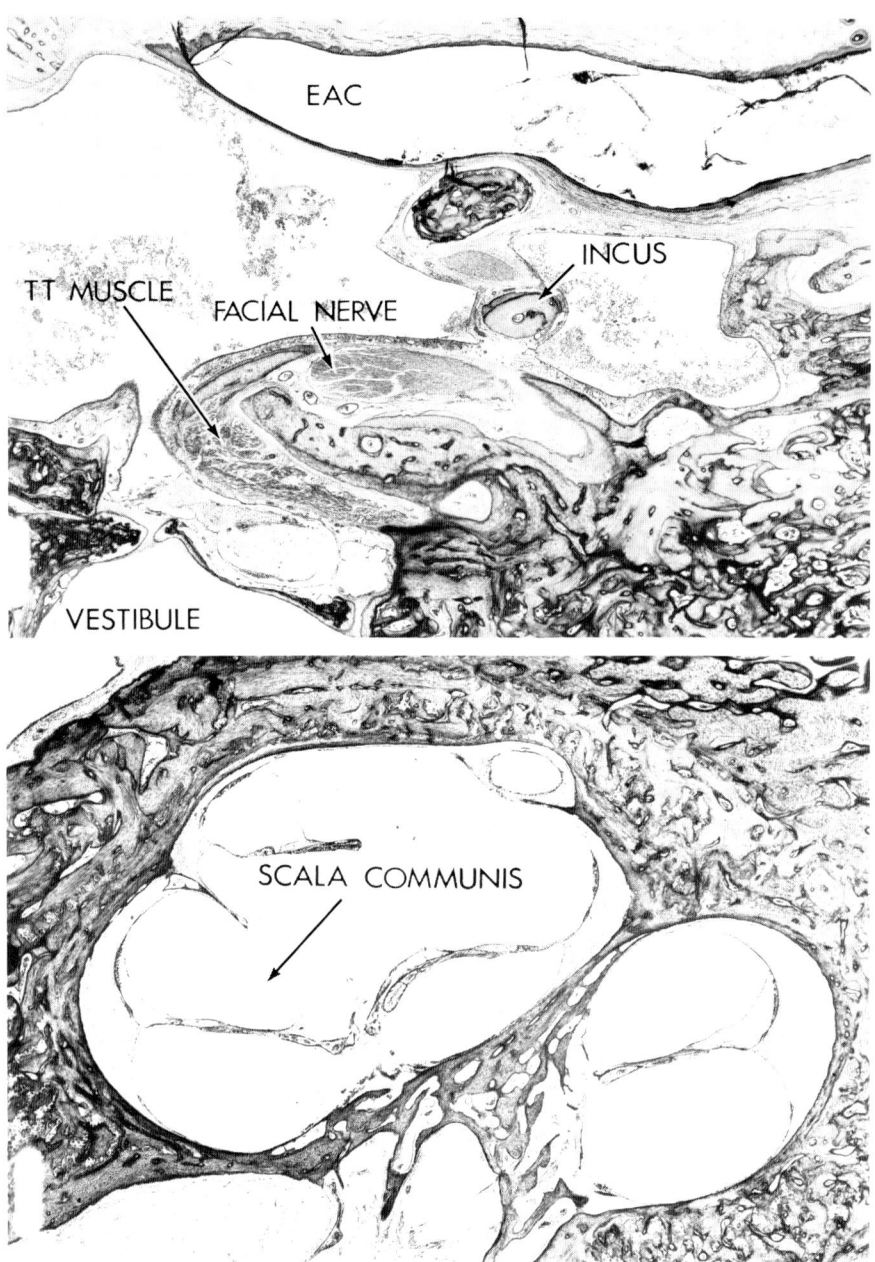

Fig. 11. Trisomy 18 showing anomalies of the middle and inner ears.

vascular defects, microcephaly, dental defects, stunted growth, and hearing loss. The inner ear shows cochleosaccular aplasia with loss of hair cells and distortion and encapsulation of the tectorial membrane.

Case 5 (Multiple Anomalies and Hearing Loss)

The mother is said to have suffered from food poisoning during the 1st trimester. The subject was born with multiple anomalies of the limbs and skin, and a malformed head. A sacrococcygeal teratoma was removed during infancy. He had a left nephrectomy for a double urinary drainage system and hydronephrosis. He was mentally retarded, appeared to have hearing loss (Fig. 12), and had recurring otitis media. Multiple hearing tests indicated a 70–90 dB threshold loss; however, testing was difficult and reliability uncertain. He died at age 19 of renal failure.

Histologic studies showed bilateral congenital fixation of the stapes. The utricle, saccule, and lateral semicircular canal were widely confluent bilaterally (Fig. 13). The sensory and neural structures were normal in both ears. There was mild fibrous proliferation in both middle ears but no active infection. It would appear that the findings are inadequate to explain the hearing loss and that a defect may have existed in the higher auditory pathways.

ISOLATED DYSPLASIAS

There is a group of dysplasias occurring in isolation — that is, without associated anomalies in other organ systems. They are caused principally by genetic factors. Hereditary deafness occurs in somewhere between 1 in 650 and 1 in 2,000 school children in the United States. The patterns of single gene inheritance are autosomal dominant, autosomal recessive, and X-linked. Most cases of hereditary profound congenital deafness are caused by dysplasia of the inner ear. According to Konigsmark and Gorlin [4], most hereditary hearing loss is recessive and has preservation of some hearing for low tones, while dominantly inherited hearing losses which have their onsets after birth do not constitute a true form of dysmorphogenesis and will not be included further in this discussion.

The isolated dysplasias are principally of 2 types: Scheibe dysplasia and Mondini dysplasia. Other types which have been mentioned in the literature are the Bing-Siebenmann type (normal bony labyrinth and underdeveloped membranous labyrinth) and the Alexander type (familial high-tone deafness with presumed underdevelopment of the basal turn). These latter types are so inadequately documented, both clinically and pathologically, that they cannot be considered as established forms of dysplasia. Furthermore, the Michel type, which is characterized by complete failure of development of the inner ear, is so rare that it is of little otologic significance.*

---

*We have so little data on the frequency of occurrence of the various forms of cochlear dysmorphology, that this statement may not be true. *R.J. Gorlin, Editor*.

Scheibe (cochleosaccular) dysplasia involves only the cochlear duct and saccule. The utricle and semicircular canals are morphologically and functionally normal. The stria vascularis shows areas of aplasia alternating with regions of hyperplasia and gross deformity. The Reissner membrane is usually collapsed and lying on the stria and on a rudimentary organ of Corti. The tectorial membrane often has a spherical shape and lies in the internal sulcus. The supporting elements of the organ of Corti are distorted and collapsed, and hair cells are sparse or missing. The appearance is nearly identical to that occurring in inherited deafness in some animals, for example Dalmatian dogs. The wall of the saccule is collapsed onto an atrophic sensory epithelium and deformed otolithic membrane. The cochlear and vestibular nerves are usually normal.

Cochleosaccular dysplasia caused by an inherited or mutant gene can be distinguished histologically from the cochleosaccular dysplasia caused by maternal viral infections occurring in the 1st trimester. The genetic type shows remarkable

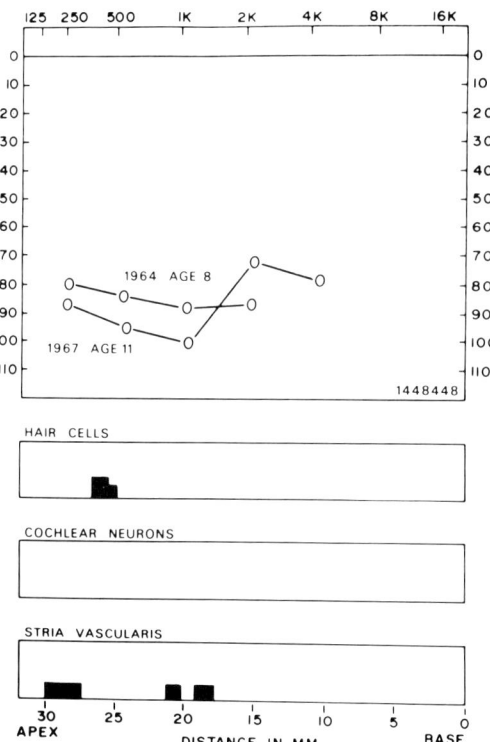

Fig. 12. Multiple congenital anomalies and hearing loss possibly associated with maternal food poisoning during the 1st trimester. See Figure 13.

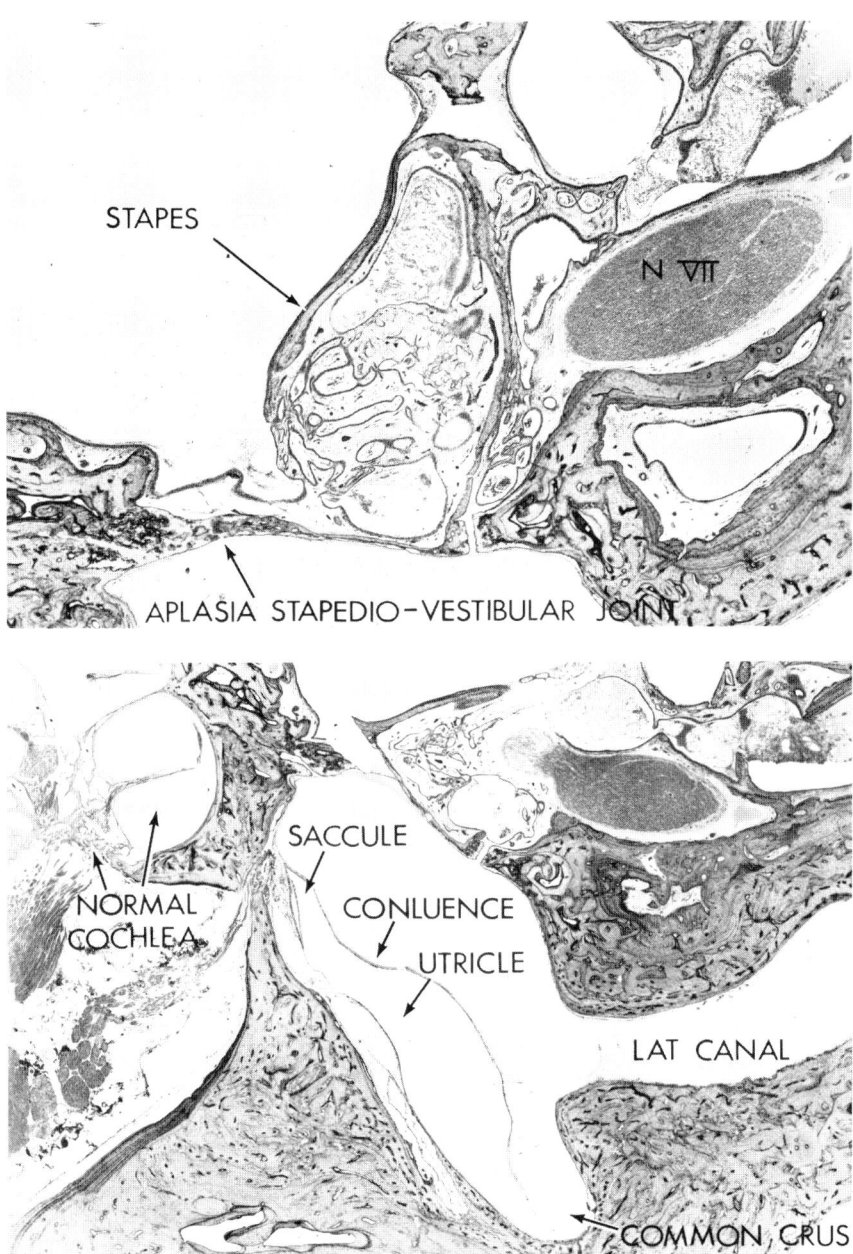

Fig. 13. Congenital fixation of the stapes and utriculosaccular confluence possibly caused by noxious prenatal influence. See Figure 12.

morphologic aberrations with preservation of the cochlear nerve fibers, while the viral type exhibits atrophic changes in both cochlear duct and nerve after the attainment of well-advanced embryologic differentiation.

Case 6 **(Scheibe Dysplasia)**

This full-term infant died of asphyxiation 10 hours after birth. The father and mother were known to be "deaf-mutes." The right ear is available for study and shows severe dysplasia of the cochlear duct and saccule. The stria vascularis is atrophic in some areas and hyperplastic in others. In some areas it forms multiple layers separated by fibrous tissue (Fig. 14). The Reissner membrane is collapsed. The organ of Corti appears atrophic but scattered hair cells can be identified. The tectorial membrane has a spherical shape and lies in the internal sulcus. The population of ganglion cells is normal. The saccular wall is collapsed and lying on an irregular distorted otolithic membrane and atrophic sensory epithelium. The utricle and semicircular canals are normal.

Case 7 **(Scheibe Dysplasia)**

This child was known to be profoundly deaf in both ears from the time of birth and died at the age of 10. One ear is available for study and shows severe dysplasia of the cochlear duct and saccule. The organ of Corti consists of a flattened mound of cells consisting of remnants of pillars mixed with other cells having no recognizable organization. The Reissner membrane is collapsed and obliterates the endolymphatic space.

The stria vascularis is atrophic in some areas and hyperplastic in others (Fig. 15). This hyperplasia appears to be characteristic of genetically induced dysplasia rather than of 1st trimester embryopathy from teratogenic drugs or maternal viral infections. The tectorial membrane has a spherical shape and lies in the internal sulcus. There is a slight loss of cochlear neurons in the basal turn but elsewhere the population is normal (Fig. 16). The saccule shows severe atrophic changes including collapse of its wall and absence of the otolithic membrane. The sensory epithelium consists of an irregular layer of supporting cells and hair cells separated by spaces containing either a homogeneous acidophilic fluid or a basophilic granular material. The utricle and semicircular canals appear normal.

Case 8 **(Scheibe Dysplasia)**

This man was born deaf and died at age 66. The left temporal bone is available for study and shows a normal bony labyrinth. The utricle and semicircular canals appear normal. The stria vascularis is atrophic in some areas and hyperplastic in others. In areas of hyperplasia it consists of an irregular mass of strial tissue located in the region of the spiral prominence.

The Reissner membrane is atrophic and lies on the stria and limbus, thus partly obliterating the endolymphatic space. The organ of Corti is missing in some areas and consists of a mound of disorganized cells in other areas. The tectorial mem-

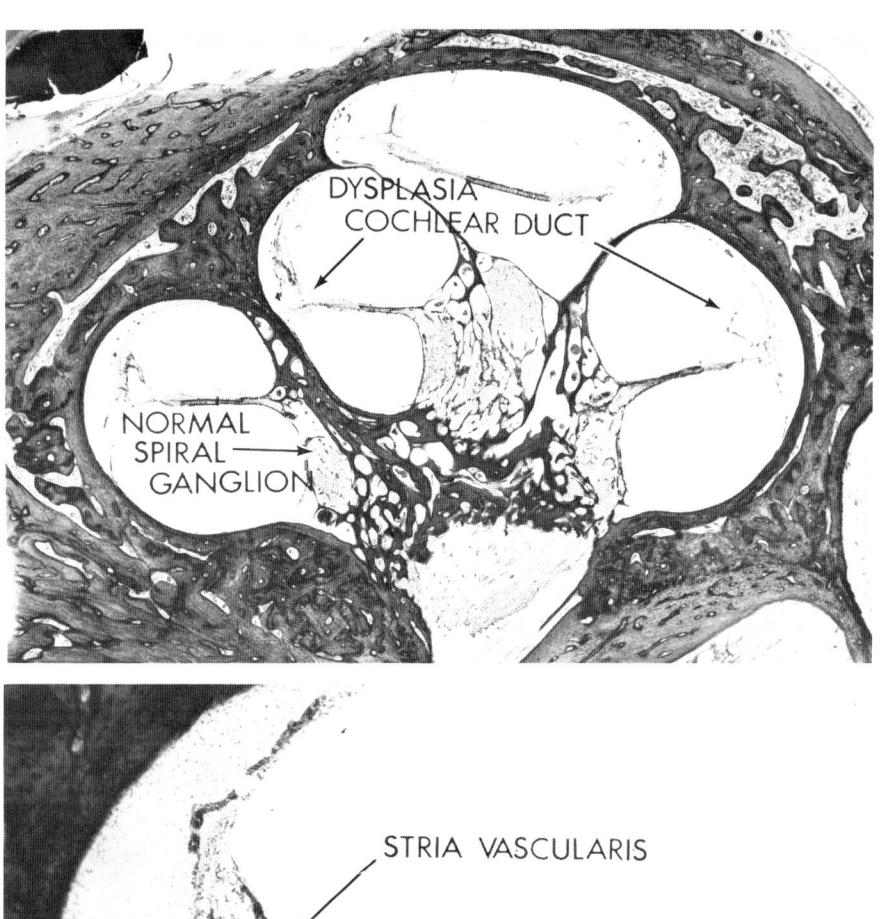

Fig. 14. Scheibe (cochleosaccular) dysplasia. (Figs. 14–19 from the Zurich Collection.)

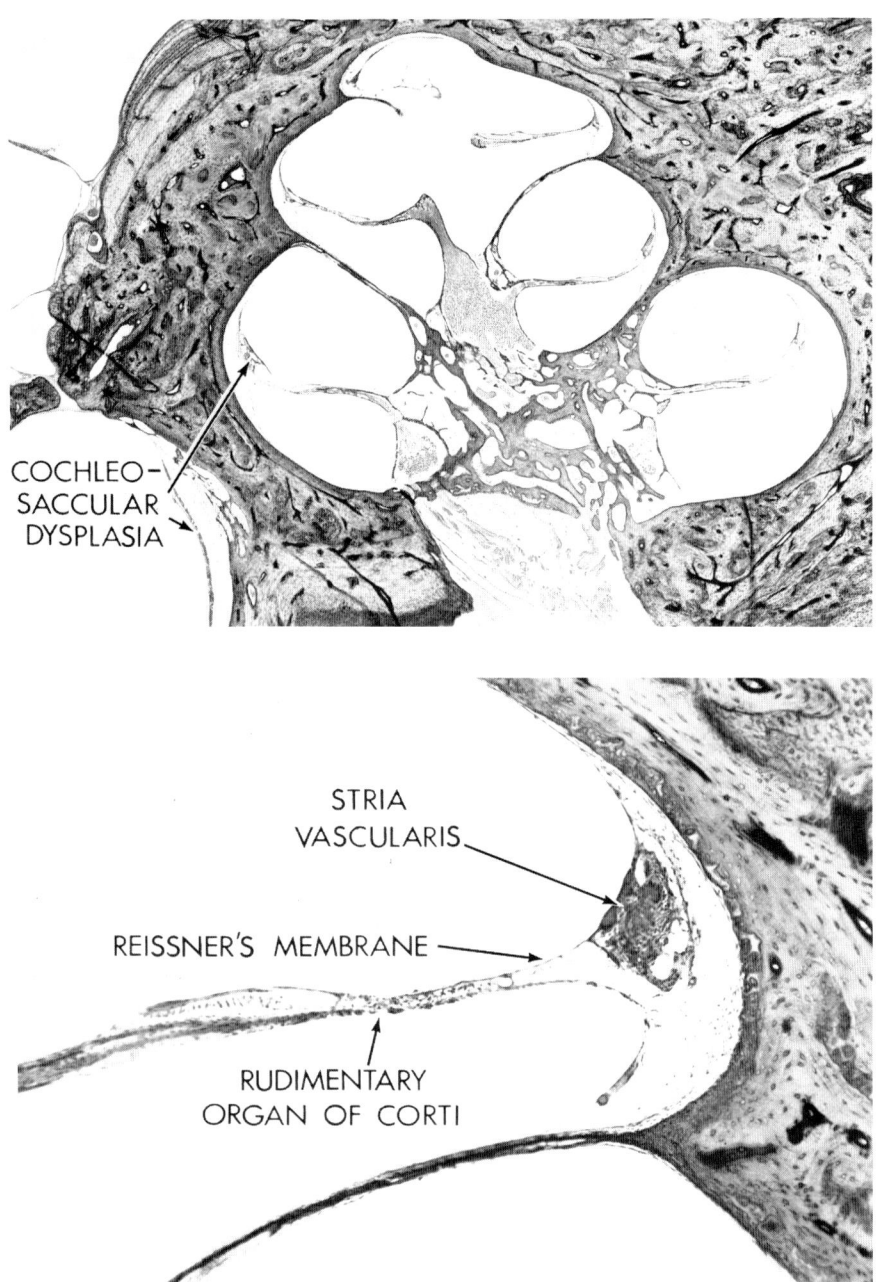

Fig. 15. Scheibe (cochleosaccular) dysplasia.

brane is shrunken and lies in the internal sulcus (Fig. 17). The population of cochlear neurons is greatly diminished. The saccule shows severe atrophy of the sensory epithelium, stroma, and otolithic membrane, and the saccular wall is collapsed onto the macula (Fig. 18).

Mondini dysplasia (dysplasia of bony and membranous labyrinth) was first described by Mondini in 1791 [14], and then by Alexander in 1904 [15], and Siebenmann in 1950 [16]. Ormerod [17] defined the condition as a "flattened

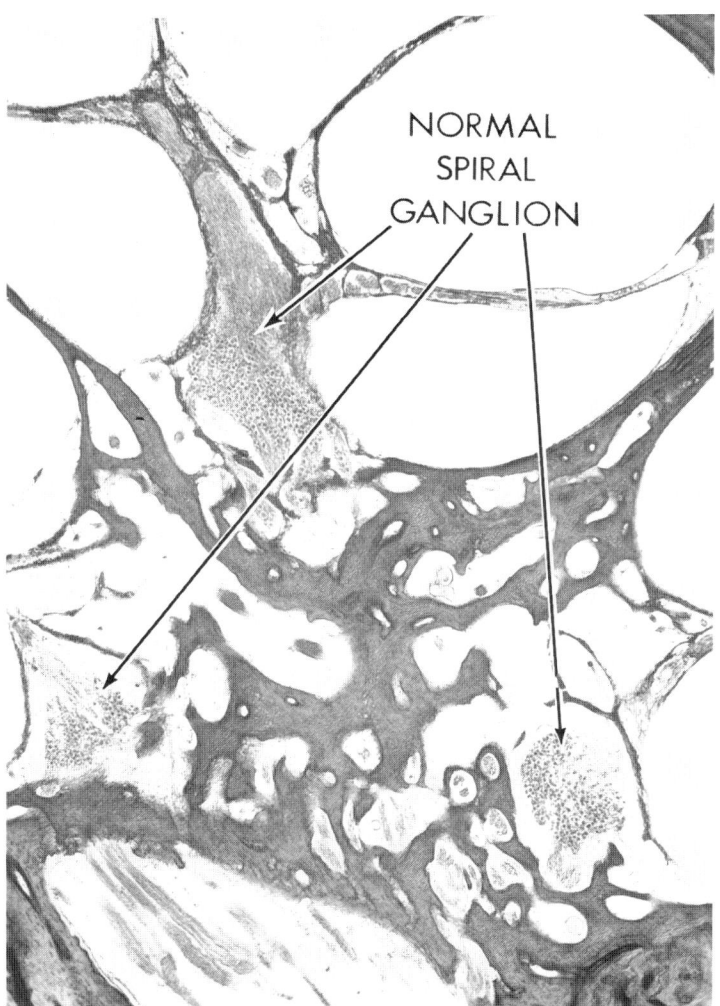

Fig. 16. Scheibe (cochleosaccular) dysplasia. In spite of severely dysplastic changes in the cochlear duct, the cochlear neuronal population is near normal.

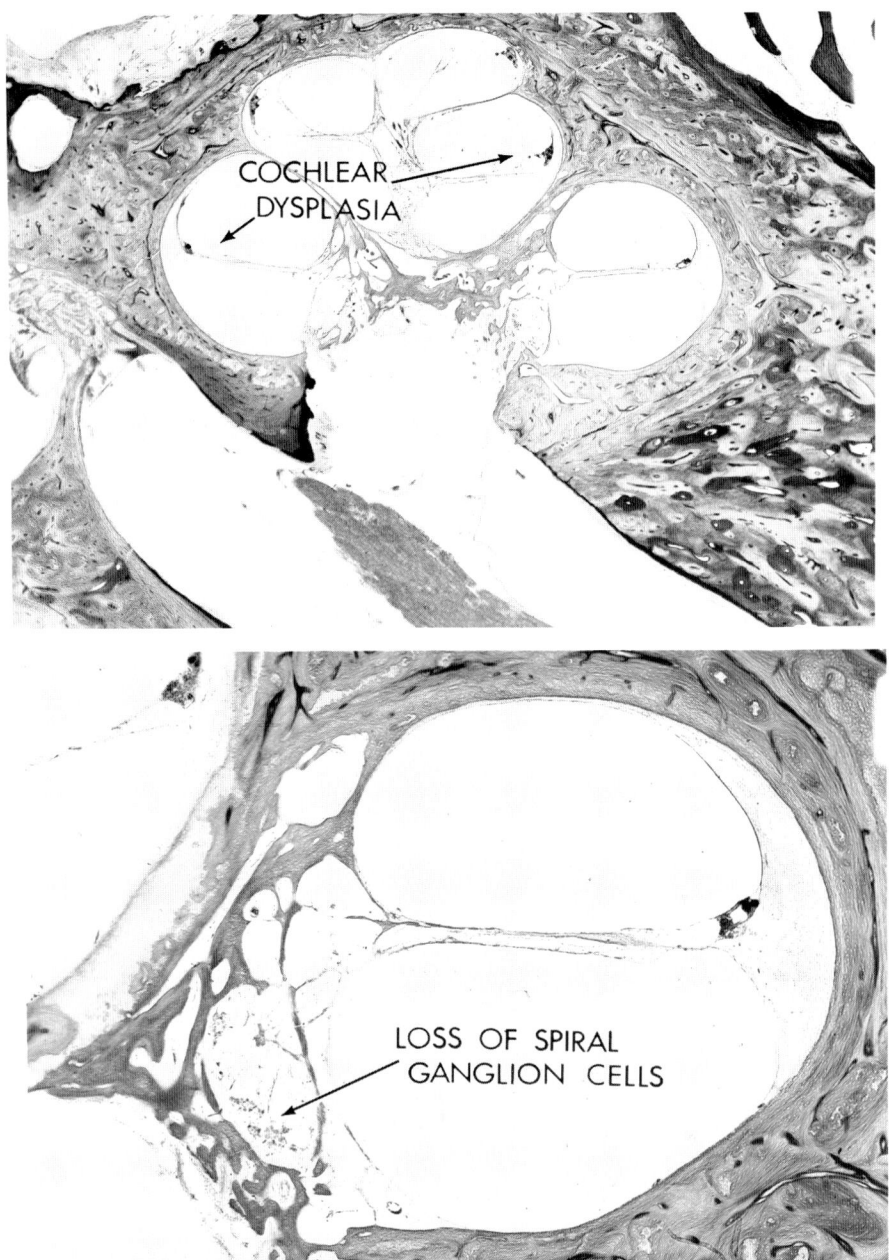

Fig. 17. Scheibe (cochleosaccular) dysplasia.

cochlea with development of the basal coil only, and with a comparable underdevelopment of the vestibular structures." Less severe deformities than those originally described by these authors might also be appropriately classified as the Mondini anomaly [18]. Altmann [2] characterized the Mondini dysplasia as a flattened bony cochlear capsule with a normal scalar arrangement only in the basal turn, and an underdeveloped bony structure in the apical part of the cochlea (defective interscalar septum, modiolus, and osseous spiral lamina), reduction in the number of cochlear turns, and dilated saccule and endolymphatic duct system. He also stated that the "extent of the changes in the stria vascularis, organ of Corti, spiral ganglion cells, and the other parts of the cochlearis system determined the degree of hearing loss, and that clinically, malformation of the Mondini-type might therefore show complete deafness or only partial loss of hearing."

Case 9 (Mondini Dysplasia)

This male subject had bilateral profound congenital deafness and died at age 5. Both ears showed severe dysplasia. The right cochlea (Fig. 19) consists of a single round space without scalar formation. Within the cochlear space, adjacent to a small cribriform area is a nest of cochlear neurons and from this core springs a single turn of the spiral lamina. The spiral ligament and cochlear duct show

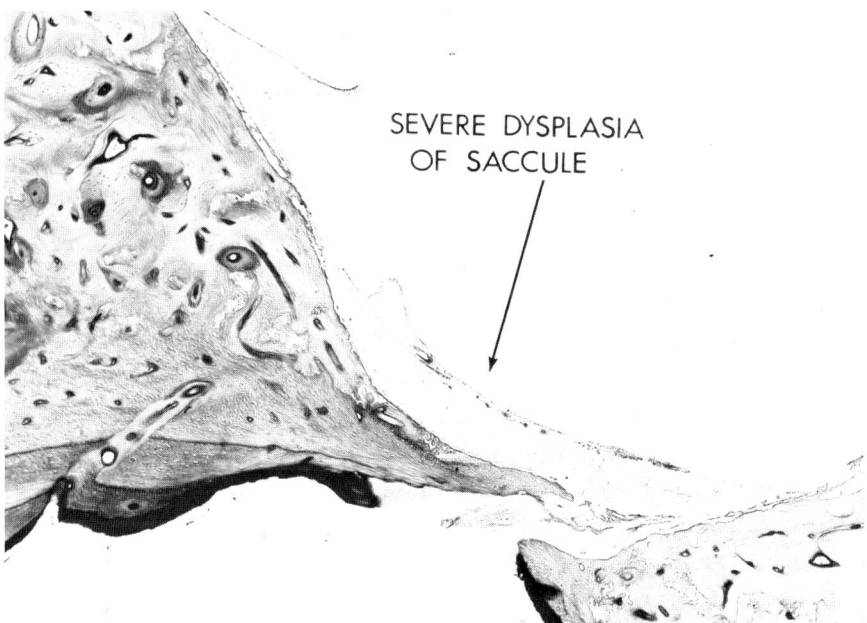

Fig. 18. Scheibe (cochleosaccular) dysplasia. The saccule shows severe dysplasia.

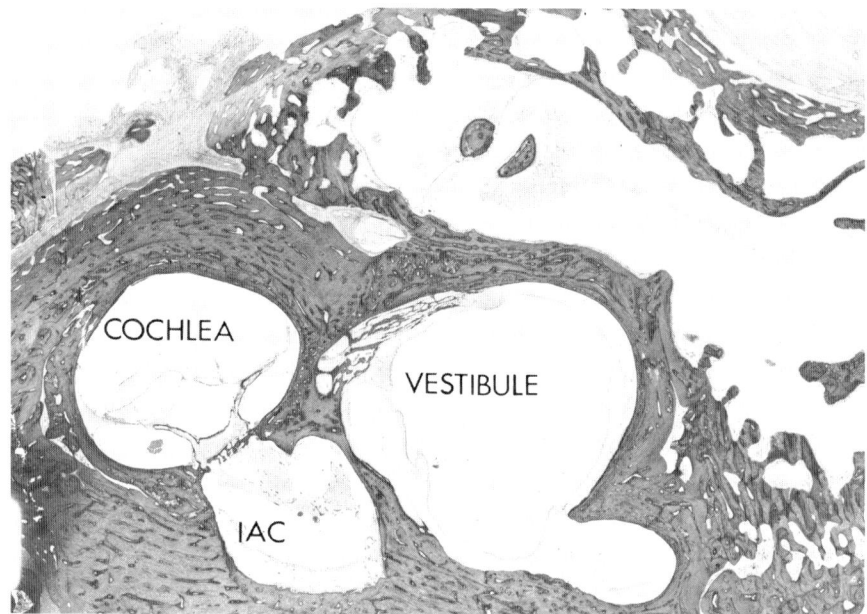
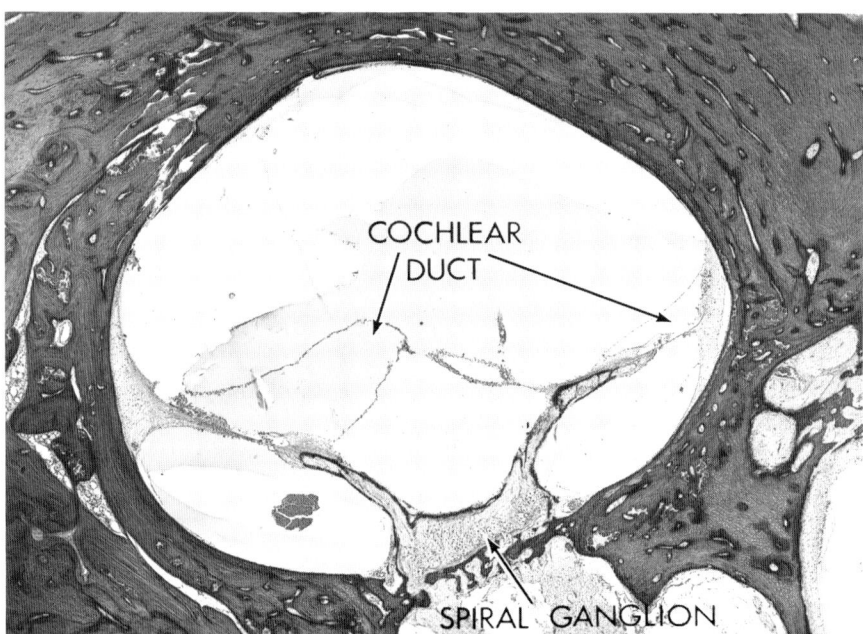
Fig. 19. Mondini dysplasia.

gross abnormalities in size and contour in some areas and the organ of Corti appears atrophic. The stria vascularis is missing in some areas. The vestibule is large and contains a large utricle, normal saccule, and a single crista. One semicircular canal, probably the lateral, is present [19].

This brief review of dysmorphology of the inner ear attempts to describe the patterns of dysplasia as observed in studies of human temporal bone. In the broad sense they may be viewed as 1) anatomic variants of little or no clinical significance, 2) dysplasias occurring in association with defects in other organ systems (syndromes), and 3) as isolated otic dysplasias. Functional deficits correlate closely with the magnitude of dysmorphogenesis and are generally fixed and unyielding to medical or surgical therapy.

REFERENCES

1. Guild S: A case of bilateral scala communis cochlea uncomplicated by other defects: An embryological interpretation of this and associated anomalies. Anat Rec 42:19, 1929.
2. Altmann F: Histologic picture of inherited nerve deafness in man and animals. Arch Otolaryngol 51:852, 1950.
3. Egami T, Sando I: Hypoplasia of the vestibular aqueduct and endolymphatic sac in endolymphatic hydrops. ORL 86:327, 1978.
4. Konigsmark B, Gorlin R: "Genetic and Metabolic Deafness." Philadelphia:WB Saunders Company, 1976.
5. Alport A: Hereditary familial congenital haemorrhagic nephritis. Br Med J 1:504, 1927.
6. Fujita S, Hayden R: Deafness and Klippel-Feil syndrome. J Laryngol 83:175, 1969.
7. Usher C: On the inheritance of retinitis pigmentosa, with notes of case. Roy London Ophthal Hosp Rep 19:130, 1914.
8. Klippel M, Feil A: Un cas d'absence des vertebres cervicales. Nouv Iconogr Saplêt 25: 223, 1912.
9. McLay K, Maran A: Deafness and Klippel-Feil syndrome. J Laryngol 83:175, 1969.
10. Kos A, Schuknecht H, Singer J: Temporal bone studies in 13-15 and 18 trisomy syndromes. Arch Pathol 82:506, 1966.
11. Lenz W, Knapp R: Die Thalidomidembryopathie. Dtsch Med Wochenschr 87:1232, 1962.
12. Hemenway W, Sando I, McChesney D: Temporal bone pathology following maternal rubella. Arch Klin Exp Ohr-, Nas Kehlk Heilk 193:287, 1969.
13. Jorgensen M, Kristensen H, Buch N: Thalidomide-induced aplasia of the inner ear. J Laryngol Otol 78:1095, 1964.
14. Mondini C: Anatomia surdi nedi sectio. De Bononiensi Scientiarum et Artium Instituto Atque Academia Commentarii, Boniesi 7:28, 419, 1791.
15. Alexander G: Zur Pathologie und pathologischen Anatomie der kongenitalen Taubheit. Arch Ohr Nas -Kehlk-Heilk 61:183, 1904.
16. Siebenmann F, cited by Altmann F: Histologic picutre of inherited nerve deafness in man and animals. Arch Otolaryngol 51:852, 1950.
17. Ormerod F: The pathology of congenital deafness. J Laryngol 74:919, 1960.
18. Beal D, Davey P, Lindsay J: Inner ear pathology of congenital deafness. Arch Otolaryngol 85:134, 1967.
19. Fraser J: A case of congenital deafness with malformation of the bony and membranous labyrinths on both sides. Proc R Soc Med 20:475, 1927.

Discussion of Inner Ear Anomalies—Reply to Dr. Schuknecht

Isamu Sando, MD, DMS

Reacting to Dr. Schuknecht's presentation, I would like to report on our recent studies of anomalies of the inner ear, and a new classification thereof, and present representative illustrations. Dr. Suehiro, who is a research associate in my laboratory, and I have carefully reviewed the literature and found that there are 43 diseases with which anomalies of the inner ear are associated (Table 1). We list diseases which include malformations due to inherited traits, prenatal infections, iatrogenic ototoxicities, environmental factors, and those of unknown etiology. As a matter of fact, we have listed as "anomalies" what Dr. Shuknecht has reported on as "variations" because they were observed to be associated with congenital anomalies and because they resemble, in most cases, stages of fetal development which were rarely observed in noncongenital cases of anomaly.

Anomalies of the cochlea were observed most frequently, being seen in 28 out of 43 diseases. Anomalies of the vestibule were less frequent, being observed in 17 diseases. Anomalies of the semicircular canals were seen in 16 diseases. Of the cochlear anomalies, anomalies of the modiolus including anomalies of the Rosenthal canal, the osseous spiral lamina, and the interscalar septum were the most commonly observed, being seen in 10 out of 28 diseases. The endolymphatic duct and sac were most commonly involved in vestibular anomalies (in 8 of 17 diseases). Anomalies of the the semicircular canals most frequently involved the lateral semicircular canal, as was seen in 13 of 16 diseases.

Figure 1 is a photomicrograph of a section of temporal bone from a 6½-week-old girl with trisomy 13 syndrome. The cochlea is incompletely developed, with absence of the interscalar osseous septum and a poorly developed modiolus. Figure 2 is a photomicrograph of a horizontal section of temporal bone from a 21-day-old girl with trisomy 13 syndrome. The wide cochlear aqueduct is shown by an arrow.

TABLE 1. Anomalies of the Inner Ear in 43 Diseases

Labyrinth	2
Cochlea	28
Vestibule	17
Canals	16
Superior canal 7	
Posterior canal 7	
Lateral canal 13	
Otic capsule	11
Internal auditory meatus	9
Nerves	6
Facial nerve 2	
Statoacoustic nerve 6	
Vessels	2
Subarcuate fossa	1

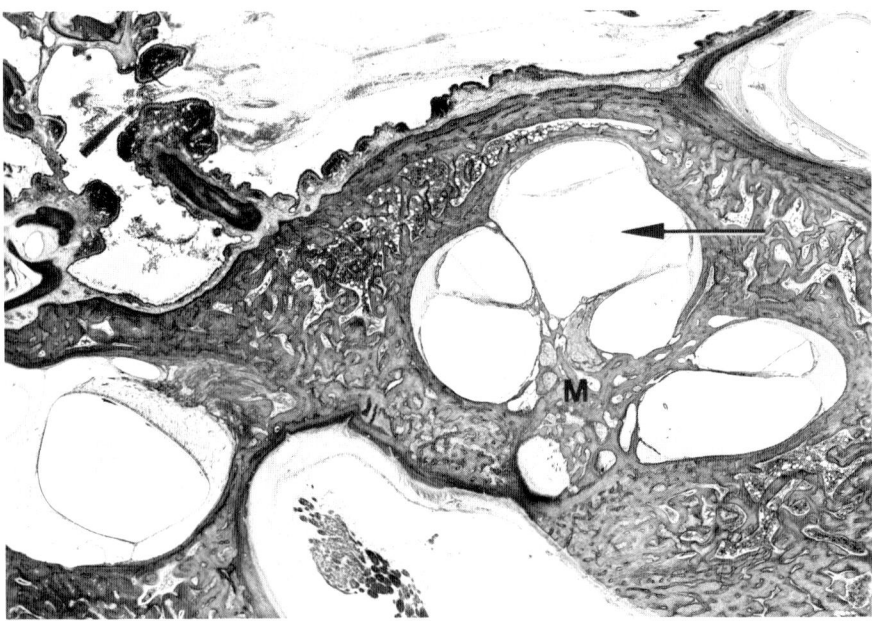

Fig. 1. Photomicrograph of histologic section of human temporal bone. In this horizontal section, the arrow shows absence of the interscalar osseous septum in the middle turn of the cochlea, while M indicates the poorly developed cochlear modiolus (H&E × 8).

Figure 3 is a photomicrograph of a section of temporal bone from a 6-week-old boy with trisomy 13 syndrome; the shortened endolymphatic valve permits direct communication between the utricle and the saccule. In Figure 4, a photomicrograph of a section of temporal bone from a 35-year-old man with congenital heart disease, simple outpouching of the lateral semicircular canal has resulted in a wide vestibule. Figure 5 is a photomicrograph of a section of temporal bone from a 13-month-old girl with congenital anomalies of the facial nerve and the stapes. The fibers of the facial nerve transverse the spiral ligament of the cochlea.

Table 2 summarizes the relationships of the anomalies of the inner ear, with or without associated anomalies in other parts of the body, to the etiologies of the diseases. In this study we noted the following trends: 1) hereditary disorders are most commonly associated with anomalies of the inner ear, diseases of unknown etiology being the next most closely associated with inner ear anomalies. 2) most of the diseases associated with anomalies of the inner ear are also associated with anomalies in other parts of the body.

Now I would like to report on our recent studies on new classifications for anomalies of the inner ear (Fig. 6). In 1960 Ormerod [1] classified the anomalies of the labyrinth which resulted in congenital deafness into the following 4 types:

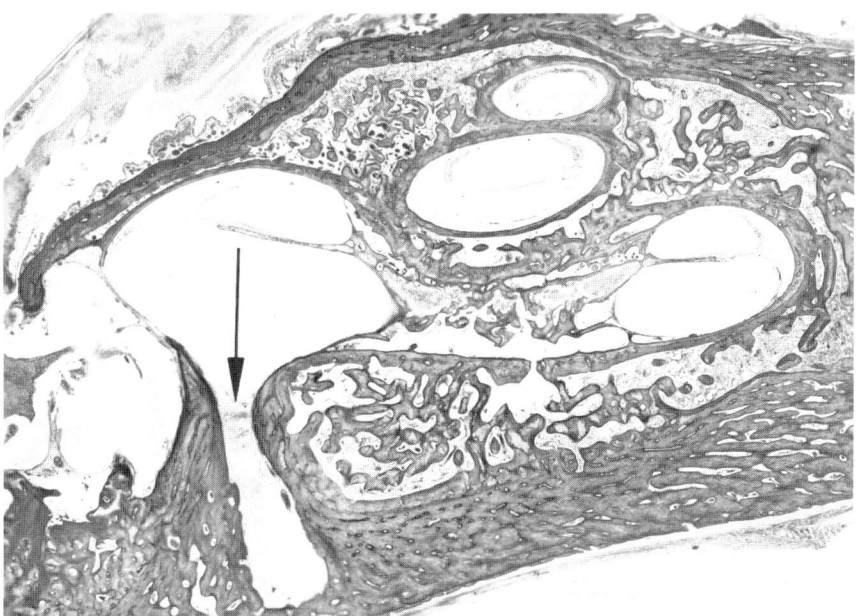

Fig. 2. Human temporal bone, histologic section. The arrow points to the unusually wide cochlear aqueduct, seen in horizontal section. (H&E × 7.8).

1) Michel (complete lack of development of the inner ear); 2) Mondini-Alexander (anomalies in which only a single curved tube representing the cochlea developed, and in which the vestibule and canals showed similar immature development); 3) Bing-Siebenmann (underdevelopment of the membranous labyrinth in the presence of well-formed bony labyrinth); 4) Scheibe (malformations restricted to the membranous cochlea and saccule).

In 1967, Schuknecht [2] classified the labyrinthine aplasia associated with deafness of genetic origin into 4 types as follows: 1) Michel (complete failure of development of the inner ear); 2) Mondini (incomplete development of the bony and membranous labyrinth); Scheibe (cochleosaccular aplasia); 4) Alexander (membranous cochlear aplasia). Within any one of these classifications, however, defects occur

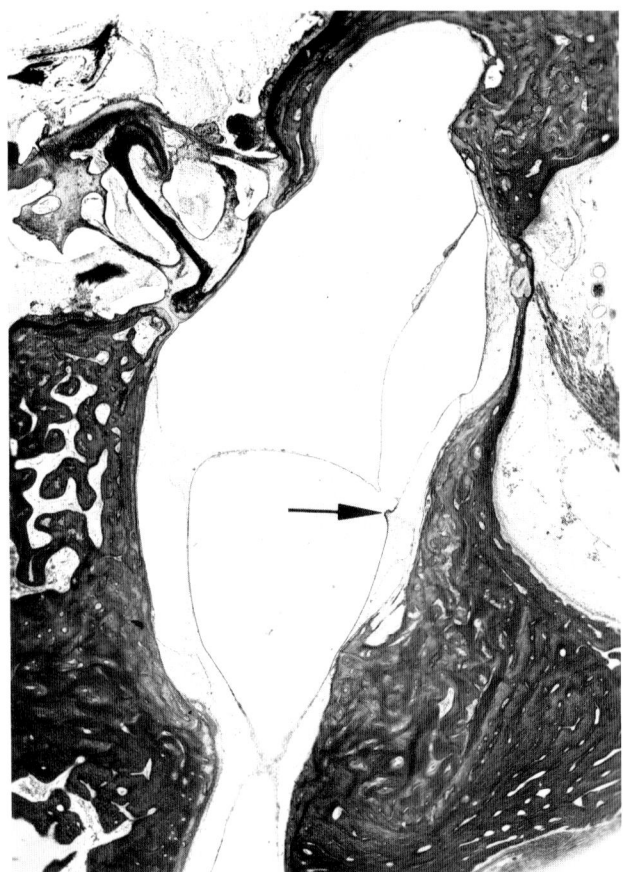

Fig. 3. Horizontal section, human temporal bone. The arrow shows the shortened endolymphatic valve. (H&E × 10).

which are not described fully by the classification. In Figure 6, we have attempted to describe our system for classifying congenital anomalies of the labyrinth. This system takes into consideration the varying degrees of pathology of the labyrinth which have been described in the literature, and also includes anomalies which have not been categorized previously. With this new system of classification, anomalies of the labyrinth can be categorized into two major types: those involving aplasia and those involving hypoplasia of labyrinthine structures. Hypoplasia may involve the bony labyrinth (bony type), membranous labyrinth (membranous type), or both (combined type). These three subtypes are further classified into 16 different groups, depending upon which structures of the labyrinth are involved in the hypoplasia.

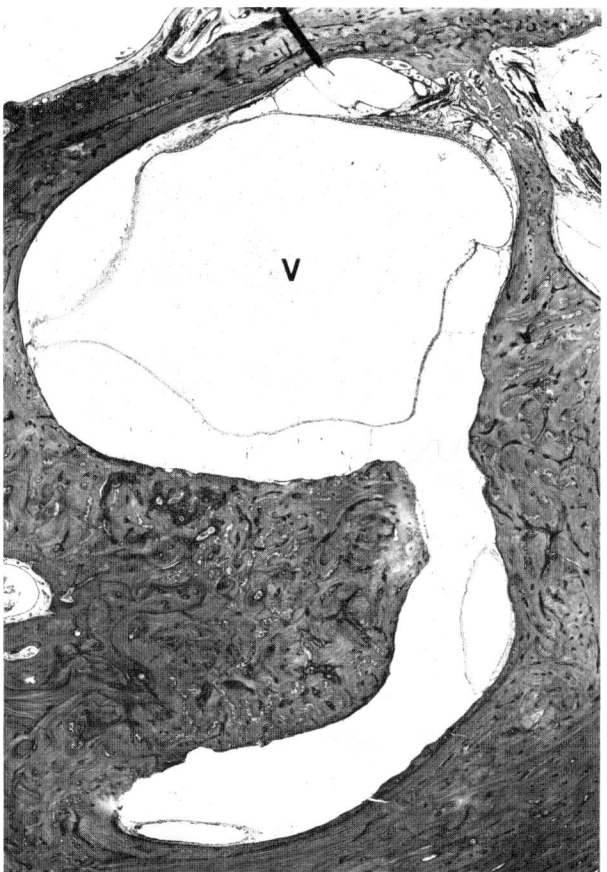

Fig. 4. Human temporal bone, horizontal section. V indicates an unusually wide vestibule. (H&E × 11).

In Figure 6, A indicates anomalies of both the cochlea and vestibule; B indicates a anomalies of the cochlea only; and C represents anomalies of the vestibule only in the *osseous* labyrinth. Anomalies of both the cochlea and the vestibule, of the cochlea only, and of the vestibule only in the *membranous* labyrinth are indicated by a (a' and a''), b, and c. a' Indicates anomalies in the cochlea and the vestibule excluding anomalies in the cochlea and the saccules (Scheibe type) which are categorized as a''. The shaded rectangles denote the areas of the labyrinth where the hypoplastic anomalies are suspected to be present in each subgroup. For example, anomalies of the Alexander type correspond to anomalies of membranous cochlear development, or b in our classification; this is shown by the shading of the rectangle for the cochlear portion of the membranous labyrinth of Figure 6.

In Figure 6 we have matched the anomalies described by Ormerod (1960) and by Schuknecht (1967) with these anomalies as we classify them. Since our classification system involves simply categorizing the area of the labyrinth involved and the type of involvement observed with each anomaly, it is clear that discrepancies in other authors' descriptions of anomalies need not concern us in this type of classification system. As long as the location and type of anomaly are described, it can be classified without having a "name" (eg "Mondini type") attached to it.

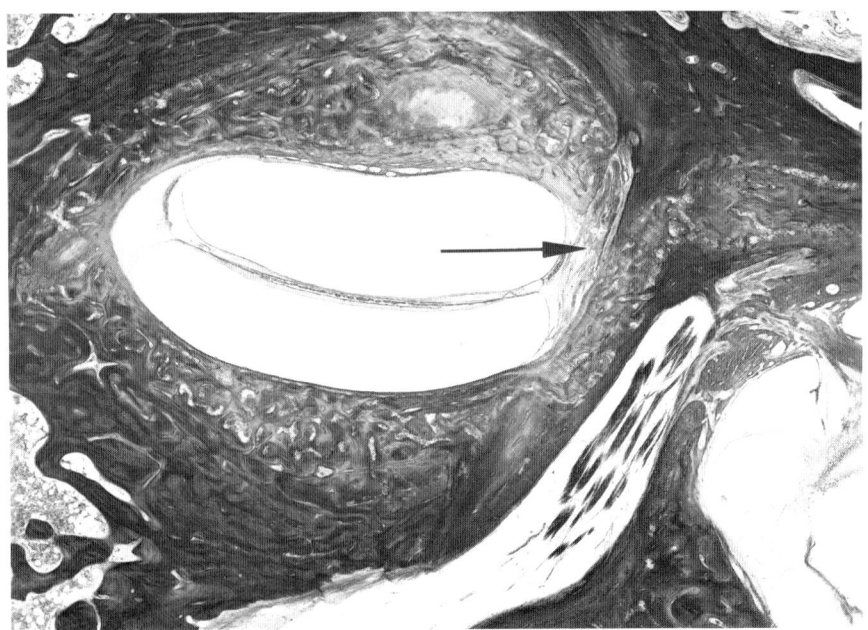

Fig. 5. Human temporal bone slide, horizontal section. The arrow indicates facial nerve fibers in the spiral ligament. (H&E×11).

TABLE 2. Relation of Anomalies of the Inner Ear to Etiologies of Diseases

Etiologies Anomalies	Unknown etiologies	Hereditary characteristics	Prenatal infections	Iatrogenic ototoxicities	Environmental factors	Total
I	1					1
M, I		1				1
E, I						0
E, M, I		1				1
I, O	2	6	1	1		10
M, I, O	2	7	1		1	11
E, I, O						0
E, M, I, O	6	12		1		19
TOTAL	11	27	2	2	1	43

E, M, I, and O indicate an anomaly or anomalies observed in the external ear, middle ear, inner ear, and other parts of the body, respectively.

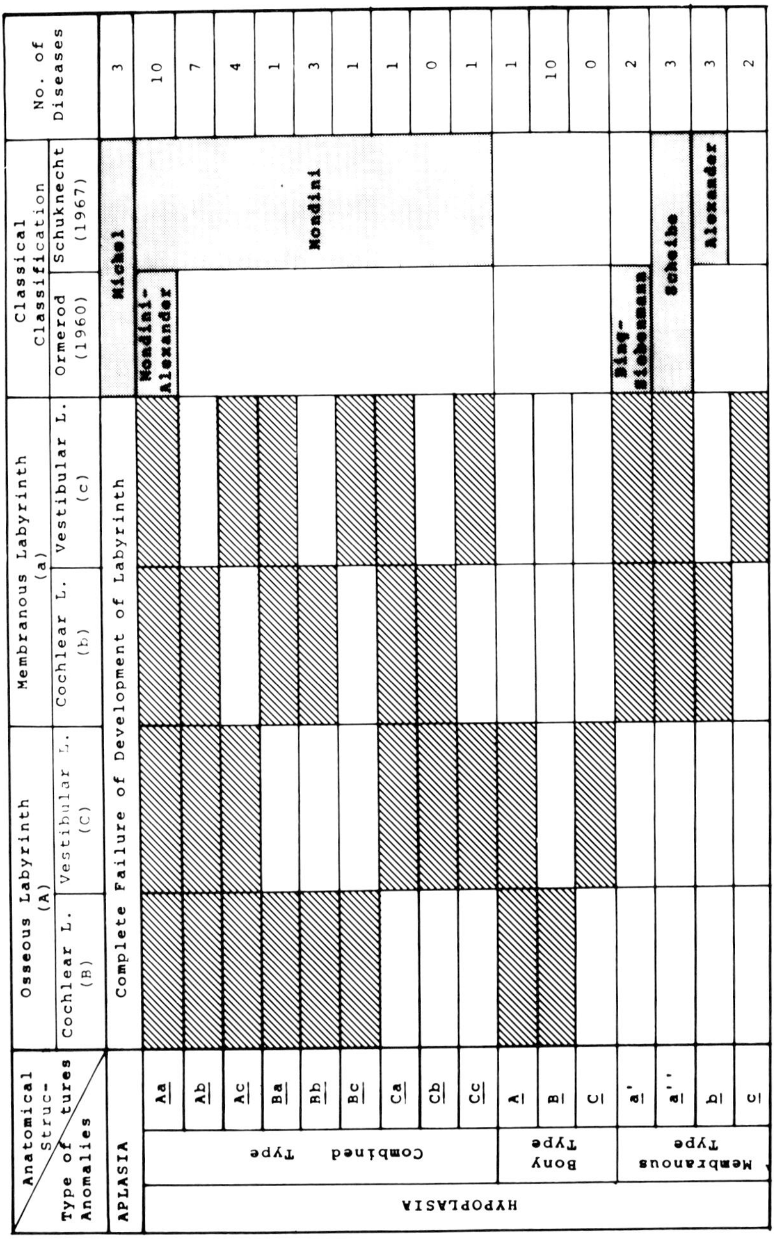

Fig. 6. A new system for classifying anomalies of the labyrinth.

We make the following observations concerning labyrinthine anomalies in our classification: 1) labyrinthine anomalies of the Michel type are the same as those classified as aplasia by our system; 2) we believe that anomalies of the Mondini-Alexander type are the same as those labeled Aa in our classification; 3) likewise, anomalies of the Bing-Siebenmann type, Scheibe type, and Alexander type are the same as those classified as a', a'', and b, respectively, in our system; 4) we found that there are suspected labyrinthine anomalies which do not fit into the classic types of anomalies described by Ormerod (1960) and/or Schuknecht (1967). They are anomalies of the bony labyrinth and those of the vestibular portion of the membranous labyrinth. Anomalies such as those we have labeled A and B of the bony type and c of the membranous type have been reported previously in the literature on the histopathology of the temporal bone, but it is difficult to determine whether or not these isolated anomalies truly exist since the information about them is so scanty. This is especially true in the case of anomalies of the membranous labyrinth, since this structure is so susceptible to postmortem changes. Further light and electron microscopic studies are needed to confirm the existence of these described anomalies; 5) anomalies indicated as Aa and B were those most frequently associated with the different diseases being studied (as they were observed to occur with 10 out of the 43 diseases studied); and 6) C and Cb represent anomalies which are suspected to exist but which have not been reported to date.

ACKNOWLEDGMENT

I appreciate the University of Colorado Medical Center making available the materials used for this discussion.

REFERENCES

1. Ormerod F: The pathology of congenital deafness. J Laryngol 74:919–950, 1960.
2. Schuknecht HF: Pathology of sensorineural deafness of genetic origin. In McConnell F, Ward PH (eds): "Deafness in Childhood." Nashville: Vanderbilt University Press, 1967, pp 69–90.

DISCUSSION

Dr. Heinrich Spoendlin: One cannot always tell whether or not there is primary degeneration in the organ of Corti and stria vascularis followed by secondary degeneration of the neurons. There is the possibility that the opposite may occur, that there may be primary degeneration of the neurons with the sensory organs remaining intact. As an example, two sisters who suffered from Friedreich ataxia and had progressive deafness died at approximately age 25. The cochlea of one of the sisters reveals an essentially normal organ of Corti in all turns, but has a great loss of ganglion cells. In spite of the fact that this sister had relatively few ganglion cells left, these were enough to give her a certain amount of hearing. The other sister had no ganglion cells and she was completely deaf.

Dr. Isabelle Rapin: I think one should be very careful when talking about Friedreich ataxia. When one says "Friedreich ataxia" one is really talking about a group of genetic diseases.

Dr. Walter Nance: My question concerns the case that Dr. Schuknecht showed earlier today of a patient with Usher syndrome. I hope someone can refresh my memory as to the previous reports concerning temporal bones of patients with Usher syndrome. I feel that there is probably a large amount of heterogeneity associated with retinitis pigmentosa and deafness. We have recently found that hearing loss is the most common extraocular symptom in patients with retinitis pigmentosa. At least 15–20% of these patients report moderate-to-severe hearing loss. If you ever lecture to a meeting of people with retinitis pigmentosa, and you look around at the audience, there are always two or three with hearing aids. I was also intrigued by the mention that the patient had progressive hearing loss, as this is not the usual set of symptoms seen in Usher syndrome. It is our experience that Usher syndrome mainly manifests itself in profound deafness at birth.

Dr. Robert Gorlin: This type of Usher syndrome is so-called Usher syndrome Type Type III. There are at least 4 types of Usher syndrome, 3 of which are definitely inherited as autosomal recessive, and one of which is inherited as an X-linked. The first type, approximately 90% of the cases, has the onset of retinitis pigmentosa prior to the age of 10. In Type II, the onset is after the age of 18. Both Types I and II are autosomal recessive and they account for 99% of the cases. Type III is associated with progressive retinitis pigmentosa. Type IV is X-linked with the phenotype of Type II. Thus, some of the Type II's may be heterogeneous. There is a tremendous problem concerning nosology when one discusses a symptom complex which has been called Friedreich ataxia or Usher syndrome. There can be many different varieties. One must describe exactly which one of the varieties one is discussing.

Dr. Robert Ruben: In the older European literature, one or two cases of temporal bones have been described from patients who presumably had Usher syndrome. However, it is not known which type of Usher syndrome this was and whether there were other confounding variables.

Biochemistry of the Inner Ear*

Ruediger Thalmann, MD, Daniel C. Marcus, DSc, and Isolde Thalmann, MA

The volume of information on biochemistry of the inner ear has exploded since 1964, when the only book covering this topic was written by Rauch [1]. It is impossible, therefore, to discuss the entire area, even superficially, in a brief review. Accordingly, our treatment of the subject will be illustrative rather than comprehensive. We will point out some fundamental biochemical features of the 2 main structures of the cochlear duct — the organ of Corti (OC) and the stria vascularis (SV) — and will rely heavily upon data obtained by a quantitative histochemical approach similar to that developed by Lowry and Passonneau [2] over the years for the study of discrete tissue units of other complex tissues, such as brain and retina.

In order to put matters into perspective, we present a brief historical review of the evolution of current concepts regarding the energetic processes involved in mammalian auditory transduction. In 1930, Wever and Bray [3] discovered a sound-evoked peripheral potential, which Adrian [4] identified as an almost exact electrical replica of the incoming sound signal; accordingly, the potential was named the cochlear microphonic (CM). Although the CM was found to be highly susceptible to hypoxia and ischemia, for a long time it was believed that the potential was the product of a passive transduction process, comparable to the piezoelectric effect [5]. However, on the basis of order of magnitude estimates, von Békésy [6] demonstrated that the energy of the CM greatly exceeds the energy contained in the incoming sound signals, and consequently he postulated a large source of biologic energy responsible for powering the generator of the CM. In searching for this source of energy, von Békésy [6], discovered a unique positive potential (80–90 mV) in scala media, which was named the endocochlear or endolymphatic potential (EP). Subsequent experiments provided strong suggestions that the SV is the (main) generator of the EP. On the basis of this in-

*Supported by NIH grant NS 06575, and NSF grant BNS 77-16842

formation, Davis [7] proposed the "battery theory" of cochlear transduction, according to which one battery in the SV and another in the hair cells cause a current to flow across the apical surface of the hair cells; the resistance across the hair cells is modulated by the sound waves, thus giving rise to the CM as an electrical replica of the sound stimulus, but with a much greater energy content.* Whereas in Davis' model the contribution of energy from the SV and the hair cells is equal, a modification of this model, proposed by Honrubia et al [8], attributes two-thirds of the power for the transduction process to the SV and one-third to the hair cells.

Shortly after the discovery of the EP, Smith et al [9] discovered the unusual ionic composition of endolymph — extremely high K^+ values and low Na^+ values. Bosher and Warren [10] confirmed the high K^+ values (140–150 meq/l) of endolymph, but found that the $[Na^+]$ of cochlear endolymph was much lower (1 mM or less) than the figure published by Smith et al [9] for (saccular) endolymph. They further proved that K^+ must be transported actively into, and Cl^- and Na^+ out of, endolymph. It was first pointed out by Johnstone [11] that the difference between the ionic composition of the fluid in contact with the endolymphatic surface, and of that bathing the remaining surface of the hair cells (most likely a perilymph-like fluid similar in ionic content to other extracellular fluids) provided the asymmetry required for a standing current flow. Furthermore, this assymmetry may contribute an additional reservoir of energy which ultimately would also depend upon power generated in the SV.

The OC per se is avascular, and the spiral vessel underneath the tunnel of Corti, which is large during embryonic development, is absent in the adult stage in many species, including the guinea pig. It would seem logical that a rich vasculature of the auditory transducer itself — the OC — would be undesirable in the interest of optimal acoustic function (eg high sensitivity, high frequency resolution, wide dynamic range, low background noise, etc). This idea is supported by the presence of a highly vascularized tissue — the SV — on the lateral wall of scala media, and early workers came to the conclusion that the SV was responsible for supplying the OC with oxygen and fuels. At that time it was not known that the SV has a very high metabolic rate of its own (to be discussed later), and that it could, therefore, hardly qualify as a provider of oxygen and fuels for the OC. Furthermore, it was not known that the basilar membrane is freely permeable and that the fluid spaces of the OC are thus continuous with perilymph. It has been established that even in the absence of the spiral vessel, the nearby vessel of the tympanic lip is invariably present. Also, there are indications (see below) that the OC has a relatively low metabolic rate.

---

*It has not been established whether the CM is a causal link in the chain of events leading to neural excitation or whether it merely represents an epiphenomenon.

Given all this, it seems that the relatively low fuel and oxygen requirements of the OC are met from sources other than the SV.* In a sense, however, the SV remains an important "provider" for the OC, not as originally thought, by transporting fuels and oxygen via the endolymph, but in a more elegant manner by the transmission of energy via the EP, and by providing the unique ionic composition of endolymph. There appears to be, then, a most favorable division of duties, by segregation of the delicate auditory transducer — the OC — from the main power plant — the SV. It may be premature to define quantitatively the amount of energy contributed by the different tissues to the transduction process on the basis of the above electrophysiologic evidence alone. Biochemical data, presented here later, suggest that the amount of power contributed to the transduction process by the SV may substantially exceed the estimates based on bioelectric techniques.

Before presenting biochemical results, it appears relevant to discuss briefly the problems associated with quantitative chemical analyses of tissues and fluids of the inner ear, and to point out the potential and limitations of the pertinent techniques. An investigator of the biochemistry of the inner ear is confronted with a dilemma: he must choose between the conflicting requirements of achieving a meaningful level of morphologic resolution, and of obtaining an adequate amount of tissue to utilize the most powerful modern biochemical methods effectively. Subcellular fractionation studies on the ear require enormous amounts of tissue; for instance, in studies concerning the stimulation of adenylate cyclase, all cochlear soft tissues from a large number of guinea pigs had to be pooled [12]. Although these studies indicate some interesting response patterns of cochlear adenylate cyclase, they do not give any indication of which tissue(s) may be responsible for the observed effects. In addition, all information on differences in any given tissue along the extent of the cochlea is lost. On the opposite end of the spectrum, techniques have been developed which afford relatively high resolution with respect to individual tissues and (in the case of the OC) cell types, but which are limited in the number and type of analytic methods which can be applied meaningfully at the microlevel. Although such subdivision of cochlear tissues and isolation of cell populations is feasible with fresh tissues, this type of material is useful only for the determination of activities of enzymes and of the concentration of other *biologically* stable compounds. If biologically labile compounds, such as adenine nucleotides, P-creatine, and various substrates and intermediates of energy metabolism are to be measured, meaningful determinations can only be made if the chemical state of the tissues is preserved as nearly as possible to that existing in vivo. A powerful method for this purpose has been developed by Lowry and Passonneau [2], based on rapid freezing, frozen sectioning,

---

*It has also been pointed out recently that the limbus spiralis is richly vascularized, and thus sufficient oxygen could conceivably diffuse across the inner sulcus to the inner hair cells.

and subsequent freeze drying at $-40°$. This is followed by microdissection at room temperature under conditions of low humidity, and weighing of the samples on quartz fiber balances. The samples are then analyzed by enzymatic fluorometric assays as developed by Lowry and Passonneau [2] or by any other sufficiently sensitive and specific technique, such as microradioimmunochemical analysis for cyclic nucleotides. In the cochlea, frozen sectioning is not readily feasible, but this cumbersome step can be avoided, since freeze drying of the cochlea in toto preserves the three-dimensional structure of inner ear tissues, which can be readily identified and isolated in this state [13, 14]. In other instances, such as in the analysis of phospholipids [15] and nucleic acids [16], it is possible to fix the tissue chemically prior to dissection and analysis.

A variety of problems are also encountered in the analysis of fluids of the inner ear. Because of the pronounced ionic gradients between the endolymph and the surrounding fluid spaces, sophisticated methods had to be developed for the determination of the ionic content of endolymph. By observing the most exacting precautions, Bosher and Warren [10, 17] were able to improve endolymphatic sampling techniques to the point that the extremely low Na^+ and Ca^{++} levels of endolymph (1 mM and 0.02 mM, respectively) could be established. Presently, techniques using ion selective glass or ion exchange resins are gradually replacing the more cumbersome sampling techniques [17, 18]. In the case of perilymph, although there is a much greater volume of fluid available for sampling (compared to endolymph), and although the levels of most of its chemical constituents are similar to the levels in other extracellular fluids, there is still confusion concerning its exact composition. One of the major problems is due to admixture of cerebrospinal fluid with perilymph, which will occur unless sample volumes are kept small, and unless precautions are observed to guard against the creation of pressure gradients due to the opening of the cochlea and aspiration of the fluid sample.

With respect to biologically labile substances in cochlear tissues, it was one of our primary objectives to determine the distribution pattern of the presumed chief substrates of energy metabolism of the OC and the SV: glycogen and glucose.*
This information, together with the corresponding values for the high energy phosphates ATP and P-creatine, allowed the calculation of the total energy reserve [20], in the manner proposed by Lowry et al [21] for other tissues dependent upon carbohydrate metabolism. The formula of Lowry et al takes into account all of the preformed high energy phosphate ($\sim$ P) present in ATP and P-creatine, and

---

*There seemed a priori to be no doubt that the OC, like other neurosensory structures, is dependent upon utilization of carbohydrates; but this was not certain for the SV, an auxiliary tissue with many features in common with kidney tissue, which is known for its preferential utilization of lipids. However, recent in vitro experiments in our laboratory indicate that the respiratory quotient of the SV is substantially higher than unity (1.2), making it highly likely that this structure also depends upon carbohydrate metabolism [19].

that potentially available by anaerobic glycolysis from endogenous glucose and glycogen ($\Sigma \sim P = 2 \times ATP + 1 \times PCr + 2 \times glucose + 2.9 \times glycogen$).

The average values of the total energy reserve for different inner ear structures obtained in this way are shown in Table 1. The energy reserve is substantially higher in the OC than in the SV. The average figures in the OC are somewhat misleading, however, since glycogen — the main contributor to the energy reserve — exhibits a pronounced longitudinal gradient, rising toward the apex (Fig. 1) [20].*
Thus the energy reserve is higher in the cochlear apex and lower in the base than the average value given.

The significance of the high energy reserve of the OC is not clear. It is possible that it represents an adaptation to an environment relatively low in oxygen, although enzymatic and other studies indicate that the energy metabolism of the OC is largely aerobic [23]. The high glycogen level may, however, present an advantage in situations in which energy must be generated on "short notice." The appropriate mechanism would be aerobic glycolysis,** because of its high temporal efficiency, although the energetic efficiency of this mode of energy generation is very poor.

The next step in our discussion concerns the dynamics of the components of the energy reserve in ischemia. The first objective is to examine whether levels of ATP correlate with the potential attributed to the OC and SV, respectively; the

TABLE 1. Total Energy Reserve and Initial Use Rate of High Energy Phosphate in Structures of the Inner Ear

	Organ of Corti	Stria vasc.	Coch. nerve	Ganglion spirale	Mac. sacc.	Mac. utric.
Total energy reserve	500–530	245	70	265	268	265
Initial use rate of $\sim P$	15–21	65–80	25–34	35–47	20	18

The total energy reserve represents the sum of high energy phosphate (in mmoles/kg dry weight) available from preformed ATP and phosphocreatine and potentially available from glycolytic breakdown of glucose and glycogen to lactate. The initial use rate (in mmoles/kg dry weight/min) of high energy phosphate (metabolic rate) represents the sum of the initial rates of change of the major energy sources in ischemia translated into fluxes of equivalents of high energy phosphate. (Adapted from reference 20).

*The glycogen level is particularly high in the outer hair cells of the upper cochlear turns in the guinea pig (Fig. 2) [22]. However, there are large differences among species in the amount of glycogen present in the OC, with very low levels in the mouse, for example.

**Aerobic glycolysis is defined as production of lactate in the presence of oxygen; in brain, for instance, aerobic glycolysis accounts for about 15% of the glucose use rate.

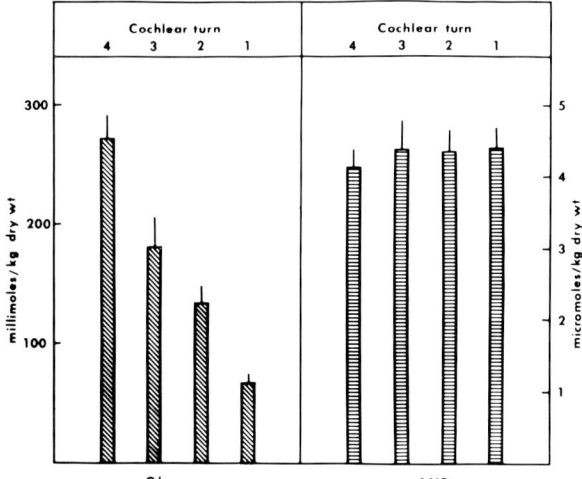

Fig. 1. Distribution of glycogen and cyclic AMP (cAMP) in different turns of the organ of Corti of the guinea pig. The vertical lines indicate the SEM for 4 ears in the case of cAMP and 7 ears in the case of glycogen. Five to 7 individual specimens were taken from each turn per ear. (Figs. 1, 2, and 7 from Thalmann R, Paloheimo S, Thalmann I: Distribution of cyclic nucleotides of the organ of Corti. Acta Otolaryngol 87:375–380, 1979, with permission.)

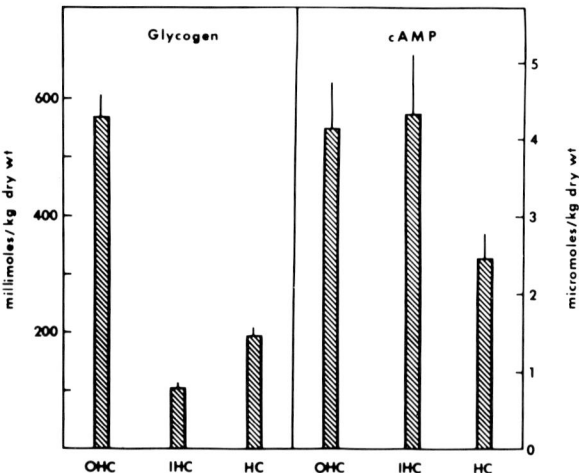

Fig. 2. Distribution of glycogen and cyclic AMP (cAMP) in different cellular layers of the organ of Corti of the apical cochlear turn in the guinea pig. Vertical lines indicate the SEM for 7 ears in all instances, except in the case of cAMP in the inner hair cell layer, for which only 4 ears were used. Five to 8 individual specimens of each layer were taken per ear. OHC = outer hair cell layer; IHC = inner hair cell layer; HC = Hensen cell layer.

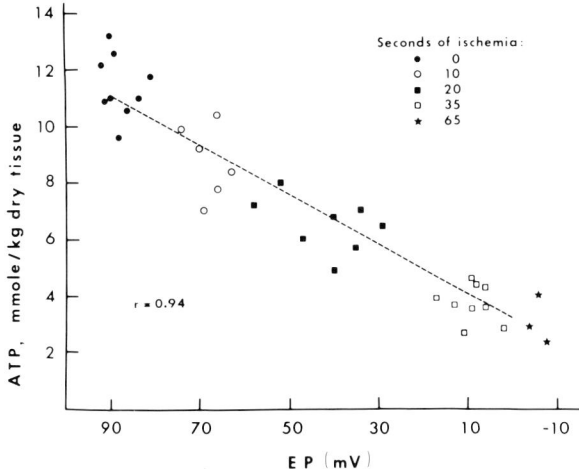

Fig. 3. Effect of ischemia upon the endolymphatic potential (EP) and the levels of ATP in the stria vascularis of the guinea pig. The EP was measured in the basal turn via the round window. Ischemia was produced by sectioning the aorta. At the indicated times, the cochleae were frozen and processed as described in the text; 12–14 samples were dissected from the 1st and 2nd turns of each ear and analyzed for ATP. Data points represent the mean results in individual ears. The line represents the least squares best fit; "r" is the correlation coefficient. (From Thalmann R, Kusakari J, Miyoshi T: Dysfunctions of energy releasing and consuming processes of the cochlea. Laryngoscope 83:1690–1712, 1973, with permission.)

second, closely related objective, is to arrive at an estimate of the initial energy use rate in ischemia (metabolic rate) according to the "closed system" method of Lowry et al [21].

Figure 3 demonstrates that the rapid decline of the EP in ischemia is closely paralleled by the decline of ATP in the SV. By contrast, ATP levels in the OC drop only slowly in ischemia; this decline correlates surprisingly well with the decline of the OC potential (Fig. 4).* These facts already appeared to indicate pronounced differences between the metabolic rates of the OC and the SV. Yet there still existed the possibility that a very rapid rate of glycogenolysis and (aerobic) glycolysis would support a potentially high metabolic rate of the OC. However, we later found that glycogen of the OC declines very slowly during ischemia, which led to the conclusion that the metabolic rate of the OC is low [20]. More complete estimates based on Lowry's "closed system" method, estimates derived from the initial rate of change of preformed and potentially available high energy

*The OC potential, measured via the approach through the round window and basilar membrane, presumably reflects the intracellular potentials only of the supporting cells of the OC. Although evidence exists that the resting potential of the hair cells is very similar to the OC potential, nothing is known about the dynamics of the hair cell potential proper in ischemia.

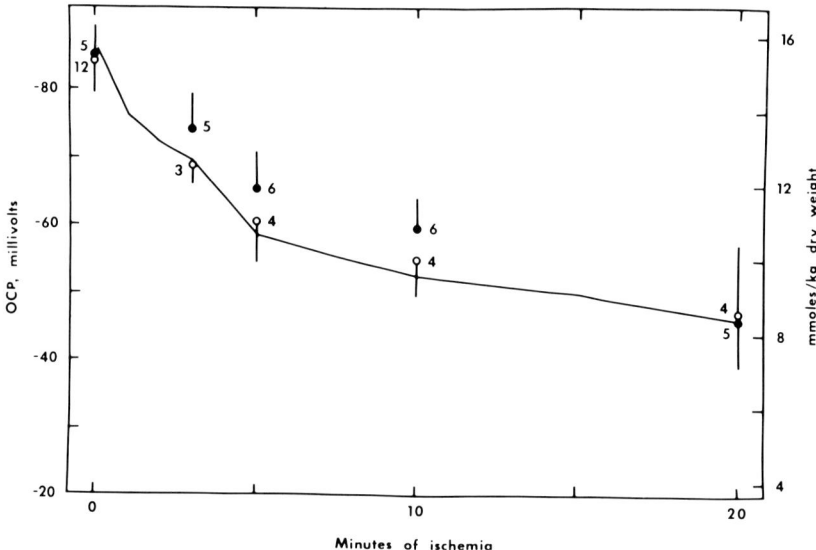

Fig. 4. Influence of ethacrynic acid upon the organ of Corti potential (OCP) under normal and ischemic conditions, and effect of ischemia upon the ATP levels of the organ of Corti. The OCP was measured via the round window and the basilar membrane using microelectrodes with tips of 2–3 μm in diameter. Ethacrynic acid was administered intravenously at a dosage of 50 mg/kg. The "zero time" OCP was measured when the endolymphatic potential had reached its maximum negative level (−25 to −40 mV), and at the indicated times during superimposed ischemia (open circles). Closed circles represent the response to ischemia in animals not treated with ethacrynic acid (controls). Vertical lines signify the means ± SD. The number of ears tested is indicated. The solid curve represents average ATP levels of the organ of Corti during ischemia (in nonintoxicated animals; control value 15.4 ± 0.9 mmoles/kg dry weight). Ischemia was induced by sectioning the aorta (zero time). (Figs. 4 and 6 from Thalmann R, Thalmann I, Ise I, Paloheimo S: Noxious effects upon cochlear metabolism. Laryngoscope 87:699–721, 1977, with permission.)

phosphate in ischemia ($\Delta_t \sim P = 2 \times \Delta_t ATP + \Delta_t PCr + 2 \times \Delta_t glucose + 2.9 \times \Delta_t glycogen$), are shown in Table 1 and indicate that the metabolic rate of the OC is about 4 times lower than that of the SV [20]. In qualitative agreement, cartesian diver studies indicate that the respiratory rate of the SV is one order of magnitude higher than that of the OC [24].

The measurements made in the OC are complicated by the fact that the system is not strictly closed in ischemia, since the large glucose reserve in the perilymph continues to be available as fuel. Studies are, therefore, in progress in which the glucose pool in the perilymph (and the major part of the oxygen pool) is removed prior to the initiation of ischemia. Although much more glycogen is present in the apical than in the basal turns, the *absolute* amount of glycogen broken down in the initial stage of ischemia is similar in different regions of the cochlea

[20]. According to preliminary experiments, the level of glycogen in the outer hair cell layer of the apical turns does not change significantly in the first 15 minutes of ischemia. The rate of decline of ATP in ischemia in the outer hair cells is as slow as that in the whole OC [25]. Recent studies indicate that the decline of ATP and the increase of 5'AMP in the inner hair cell layer (which contains only comparatively small amounts of glycogen) are not significantly faster than in the outer hair cell layer (I. Thalmann and R. Thalmann, unpublished data). Therefore, it is not likely that the metabolic rate of the hair cells proper is significantly higher than that determined for the whole OC.

On the other hand, we have reason to believe that the metabolic rate of the SV is even higher than is shown in Table 1. This assumption is based on the fact that when a bolus of nitrogen-saturated oxygen-free "simplified blood" is injected by rapid vascular perfusion, the EP drops much faster than in ischemia induced by sectioning the aorta. This is consistent with the existence of a substantial reservoir of oxygen in the large vascular space of the SV. It will now be of interest to determine whether the rate of decline of high energy phosphates is as fast as the decline of the EP, when the oxygen reserves are almost instantaneously removed.

In summary, the dynamic electrophysiologic and biochemical features presented would suggest that the energy required for the maintenance of the EP and/or contributed by the SV to the auditory transduction process substantially exceeds that contributed by the OC or the hair cells proper.

A topic of particular interest in cochlear physiologic chemistry is the mode of generation of the EP. It is the present consensus that the EP is the algebraic sum of 2 potentials of opposite polarity (+ 120 mV and −40 mV, respectively) [8, 18, 26, 27]. The positive component is ascribed to electrogenic K^+ transport into scala media, and is extremely sensitive to anoxia and other metabolic interferences. There is no consensus about the nature of the negative component, but it is most likely a K^+ diffusion potential across some as yet unidentified structure bounding the cochlear duct. The negative component is not directly sensitive to anoxia and other interferences with energy metabolism. The relative insensitivity of the negative component to oxygen lack is the reason that the (composite) EP drops to negative levels in anoxia. The (composite) EP returns only gradually towards zero mV as the ionic gradients equilibrate.

Kuijpers [26] proposed that the Na^+K^+-ATPase system of the SV is responsible for the generation of the positive component of the EP. This theory was based on 2 lines of evidence: first, the SV has an extremely high activity of Na^+K^+-ATPase (an order of magnitude higher than other cochlear tissues). Second, the inhibition curves of the EP and of strial Na^+K^+-ATPase with respect to ouabain virtually overlap. Although Kuijpers [26] suggested that the (positive) EP is due to electrogenic K^+ transport, he did not elaborate on how the coupled Na^+/K^+ exchange pump could lead to the large net movement of K^+ required. If the basal-lateral surfaces of the marginal cells of the SV are assumed impermeable to Na^+, the

K^+/Na^+ transfer ratio would be about 90 [28, 29], whereas in all other tissues the ouabain-sensitive Na^+/K^+ pump has been found to exhibit a ratio close to unity. In endolymphatic perfusion experiments, Sellick and Bock [28] presented evidence that the EP is, indeed, due to transport of K^+ into scala media. However, they ascribed this effect to an independent K^+ pump similar to that found in the midgut of the silkworm and in other insects.

In addition to the rheogenic transport of K^+ into endolymph that results in the positive component of the EP, Na^+ and Cl^- are actively transported out of endolymph. This predominantly electroneutral transport modifies the composition of endolymph without affecting the EP. It is difficult to explain the apparent paradox that the characteristic Na^+-K^+ profile of endolymph in the rat is already present at birth, at a time when the EP is still absent [30]. The EP develops rather abruptly during the 13th to 14th postnatal day, during the same time in which a drastic increase of Na^+K^+-ATPase occurs in the SV [31]. Whether the increase of Na^+K^+-ATPase is a causal or merely coincidental phenomenon cannot yet be decided. It is possible that the sudden appearance of the EP could be due to an increase of the resistance of the membranes surrounding the cochlear duct occurring during maturation.

There has been much debate about the source(s), flow, and resorption of endolymph. Essentially, 2 theories, the theories of "radial" flow and of "longitudinal" flow have been proposed [32]. It appears that neither of these theories tells the whole story. There exist several lines of evidence that we are not dealing with a large bulk-flow of endolymph, but rather that the ions are transported with little concomitant movement of water. However, on a long time scale, there is undoubtedly some degree of longitudinal flow toward the endolymphatic sac. This is indicated by the fact that cell debris and other particulate matter are carried in the direction of the endolymphatic sac, where they are broken down further and resorbed [33]. In addition, obstruction of the endolymphatic duct and sac leads to endolymphatic hydrops ("a" or "the" pathologic substrate of Ménière disease) in experimental animals. Hydrops develops particularly rapidly (in a matter of days or weeks) in the guinea pig [34] but far more slowly in the cat [35].

We have mentioned the high activity of Na^+K^+-ATPase in the SV, which undoubtedly plays an important role in the maintenance of the ionic profile of endolymph. Another enzyme frequently associated with ion transport — carbonic anhydrase — is present at substantial levels in the SV. However, the reason for the extremely high level of this enzyme in the spiral ligament, a structure which is not thought to play a significant role in the production of endolymph, is obscure [36]. Adenylate cyclase, which also exhibits a substantial activity in the SV, may be another enzyme important in the homeostasis of endolymph [37, 38]. In fact, on the basis of experiments involving the endolymphatic application of cholera toxin, Feldman and Brusilow [39] proposed that a dysfunction of this enzyme may be the pathologic basis for endolymphatic hydrops (or Ménière disease).

Although studies on perilymph would seem less complicated than those on endolymph, experimental results do conflict and there is no consensus about the exact composition and dynamics of perilymph. It has been proposed that the perilymph is essentially an ultrafiltrate of serum [40]. However, recently it has been shown that the biochemical profile of low molecular weight substances in perilymph differs significantly from that of serum in several ways. Therefore, the existence of a selective blood-perilymph barrier has been postulated [41]. In spite of the presence of the perilymphatic duct, the biochemical profile of perilymph also differs significantly from that of cerebrospinal fluid (CSF). It has recently been estimated that in the guinea pig, no more than 25% of the perilymph could be derived from CSF [42].

In view of the differences in experimental approaches, analytic techniques, and species used, it is difficult to integrate the presently available information on perilymph. However, it appears certain that early estimates of the rate of turnover of perilymph based on dye dilution techniques were too high [40]. Recent evidence suggests that one cannot speak of a turnover rate of the perilymph as a whole, but that each substance must be considered individually. For instance, in the case of Na^+, the half times of entry into perilymph [43] and of disappearance from the cochlea [44] have been found to be on the order of 3 hours. Much shorter half times have been found for Cl^- and far longer times for Ca^{++} (W.K. Jung, personal communication). To our knowledge, no information is available about the rate of turnover of perilymphatic water or whether there exists a significant bulk flow. Experiments with tritiated water should answer this important question.

Apart from its mechanical role in transmitting acoustic vibrations, the perilymph is the main medium of metabolic exchange of the OC. Perilymph (modified to some extent by the spiral vessel and the vessel of the tympanic lip and by the absorption and excretion of metabolites by the OC) pervades the fluid spaces of the OC as the so-called "Cortilymph." Any drug or toxic substance must diffuse through perilymph and Cortilymph over a considerable distance in order to reach the OC. Certain substances have a tendency to persist in the perilymph for extended periods, long after the levels in the serum have declined. Such a delayed clearance is, inter alia, present in the case of aminoglycoside antibiotics, and this has been suggested as one of the reasons why the OC is particularly vulnerable to these substances [45].

The aminoglycoside antibiotics are undoubtedly the most dangerous ototoxic drugs currently in clinical use. Their primary pathohistologic effects are manifested by degeneration of the hair cells of the OC and of the vestibular end-organs [46]. In contrast to the other main categories of ototoxic drugs in current use (the salicylates and the "loop" diuretics), the hearing loss and decrease of vestibular sensitivity incurred by aminoglycosides are largely irreversible. Many theories about the selective vulnerability of the inner ear to aminoglycosides have been forwarded. The slow clearance of these drugs from the inner ear fluids, alluded to above, may be one of the contributing factors [45]. However, a systematic series of studies by Schacht [15] has led to the first solid theory regarding the mechanism of toxic action of aminoglycosides upon the inner ear and the kidney.

Schacht [15] has presented several lines of evidence which indicate that the polyphosphoinositides are in vivo receptors of aminoglycoside antibiotics. He first demonstrated that chronic treatment of guinea pigs with neomycin impairs the metabolism of polyphosphoinositides, a class of acidic phospholipids, both in the kidney and in the inner ear. When the drug is applied locally, via perilymphatic perfusion, the neomycin-induced inhibition of polyphosphoinositide metabolism parallels the decline of the CM. Furthermore, in experiments involving isolation of polyphosphoinositides from cell extracts of the inner ear and kidney, it was found that the highest affinity towards neomycin is displayed by phosphatidyl inositol diphosphate. This lipid could not be eluted efficiently at neutral pH by increasing the ionic strength of the solvent, but required acid or base for its displacement from neomycin. Binding of aminoglycosides to polyphosphoinositides displaces Ca^{++} and inhibits the turnover of these lipids, which play an essential role in the control of membrane permeability. Apart from this primary effect of the drug, the disruption in the structure of the membrane resulting from the binding may facilitate the entry of neomycin into the cell, where it may exert further toxic effects. In addition, one could speculate that such a disturbance of membrane permeability may be the reason for the well-documented potentiative interaction of aminoglycosides with noise and "loop" diuretics.

Jarlstedt and Bagger-Sjöbäck [16] demonstrated that application of gentamicin resulted in a substantial reduction of the RNA content of sensory and ganglion cells of the hearing organ of the lizard at a time when ultrastructural signs of cellular damage were not yet apparent. It needs to be decided whether this effect occurs at a stage of intoxication which precedes, parallels, or follows the above-mentioned effects upon the phospholipids. Tachibana et al [47] found that treatment of guinea pigs with kanamycin results in a substantial reduction of the activity of the glycolytic enzymes phosphofructokinase and hexokinase in the OC and the kidney. No inhibition of the enzymes of the pentose phosphate shunt was found in the same structures. Again, it is conceivable that this effect is secondary to the impairment of metabolism of phospholipids and damage to membrane structures.

The second major category of ototoxic drugs in current use is the salicylates. In fact, the first subjective ototoxic side effect, the occurrence of tinnitus, is still being used clinically as an index of the maximum tolerable dosage. Salicylates have several different modes of action, an important one of which is an uncoupling of oxidative phosphorylation. In view of the extremely high respiratory rate of the SV, it seemed natural to assume that salicylates would act via interference with strial energy metabolism. However, neither the EP nor the content of high energy phosphates in the SV changed following application of the highest tolerable dosage of the drug in the guinea pig. Also, the CM and the high energy phosphates of the OC remained normal. Only the compound action potential showed a characteristic change, namely a progressive steepening of the input/output curve with little or no reduction of the peak values [48]. It is possible that this effect is due to an impaired energy metabolism in the nerve endings at the base of the hair cells, which are extremely rich in mitochondria. There is no way that such a localized biochemical change could be detected with presently available quantitative histochemical techniques. Interference with the synthesis of prostaglandins is another important action of salicylates, but no pertinent studies have, to date, been carried out on the cochlea. Of the 3 major categories of ototoxic drugs discussed here, only the salicylates do not seem to interact with noise [49].

Following several reports of temporary impairment of hearing due to application of the powerful salidiuretic drug ethacrynic acid, intensive experimentation on animals with this drug and the other "loop" diuretics, furosemide and bumetanide, was initiated. The term "loop" diuretics refers to the fact that the primary site of action of these drugs is the loop of Henle. According to a large number of animal studies, the main target of ototoxic action of these drugs seems to be the SV and the EP. In fact, loop diuretics are the only chemical agents known to date which produce a maximal depression of the EP (-30 mV) when administered systemically at sublethal dosages [50, 51]. This effect is accompanied by intense edema of the SV and shrinkage of the intermediate cells.

Upon IV administration of 50 mg/kg of furosemide, the EP starts to decline immediately and reaches maximally negative levels within 2 minutes. This is followed by a complete recovery within about 60 minutes (Fig. 5). In the case of ethacrynic acid, the reaction is distinctly slower (maximum depression following 50 mg/kg within about 10 minutes). This is followed by a biphasic, initially rapid, and subsequently very slow but eventually complete recovery (24–48 hours) [52].

Because of the profound decline of the EP with attainment of extreme negative values, we assumed that ethacrynic acid acted upon the EP by the same mechanism as does ouabain, namely by interference with Na^+K^+-ATPase. However, in contrast to those of ouabain, the inhibition curves of the EP and of strial Na^+K^+-ATPase with respect to ethacrynic acid are markedly out of line; half-maximal inhibition of the enzyme is attained only by concentrations 500 times higher than those required to produce half-maximal inhibition of the EP (Fig. 6) [51]. In the case of furosemide, no inhibition of Na^+K^+-ATPase was achieved with highest possible concentrations of the drug (10 mM). This makes it very unlikely that Na^+K^+-ATPase is the target of the toxic action of loop diuretics upon the ear. By contrast, ethacrynic acid and furosemide interfere with strial adenylate cyclase at

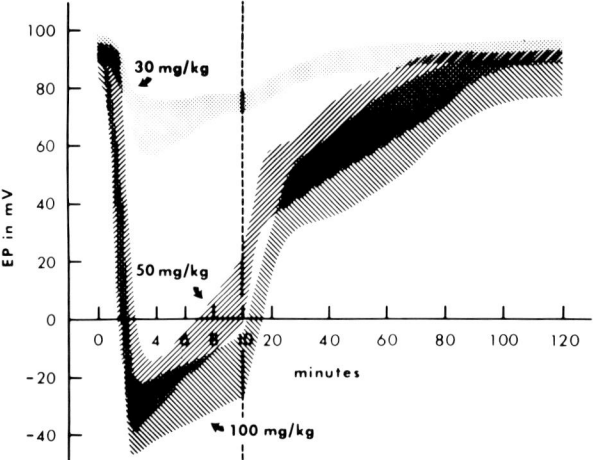

Fig. 5. Effect of intravenously applied furosemide upon the endolymphatic potential in the guinea pig. The dosages are indicated. The shaded areas represent the mean ± SD of five 30 mg/kg, eight 50 mg/kg, and nine 100 mg/kg experiments. Note the change in the time scale at the 10 min mark. (From Kusakari J, Ise I, Comegys TH, Thalmann I, Thalmann R: Effect of ethacrynic acid, furosemide, and ouabain upon the endolymphatic potential and upon high energy phosphates of the stria vascularis. Laryngoscope 88:12–37, 1978, with permission.)

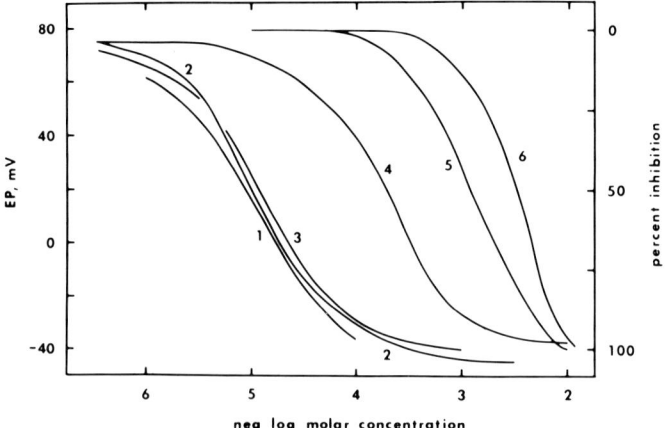

Fig. 6. Curves 2 and 3, respectively, are the inhibition curves of the endolymphatic potential (left ordinate) and strial adenylate cyclase (7 min preincubation: right ordinate) with respect to ethacrynic acid. Curves 4 and 1, respectively, are the inhibition curves of the endolymphatic potential (left ordinate) and strial adenylate cyclase (15 min preincubation: right ordinate) with respect to furosemide. Curves 5 and 6, respectively, represent the inhibition of strial Na^+K^+-ATPase with regard to ethacrynic acid, with and without 30 min of preincubation. All data are from the guinea pig.

concentrations similar to those which cause inhibition of the EP (Fig. 6) [38]. Adenylate cyclase has been shown to play an essential role in the control of ion movements in kidney tubules and in other transport epithelia. Although the inhibition characteristics of strial adenylate cyclase are consistent with the possibility that this enzyme is the target of the toxic action of ethacrynic acid and furosemide upon the SV, more evidence would be required to establish a causal relationship. The next logical step here would be the determination of steady state levels of cyclic AMP under comparable conditions. Supportive evidence that transport enzymes are impaired by ethacrynic acid is provided by the dynamics of the high energy phosphates ATP and P-creatine, which indicate that the drug causes a massive interference with strial energy utilization [51]. Using another experimental approach, Bosher [53] arrived at the conclusion that the decline of the EP in the early phase of ethacrynic acid intoxication is due to interference with strial enzymes, whereas subsequent events are dominated by a massive change in the membrane permeability in the cochlear duct.

Ethacrynic acid is also known to interfere with energy generation, both glycolytic and respiratory. Interference with glycolysis in cell-free kidney preparations occurs at unphysiologically high concentrations. The same is true for effects upon respiration of renal mitochondria. However, in long-term experiments on preparations of rabbit renal cortex, Case et al [54] found that reductions of the P:O ratio occur at considerably lower concentrations than do changes in mitochondrial respiration, ie in the approximate range in which first alterations of the EP occur. It is, therefore, surprising that even when the EP is maximally depressed by ethacrynic acid, the ATP levels of the SV are only moderately reduced, and P-creatine levels are completely normal [51]. In the case of furosemide, no changes in high energy phosphate levels are present when the EP is maximally reduced.

It appears that the ototoxic action of loop diuretics is far from being understood, and that most likely several different factors contribute to the observed effects. Of the loop diuretics discussed, ethacrynic acid is most prone to cause temporary hearing problems in patients. Furosemide is much less toxic, and the safest of all seems to be the relatively new agent bumetanide. However, considerable caution must be exerted if loop diuretics are given concurrently with aminoglycoside antibiotics, since a potentiative interaction of these drugs has been observed, both clinically and in animal experiments.

Another topic of primary interest in cochlear pathobiology is the question of whether noise damage is mediated biochemically. There exists a large body of indirect evidence that biochemical changes are ultimately responsible for the damage to the inner ear incurred by exposure to levels of noise below those causing direct mechanical disruptions. It has been known for a long time that hypoxia markedly increases the susceptibility of the CM to sound-induced damage

[55]. The same is true when the CM is partially damaged by local application of metabolic inhibitors. The susceptibility to damage by sound is increased most drastically following application of iodoacetate, an inhibitor of glycolysis [56]. This finding is of interest in view of the above-mentioned high glycogen levels in the OC. Drescher [57] demonstrated that the rate of threshold shift during exposure to noise is drastically increased by elevating the body temperature of the experimental animals from 37° to 39°.

More direct evidence for a biochemical basis of noise damage is provided by several qualitative histochemical studies, particularly that by Ishii et al [58] which demonstrates a reduction and redistribution of glycogen in the outer hair cells following moderate exposure to noise. However, a series of quantitative histochemical studies conducted in our laboratory using two types of noise exposure with the guinea pig and the chinchilla, have so far failed to demonstrate significant changes in key substances involved in energy metabolism and in other essential biochemical compounds. Specifically, no significant differences between exposed and control ears were found in the outer and inner hair cell layers in the case of ATP and 5'AMP [59]. In preliminary experiments, we were also unable to detect any changes in cyclic AMP levels due to noise. The behavior of cyclic GMP during noise exposure has not yet been studied.

Although these quantitative histochemical studies yielded negative results, this does not necessarily imply that there are not changes in functionally critical compartments within the cells, because the limit of resolution of the presently used technique is at the level of whole cells. Further methodologic refinements may be required to arrive at more definite conclusions. It also needs to be decided whether the recent finding by Flock and Cheung [60] of actin filaments in the stereocilia, and experiments by Kilian and Schacht [61] on the effects of sound stimulation upon certain phospholipids in the hearing organ of the noctuid moth will shed light upon the biochemical mechanisms of noise damage.

The fact that cyclic AMP levels in the cochlear hair cells do not seem to be affected by exposure to noise is surprising, since cyclic AMP levels in the retina vary drastically, dependent upon the presence or absence of light. In certain layers of the retina, dark adaptation causes a sharp rise in cyclic AMP levels [62]. Still, cyclic AMP levels in the OC are sizeable, and from a teleological standpoint, one would assume that it serves some important function [63]. It is well established that cyclic AMP acts as "second messenger" in the control of glycogen metabolism in the liver and other organs. Because of the highly polarized distribution of glycogen within the OC, we thought that a comparison with the distribution pattern of cyclic AMP could give us a clue as to whether this nucleotide is involved in the regulation of glycogen metabolism in the OC. However, as is shown in Figures 1 and 2, the distribution of cyclic AMP does not correspond at all with the pronounced longitudinal or transverse gradients of glycogen, and it is therefore unlikely that cyclic AMP is involved in the regulation of glycogen metabolism in

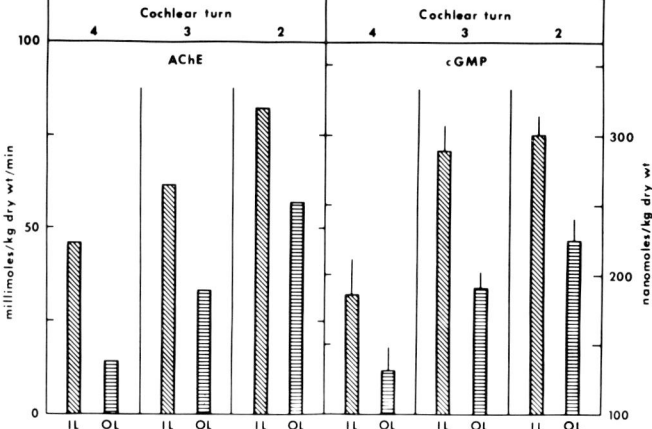

Fig. 7. Distribution of acetylcholinesterase (AChE) and cyclic GMP (cGMP) in the inner and outer layer (IL and OL) of the organ of Corti in different cochlear turns in the guinea pig. The inner layer contains the inner hair cells with their supporting cells, as well as part of the inner pillars. The outer layer contains the outer hair cells, the Hensen cells and the Deiters cells. Vertical lines shown in the case of cGMP represent the SEM for 9 ears. Four to 5 individual specimens of both layers were taken in each turn per ear. Due to technical difficulties, the cGMP values for the basal cochlear turn are not available. The differences in cGMP levels between the inner and outer layers are statistically significant in all 3 turns ($P < 0.05$ or less). In the outer layer, differences between turns are also statistically significant. In the inner layer only the difference between the 3rd and 4th turns is significant. Note that for better visualization of trends, the base line for cGMP was set at 100 nanomoles/kg dry weight.

the OC. Neither do our studies provide any evidence that cyclic AMP may be involved in neural transmission in the OC.*

As mentioned, the effects of noise upon cyclic GMP levels in the OC have not been determined to date; however, judging from the comparatively low concentration of cyclic GMP in the OC (Fig. 7) [63], one would expect that this nucleotide does not play nearly as important a role in the OC as it does in the retina, where it is an essential link in optical transduction [62, 64]. Of all tissues studied to date, by far the highest levels of cyclic GMP are found in the retina. Within the retina, steep gradients (40-fold) are present, with the maximum accumulation in the outer segments of the photoreceptor cells, where (in the dark-adapted state) the enormously high concentration of 142 μmoles/kg dry weight is reached [62]. The values in the OC are roughly 500 times lower, but these low levels are still of the same order as those found in most parts of the central nervous system.

*There exists a solid body of evidence that cyclic AMP plays the role of mediator in the synaptic processes of the adrenergic and dopaminergic systems and of adenosine.

Noteworthy is the distribution pattern of cyclic GMP in the OC. The levels in the inner layer are consistently higher than those in the outer layer, and the concentration increases toward the basal turn (Fig. 7) [63]. This pattern is conspicuously similar to that of acetylcholinesterase, as determined by Godfrey et al [65]. This similarity of distribution patterns would represent supportive evidence for the early concept that cyclic GMP plays the role of a mediator in the (muscarinic) cholinergic system. In recent years, however, the alleged role of cyclic GMP in cholinergic transmission has been strongly challenged, and thus the similarity of distribution patterns of cyclic GMP and acetylcholinesterase in the OC may be merely coincidental [64].

Based on many histologic, qualitative histochemical, and neuropharmacologic studies, it appears virtually certain that acetylcholine is the neurotransmitter of the efferent neurons traveling in the olivocochlear bundle. The above-mentioned quantitative histochemical studies on the distribution of enzymes of the cholinergic system in the OC are in agreement with these earlier findings [65]. Strongest support for a cholinergic nature of the efferent system was provided by Fex [66] and Norris and Guth [67] who demonstrated that acetylcholine is released into perilymph during stimulation of the olivocochlear bundle.

In contrast to the efferent system, no solid evidence on the nature of the afferent transmitter(s) is available. The only quantitative analytic studies concern the distribution of putative amino acid transmitters in the OC. Godfrey et al [68] found substantial levels of glutamate, aspartate, and glycine in the OC. However, because of the dual function of these substances in general metabolism and in neural transmission, the presence of these compounds in the OC does not in any way imply that they are involved in auditory transmission. Moreover, a detailed study of the distribution of aspartate, in which the different cell layers of the OC were analyzed, did not show preferential accumulation in the sensory cells [69]. In fact, highest concentrations were found in the Hensen cells and Claudius cells, which certainly have nothing to do with auditory transmission.

Felix and Ehrenberger [70] recently presented evidence that γ-aminobutyric acid (GABA) may act as an excitatory transmitter in the sacculus of the cat. This finding is at odds with numerous neuropharmacologic studies in the cochlea which exclude the possibility of a transmitter action of GABA, whether excitatory or inhibitory. In addition, the concentration of GABA in the vestibular sensory epithelia of the guinea pig is very low (1 mmole/kg dry weight or less) (I. Thalmann, R. Thalmann, T.H. Comegys, unpublished data). Of considerable interest is the recent observation by Sewell et al [71] that (cochlear) perilymph collected during exposure to sound is able to increase the firing rate of primary auditory fibers. No such effect is present with perilymph collected in silence. However, the nature of the substance(s) causing the increased neural firing rate has not yet been identified.

In order to round out this discussion of the biochemistry of the inner ear, which up to this point has been centered on the cochlea, a short review of some essential biochemical features of the peripheral vestibular system should be included. As the phylogenetically older system, the vestibular labyrinth is simpler in design, both anatomically and biochemically. Unlike the OC, the sensory epithelia of the vestibular system are in immediate contact with the vasculature. This is probably the reason why the function of the sensory epithelia is not dependent upon elaborate auxiliary tissues. No true equivalent of the SV is present in the vestibular system, although the tissue in the vicinity of the macula utriculi and of the cristae ampullares contains numerous cells resembling the dark cells found in the SV.

While the $[K^+]$ of vestibular endolymph is of the same order as that of cochlear endolymph, the $[Na^+]$ is considerably higher in the vestibular endolymph (about 15 mM) [18]. In addition, the resting potentials of the endolymphatic space of the vestibular labyrinth are very low (zero mV or slightly positive). However, during hypoxia or application of ethacrynic acid, all potentials drop to substantial negative values (-20 to -30 mV). Sellick and Johnstone [18] demonstrated that the EP of the sacculus is a remote manifestation of the cochlear EP, while the utricular EP was found to be an independent potential; the same holds true for the ampullar EP [72]. Sellick and Johnstone theorized that the vestibular EP is basically structured in the same way as the cochlear EP, namely by the combination of a positive electrogenic potential sensitive to hypoxia and a negative diffusion component not directly sensitive to hypoxia. The basic difference between the two systems is an extremely high positive component in the cochlea ($+100-120$ mV) as opposed to a low positive component in the vestibular system ($+20-30$ mV) which just offsets the negative diffusion potential. Quantitative biochemical analyses indicate that the specialized portion of the ampullar wall (that containing a high proportion of dark cells) exhibits a considerably higher activity of Na^+K^+-ATPase than the undifferentiated portion (2.9 vs 1.2 moles/kg dry weight/hr, respectively) [72]. Moreover, in ischemia the ATP levels in the specialized portion drop substantially faster than in the nonspecialized parts. These biochemical findings are in agreement with the concept that the maintenance of the ionic profile of the vestibular endolymph and/or the generation of the positive component of the vestibular endolymphatic potential is a function of the specialized regions of the ampullar wall and by extrapolation, of the utricular wall. In line with their proximity to the vascular supply, the vestibular sensory epithelia exhibit enzymatic patterns which suggest a considerably higher reliance upon oxidative metabolism than is true for the OC [73]. Accordingly, the levels of glycogen and the total energy reserve are lower, and the metabolic rate distinctly higher, than in the OC (Table 1) [74]. As yet, no attempts have been made to extend these studies to the cellular level.

REFERENCES

1. Rauch S: "Biochemie des Hörorgans: Einführung in Methoden und Ergebnisse." Stuttgart: Georg Thieme Verlag, 1964.
2. Lowry OH, Passonneau JV: "A Flexible System of Enzymatic Analysis." New York: Academic Press, 1972.
3. Wever EG, Bray CW: Action currents in the auditory nerve in response to acoustic stimulation. Proc Natl Acad Sci USA 16:344–350, 1930.
4. Adrian ED: The microphonic action of the cochlea in relation to theories of hearing. Report of a discussion on audition. Physical Society of London, June, 1931, pp 5–9.
5. Stevens SS, Davis H: "Hearing: Its Psychology and Physiology." New York: John Wiley & Sons, 1938.
6. von Békésy G: "Experiments in Hearing." New York: McGraw-Hill, 1960.
7. Davis H: A model for transducer action in the cochlea. Cold Spring Harbor: Symp Quant Biol 30:181–190, 1965.
8. Honrubia V, Strelioff D, Sitko ST: Physiological basis of cochlear transduction and sensitivity. Ann Otol 85:697–710, 1976.
9. Smith CA, Lowry OH, Wu ML: The electrolytes of the labyrinthine fluids. Laryngoscope 64:141–153, 1954.
10. Bosher SK, Warren RL: Observations on the electrochemistry of the cochlear endolymph of the rat: A quantitative study of its electrical potential and ionic composition as determined by means of flame spectrophotometry. Proc R Soc (Biol) 171:227–247, 1968.
11. Johnstone BM: Ion fluxes in the cochlea. In: Bittar EE (ed): "Membranes and Ion Transport." New York: Wiley-Interscience, 1971, vol 3.
12. Zenner HP, Zenner B: Vasopressin and isoproterenol activate adenylate cyclase in the guinea-pig inner ear. Arch Otorhinolaryngol 222:275–283, 1979.
13. Matschinsky FM, Thalmann R: Quantitative histochemistry of the organ of Corti, stria vascularis, and macula sacculi of the guinea pig. I. Sampling procedure and analysis of pyridine nucleotides. Laryngoscope 77:292–305, 1967.
14. Thalmann R: Quantitative histo- and cytochemistry. In Smith CA, Vernon J (eds): "The Handbook of Auditory and Vestibular Research Methods." Part III Biochemistry. Springfield: Charles C Thomas, 1976, pp 359–419.
15. Schacht J: Isolation of an aminoglycoside receptor from guinea pig inner ear tissues and kidney. Arch Otorhinolaryngol 224:129–134, 1979.
16. Jarlstedt J, Bagger-Sjöbäck D: Gentamicin-induced changes in RNA content in sensory and ganglionic cells in the hearing organs of the lizard Calotes versicolor. Acta Otolaryngol 84:361–369, 1977.
17. Bosher SK, Warren RL: Very low calcium content of cochlear endolymph, an extracellular fluid. Nature 273:377–378, 1978.
18. Sellick PM, Johnstone BM: Production and role of inner ear fluid. Progr Neurobiol 5:337–362, 1975.
19. Marcus DC, Thalmann R, Marcus NY: Respiratory quotient of stria vascularis of guinea pig in vitro. Arch Otorhinolaryngol 221:97–103, 1978.
20. Thalmann R, Miyoshi T, Thalmann I: The influence of ischemia upon energy reserves of inner ear tissues. Laryngoscope 82:2249–2272, 1972.
21. Lowry OH, Passonneau JV, Hasselberger FX, Schultz DW: Effect of ischemia on known substrates and cofactors of the glycolytic pathway in the brain. J Biol Chem 239:18–30, 1964.

22. Thalmann R, Thalmann I, Comegys TH: Dissection and chemical analysis of substructures of the organ of Corti. Laryngoscope 80:1619–1645, 1970.
23. Thalmann R: Recent refinements of quantitative chemical analysis of tissues and cells of the inner ear. Acta Otolaryngol 73:160–174, 1972.
24. Chou JTY, Rodgers K: Respiration of tissue lining the mammalian membranous labyrinth. J Laryngol Otol 76:341–351, 1962.
25. Thalmann R, Thalmann I, Comegys TH: Quantitative cytochemistry of the organ of Corti. Dissection, weight determination and analysis of single outer hair cells. Laryngoscope 82:2059–2078, 1972.
26. Kuijpers W: "Cation Transport and Cochlear Function." Thesis, Univ of Nijmegen, 1969.
27. Konishi T, Kelsey E, Singleton G: Negative potential in scala media during early stages of anoxia. Acta Otolaryngol 64:107–118, 1967.
28. Sellick PM, Bock GR: Evidence of an electrogenic potassium pump as the origin of the positive component of the endocochlear potential. Pflügers Arch 352:351–361, 1974.
29. Konishi T, Hamrick PE, Walsh PJ: Ion transport in the cochlea of guinea pig. I. Potassium and sodium transport. Acta Otolaryngol 86:22–34, 1978.
30. Bosher SK, Warren RL: A study of the electrochemistry and osmotic relationships of the cochlear fluids in the neonatal rat to the time of development of the endocochlear potential. J Physiol 212:739–761, 1971.
31. Kuijpers W: Na/K-ATPase activity in the cochlea of the rat during development. Acta Otolaryngol 78:341–344, 1974.
32. Lawrence M, Wolsk D, Litton WB: Circulation of the inner ear fluids. Ann Otol Rhinol Laryngol 70:753–776, 1961.
33. Lundquist PG: The endolymphatic duct and sac in the guinea pig. Acta Otolaryngol 201(Suppl): 1, 1965.
34. Kimura RS, Schuknecht HF: Membranous hydrops in the inner ear of the guinea pig after obliteration of the endolymphatic sac. Pract Otorhinolaryngol 27:343–354, 1965.
35. Schuknecht H, Northrop C, Igarashi M: Cochlear pathology after destruction of the endolymphatic sac in the cat. Acta Otolaryngol 65:479–487, 1968.
36. Drescher DG: Purification of a carbonic anhydrase from the inner ear of the guinea pig. Proc Natl Acad Sci USA 74:892–896, 1977.
37. Ahlström P, Thalmann I, Thalmann R, Ise I: Cyclic AMP and adenylate cyclase in the inner ear. Laryngoscope 85:1241, 1975.
38. Paloheimo S, Thalmann R: Influence of "loop" diuretics upon Na^+K^+-ATPase and adenylate cyclase of the stria vascularis. Arch Otorhinolaryngol 217:347–357, 1977.
39. Feldman AM, Brusilow SW: Effects of cholera toxin on cochlear endolymph production: Model for endolymphatic hydrops. Proc Natl Acad Sci USA 73:1761–1764, 1976.
40. Schnieder EA: A contribution to the physiology of perilymph. Part I: The origins of perilymph. Ann Otol Rhinol Laryngol 83:76–83, 1974.
41. Juhn SK: Experimental alteration of physiologic state of inner ear fluids. Ann Otol Rhinol Laryngol 86:689–697, 1977.
42. Kellerhals B: Perilymph production and arterial blood supply. In Portman M, Aran J-M (eds): "Inner Ear Biology." INSERM 68:279–288, 1977.
43. Juhn SK, Pearce J, Guzowski J: Sodium exchange time of perilymph. Arch Otorhinolaryngol 212:213–214, 1976.
44. Jung WK: Zur Resorptionskinetik der cochleären Perilymphe, gemessen mit Radionucliden nach minimaler Störung. Arch Otorhinolaryngol 211:113–127, 1975.

45. Stupp H, Küpper K, Lagler F, Sous H, Quante M: Inner ear concentrations and ototoxicity of different antibiotics in local and systemic application. Audiology 12: 350–363, 1973.
46. Hawkins JE, Jr: Drug ototoxicity. In Keidel WD, Neff WD (eds): "Handbook of Sensory Physiology." Part III, Clinical and Special Topics. New York: Springer-Verlag, 1976, vol V, pp 707–748.
47. Tachibana M, Mizukoshi O, Kuriyama K: Inhibitory effects of kanamycin on glycolysis and cochlea and kidney–Possible involvement in the formation of oto- and nephrotoxicities. Biochem Pharmacol 25:2297–2301, 1976.
48. Thalmann R, Miyoshi T, Kusakari J, Thalmann I: Quantitative approaches to the ototoxicity problem. Audiology 12:364–382, 1973.
49. Woodford CM, Henderson D, Hamernik RP: Effects of combinations of sodium salicylate and noise on the auditory threshold. Ann Otol Rhinol Laryngol 87:117–127, 1978.
50. Prazma J, Thomas WG, Fischer ND, Preslar MJ: Ototoxicity of the ethacrynic acid. Arch Otolaryngol 95:448–456, 1972.
51. Kusakari J, Ise I, Comegys TH, Thalmann I, Thalmann R: Effect of ethacrynic acid, furosemide, and ouabain upon the endolymphatic potential and upon high energy phosphates of the stria vascularis. Laryngoscope 88:12–37, 1978.
52. Brummett R, Smith CA, Ueno Y, Cameron S, Richter R: The delayed effects of ethacrynic acid on the stria vascularis of the guinea pig. Acta Otolaryngol 83:98–112, 1977.
53. Bosher SK: The implications of the changes produced by ethacrynic acid in the cochlear endolymph. 5th International Symposium on Cochlear Research. Halle, German Democratic Republic, June 1977. (In press).
54. Case DB, Gunther SJ, Cannon PJ: Ethacrynate-induced depression of respiration in transport systems and kidney mitochondria. Am J Physiol 224:769–780, 1973.
55. Tonndorf J, Hyde RW, Brogan FA: Combined effect of sound and oxygen deprivation upon cochlear microphonics in guinea pigs. Ann Otol Rhinol Laryngol 64:392–405, 1955.
56. Thalmann R, Thalmann I, Ise I, Paloheimo S: Noxious effects upon cochlear metabolism. Laryngoscope 87:699–721, 1977.
57. Drescher DG: Noise-induced reduction of inner ear microphonic response: Dependence on body temperature. Science 185:273–274, 1974.
58. Ishii D, Takahashi T, Balogh K: Glycogen in the inner ear after acoustic stimulation. Acta Otolaryngol 67:573–582, 1969.
59. Thalmann R: Noise and chemical agents. Proc International Commission on Biological Effects of Noise, Freiburg, Germany, September, 1978, ASHA Reports Series. (In press).
60. Flock A, Cheung HC: Actin filaments in sensory hairs of inner ear receptor cells. J Cell Biol 75:339–343, 1977.
61. Kilian PL, Schacht J: Sound stimulation increases polyphosphoinositide labeling in an acoustic receptor. Soc Neurosci (Abstract) 4:245, 1978.
62. Orr HT, Lowry OH, Cohen AI, Ferrendelli JA: Distribution of 3':5'-cyclic AMP and 3':5'-cyclic GMP in rabbit retina in vivo: Selective effects of dark and light adaptation and ischemia. Proc Natl Acad Sci 73:4442–4445, 1976.
63. Thalmann R, Paloheimo S, Thalmann I: Distribution of cyclic nucleotides in the organ of Corti. Acta Otolaryngol 87:375–380, 1979.

64. Ferrendelli JA: Distribution and regulation of cyclic GMP in the central nervous system. In George WJ, Ignarro LJ (eds): "Advances in Cyclic Nucleotide Research." New York: Raven Press, 1978, vol 9, pp 453–464.
65. Godfrey DA, Krzanowski JJ, Jr, Matschinsky FM: Activities of enzymes of the cholinergic system in the guinea pig cochlea. J Histochem Cytochem 24:470–472, 1976.
66. Fex J: Discussion. In de Reuck AVS, Knight J (eds): "Ciba Foundation Symposium on Hearing Mechanisms in Vertebrates." London: J & A Churchill Ltd, 1968, p 186.
67. Norris CH, Guth PS: The release of acetylcholine (ACh) by the crossed olivo-cochlear (COCB) bundle. Acta Otolaryngol 77:318–326, 1974.
68. Godfrey DA, Carter JA, Berger SJ, Matschinsky FM: Levels of putative transmitter amino acids in the guinea pig cochlea. J Histochem Cytochem 24:468–470, 1976.
69. Thalmann R: Biochemical studies of the auditory system. In Tower DB (ed): "Human Communication and Its Disorders." New York: Raven Press, 1975, vol 3, pp 31–44.
70. Felix D, Ehrenberger K: The action of GABA and acetylcholine in the labyrinth of the cat. Supra #42, pp 147–153.
71. Sewell WF, Norris CH, Tachibana M, Guth PS: Detection of an auditory nerve-activating substance. Science 202:910–912, 1978.
72. Kusakari J, Thalmann R: Effects of anoxia and ethacrynic acid upon ampullar endolymphatic potential and upon high energy phosphates in ampullar wall. Laryngoscope 86:132–147, 1976.
73. Thalmann R: Metabolic features of auditory and vestibular systems. Laryngoscope 81:1245–1260, 1971.
74. Thalmann R, Stroud MH, Anshutz LE: Energy metabolism of vestibular sensory structures. Adv Otorhinolaryngol 19:179–194, 1973.
75. Thalmann R, Kusakari J, Miyoshi T: Dysfunctions of energy releasing and consuming processes of the cochlea. Laryngoscope 83:1690–1712, 1973.

Glutamate Mimics the Afferent Transmitter in the *Xenopus laevis* Lateral Line*

Richard P. Bobbin, PhD, and Dorothy N. Morgan, MS

One point of malfunction, or genetic abnormality, in the ear may be at the level of the transmitting substance released by vestibular or cochlear hair cells. The absence of transmitter or an abnormal transmitter may cause degeneration of nerve fibers, leaving the organ of Corti intact, as described by several previous speakers. What is the transmitter? At present the identity of the chemical substance is unknown and one must emphasize that many criteria have to be met before a substance is proven to be a transmitter: for example, release of the chemical, presence of the chemical, enzymes for synthesis, etc. However, there is evidence that should be discussed which suggests that glutamate may be the transmitter.

Godfrey et al [1] showed that glutamate is present in the organ of Corti, thus fulfilling one criterion. Klinke and Oertel [2], and Bobbin and Thompson [3] showed that glutamate instilled into the perilymph reduced the compound action potential (CAP) of the cochlear nerve. The reduction in the CAP was interpreted to mean that the chemical was inducing an increase in spontaneous activity, with a corresponding decrease in sound-evoked synchronous firing. This was suggested to be the probable case [4] when we showed that glutamate, when placed in perilymph, stimulated fibers of the cochlear afferent nerve. One problem with this last study was the high concentration of glutamate which had to be used. Therefore, we studied the lateral line of *Xenopus laevis* to see if lower concentrations would be effective, as described by Steinbach and Bennett [5] for the afferents that are electroreceptors.

The activity of a single stitch from the lateral line of *Xenopus laevis* was studied using methods similar to those described by, for example, Bauknight et al [6].

---

*Supported in part by a grant from the NIH (USPHS NS-11647 Clinical Research Center Grant) and the Kresge Foundation.

Differences in method included placing the isolated skin with end-organ and surface of cupula on moistened filter paper and recording, with suction-electrode, the activity of a single stitch from the trunk of the nerve. Frog Ringer's solution was continually washed over the upper surface of the skin, except for a few moments before and during testing of the drugs (Fig. 1). Drugs were applied to the upper surface of the end-organ by ejection from a microliter syringe. The results indicate that glutamate at 1 mM produced an increase in spontaneous activity, although higher concentrations of 2, 5, and 10 mM produced increases followed by decreases that occasionally resulted in total abolishment of spiking activity, as shown for 5 mM in Figure 1. Recovery usually occurred during wash with Ringer's. How or where the glutamate is acting while we use these techniques is unknown; however, the results are similar to those obtained by others where glutamate is thought to be a transmitting substance [7].

In summary, preliminary results indicate that two criteria have been met which are necessary to prove that glutamate is the transmitter at the hair cell: 1) presence in the hair cell, and 2) mimicking of the endogenous transmitter. On the other hand, glutamate does not appear to be the substance detected by Sewell et al [8] in perilymph during acoustic stimulation (Guth, personal communication).

ACKNOWLEDGMENT

We thank Mark Lotz for the technical assistance he provided.

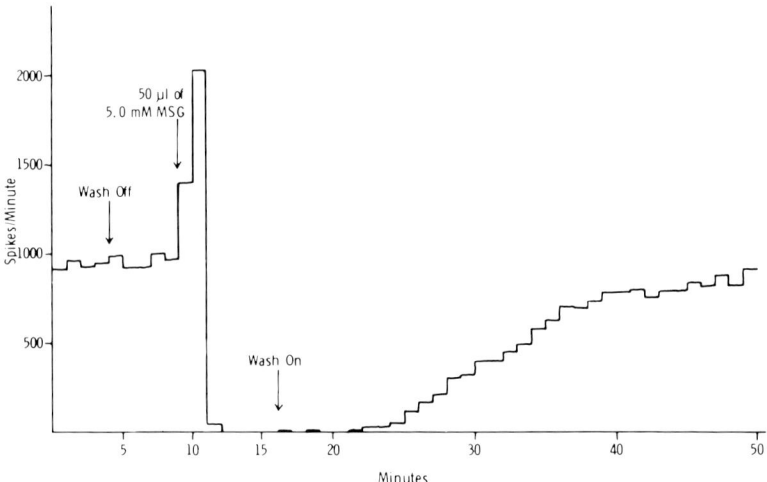

Fig. 1. Spontaneous spike-rate response of two nerves from a single end-organ from the lateral line observed during the application of glutamate to the surface of the end-organ.

REFERENCES

1. Godfrey DA, Carter JA, Berger SJ, Matschinsky FM: Levels of putative transmitter amino acids in the guinea pig cochlea. J Histochem Cytochem 24:468–470, 1976.
2. Klinke R, Oertel W: Amino acids – putative afferent transmitter in the cochlea. Exp Brain Res 30:145–148, 1977.
3. Bobbin RP, Thompson MH: Effects of putative transmitters on afferent cochlear transmission. Ann Otol Rhinol Laryngol 87:185–190, 1978.
4. Bobbin RP, Thompson MH: Glutamate stimulates cochlear afferent nerve fibers. J Acoust Soc Am 63(1):S66, 1978.
5. Steinbach AB, Bennett MVL: Effects of divalent ions and drugs on synaptic transmission in phasic electroreceptors in a mormyrid fish. J Gen Physiol 58:580–598, 1971.
6. Bauknight RS, Strelioff D, Honrubia V: Effective stimulus for the *Xenopus laevis* lateral-line hair-cell system. Laryngoscope 86:1836–1844, 1976.
7. Takeuchi A, Takeuchi N: The effect on crayfish muscle of iontophoretically applied glutamate. J Physiol (Lond) 170:296–317, 1964.
8. Sewell WF, Norris CH, Tachibana M, Guth PS: Detection of an auditory nerve-activating substance. Science 202:910–912, 1978.

Morphogenesis and Malformation of Otoconia: A Review*

David J. Lim, MD

INTRODUCTION

Very little information is available concerning the pathology of otoconia, due partly to the difficulty of studying microscopic organic crystals, partly to the inadequacy of the conventional process for decalcification used in histopathologic study of temporal bone for studying details of otoconia, and partly to the difficulty of assessing dysfunction of the gravity receptors. Numerous mutant mice have been reported by Deol [1] to have hyperactivity (waltzing or circling behavior), and many of these mutants are also known to have dysgenesis or agenesis of the vestibular sensory organ. While hyperactive behavior may be related to a central neurologic problem, it is also possible that vestibular disorder contributes to this behavior [2]. Several mutants which have head-cocking behavior (pastel mink, mocha mouse, pallid mouse, tilted-head mouse, muted mouse, grey-loco chukar partridge), and its related absence or malformation of otoconia without obvious sensorineural anomaly have been reported [3–6]. Of particular interest in these animal models is that certain mineral supplementation of the diet (manganese, zinc) during the critical period of gestation (during otoconial formation) can prevent the otoconial deficiency [4, 7]. Conversely, deprivation of these minerals during this period causes an otoconial deficiency mimicking genetic disorder [8–11]. These animal models provide an important clue to the mechanisms of morphogenesis and malformation of the otoconia.

In addition, the availability of the transmission and scanning electron microscopes, with x-ray diffraction capability and the x-ray analyzer, have added a new dimension to the understanding of the ultrastructure, morphology, morphogenesis, and pathology of the otoconia. Because of this improved ultrastructural information, we have begun to interpret the light microscopic findings on the otoconia with a certain confidence, as light microscopic findings can be correlated well with electron microscopic observations of the same specimen. Furthermore, behavioral

---

*Supported by a grant from NASA (NSG-2220) and The Deafness Research Foundation.

(such as capability for swimming) and physiologic (such as air-righting reflex and electronystagmus induced by rotatory stimulus) tests have been developed. These results can be correlated with the degree of otoconial deficiency [6, 12], providing a great opportunity to study function in the gravity receptors. Some information which may be vital in understanding the aplasia and dysplasia of otoconia, mainly in animals, will be reviewed in the hope that this will stimulate research in human otoconial pathology, which remains a virtually untouched area in otoneurology.

TERMINOLOGY

Otoconia (statoconia) and otoliths (statoliths) in the animal kingdom vary in their mode of formation. For example, lobsters and rays take up grains of sand (foreign particles) through the open endolymphatic duct and deposit them on the gelatinous layer of the statoconial membrane. This type of otoconium is called the *exogenous type*, in contrast to the *endogenous type*, which is formed in situ by the organism. Bony fish, on the other hand, form a single large crystal; reptiles and mammals have numerous sandy crystals (calcium carbonate in the form of aragonite or calcite) covering the gravity receptors. The former (in fish) is called the *otolith*, and the powdery crystals are called *otoconia* (singular: *otoconium*) [13]. In the fish otolith (ear stone), alternating bands which coincide with seasonal patterns of growth are known as *annular rings* [14, 15] and are used in determining the age of a fish.

MORPHOLOGY

Since the time when detailed morphology of mammalian gravity receptors was first described [16–21], various terminologies have been used to denote specific structures. In order to minimize confusion in terminology, the following are definitions of terms used here. The whole membrane is called the *statoconial membrane* (synonymous with *otolithic membrane* in bony fish). It is composed of the *otoconial layer, gelatinous layer,* and *subcupular meshwork*, as shown in Figure 1. Some otoconia are partly embedded in the gelatinous layer, and the rest are loosely held together by the gelatinous matrix. The gelatinous layer, when fixed with osmic acid, is formed of amorphous and fibrillar material [20, 22]. The gelatinous layer, particularly near the *striolar* zone, is perforated. The gelatinous layer is formed of 2 distinct parts: the upper layer, on which otoconia are placed, and the honeycomb layer. Each chamber of the honeycomb houses the top portion of a tall ciliary bundle of sensory cells [23]. The basal end of the honeycomb is attached to the supporting cells of the sensory epithelium by the gelatinous meshwork (Fig. 1) and is called the *subcupular meshwork* by Dohlman [24]. The meshwork often is missing in fixed specimens, leaving a wide space, which is called the *subcupular space* by Igarashi and Kanda [16]. Histochemical [25, 26] and autoradiographic

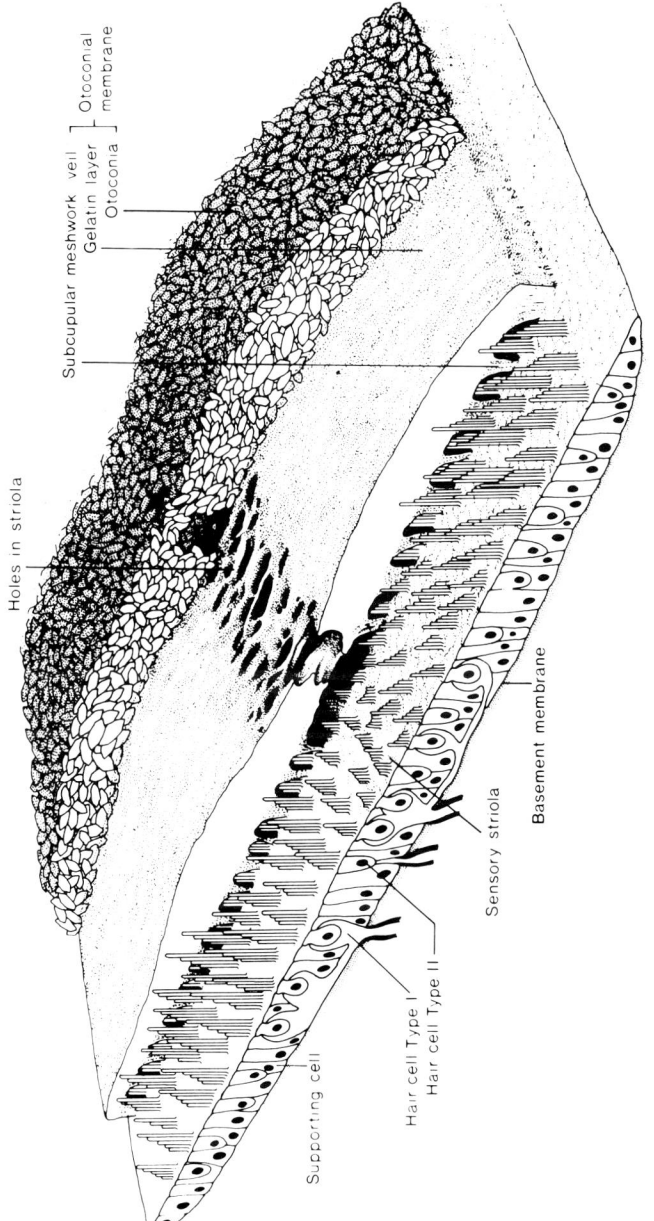

Fig. 1. Schematic diagram of the mammalian utricle shows 3 layers of the otoconial membrane. Illustration by Nancy Sally.

investigations using ^{3}H-glucose [27] have shown that the gelatinous layer and meshwork are formed of mucopolysaccharide and/or glycoprotein, which may be secreted by the supporting cells.

The composition, shape, and size of the otoconia vary considerably among species. For example, according to the x-ray diffraction investigation of Carlström and Engström [28], the otoconia consist of calcium carbonate crystallized in the form of calcite in mammals, birds, and sharks; of calcium carbonate in the form of aragonite in amphibia; and of calcium phosphate in the lamprey. The otoconia of the salamander contain carbonate hydroxyapatite as well as aragonite [29]. In the frog, the otoconia are platelike [30], but in most mammals the otoconia resemble hexagonal prisms. The mammalian otoconium has a rounded body with pointed tips, each consisting of 3 sharp surfaces (Fig. 2). The size of these otoconia ranges from 0.1 μ to 25 μ in length in guinea pigs and up to 30 μ in humans. The distribution of the different sizes of crystals has a distinct pattern in that the small crystals are located mainly on the surface and outer margin, as well as in the striolar zone of the statoconial membrane. The latter area is described as the "snow-

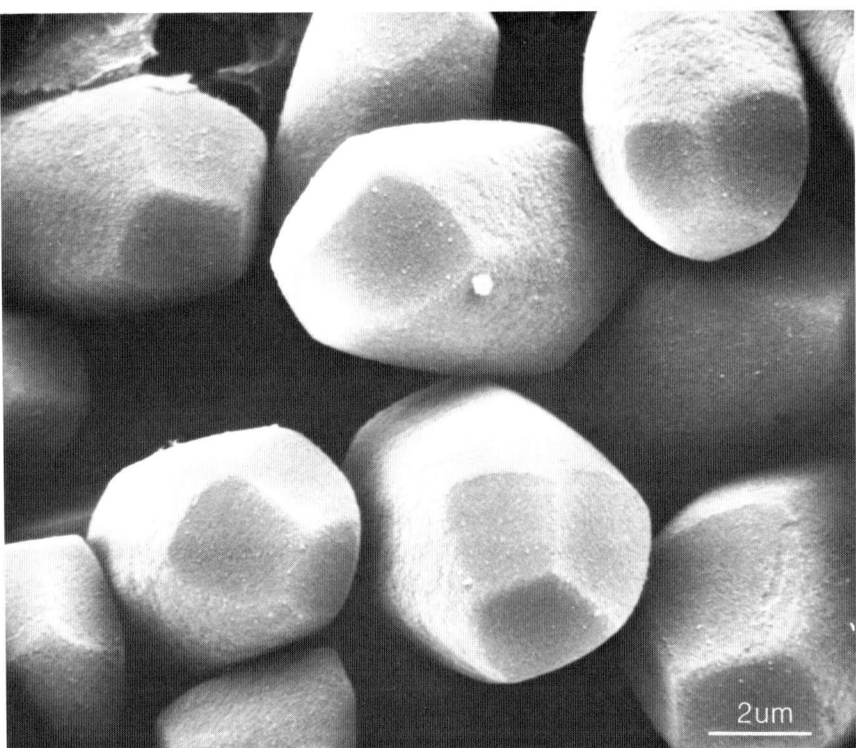

Fig. 2. Close-up view of human otoconia showing pointed tips and rounded bodies.

drift" zone, as the statoconia are piled up higher, giving the impression of drifted snow, particularly in the saccule [31].

Recently, electron microscopic study demonstrated that the otoconia in mammals are formed with a dense organic nucleus and body, which also incorporate organic materials. The fish's otolith is formed by alternating calcium-rich and gelatin-rich layers representing fast- and slow-growing zones (Fig. 3). The ground substances of the crystals (after decalcification) are essentially similar, if not identical, to the ground substance of the gelatinous layer of the statoconial membrane, and histochemical study has shown that it is PAS-positive, indicating it is made up of glycoprotein and mucopolysaccharide. The histochemical staining properties of these structures are similar to those of the cupula [25].

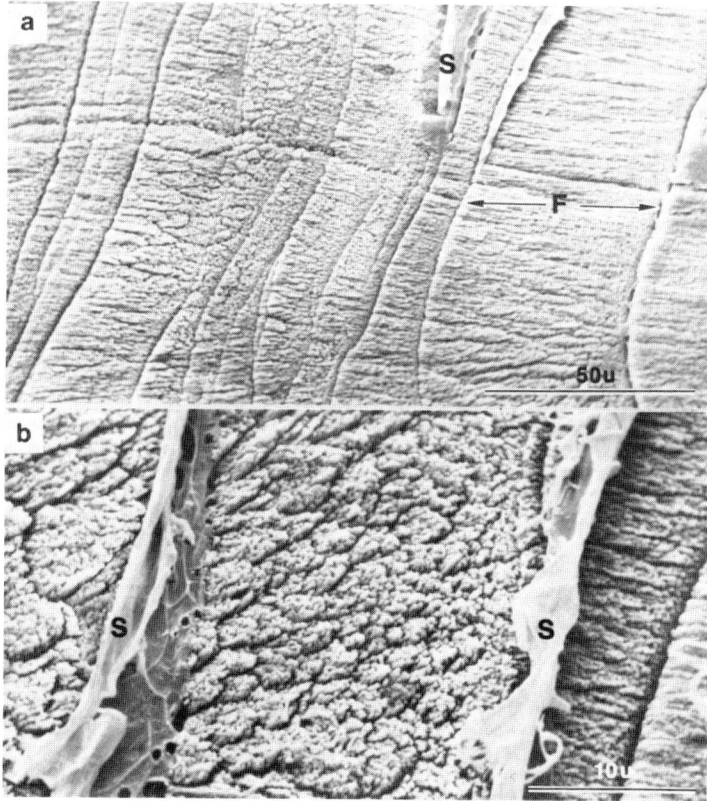

Fig. 3. a) An SEM photograph of acid-etched surface of an otolith from a bony fish (Carassium) shows bands of fast growth (F) and bands of slow growth (S). b) A close-up view of the above specimen shows bands of slow growth are rich in gelatin and bands of fast growth are rich in calcium. (From Lim DJ: The statoconia of the non-mammalian species. Brain Behav Evol 10:37–41, 1974, with permission.)

According to Iurato and de Petris [32], the density of otoconia that are composed of a calcite is 2.71, while the density of those composed of aragonite is 2.93. Therefore, the otoconia increase the specific weight (gravity) of the statoconial membrane, which has the density of 1.9–2.2. This value is higher than that of the cupula and twice as high as that of endolymph (1.02–1.04), as measured by Trincker [33].

Besides providing the specific weight and mass necessary for making gravity receptors sensitive to the force of gravity, calcium salts of the otoconia may take part in the process of calcification of bone and also may act in the storage of calcium in certain species [34]. In amphibia, a large number of crystals resembling otoconia are contained in the paravertebral calcareous sac at the level of the intervertebral foramina [35]. The calcium content of the amphibian statoconia undergoes variations depending on differences in experimental conditions. Whether the same phenomenon occurs in mammals is unknown.

MORPHOGENESIS OF OTOCONIA

Little is known of the mechanism for formation of otoconia or of the factors regulating their growth and final dimensions. As for the endogenous statoconia, there are 3 schools of thought: 1) the otoconia are formed in situ in the statoconial membrane in mammals [36–38]; 2) the statoconia are secreted by the supporting cells of the gravity receptor organs in the statocyst of *Aplysia* [39, 40]; and 3) the otoconia are formed in the endolymphatic sac and transported to the gravity receptor organs in the chick [41] and the shark [42].

Veenhof [26], using autoradiography, cytochemistry, and electron microscopy, studied the formation of otoconia in the mouse. He reported that the otoconia start to form between 13 days of gestation and a few days after birth, and the maximum activity in formation of crystal appears to be between the 15th and 16th days of gestation. The transient increase in PAS staining and transient decrease in intensity of staining of the statoconial membrane (gelatinous) during the critical period of otoconial formation occurred during gestational days 13 through 15, as shown in Figure 4 [26]. Since PAS stains neutral sugars, and toluidine blue and Alcian blue stain acid protein polysaccharide, the above results indicate that there are transient changes in composition of carbohydrates and related substances which may be critical for initiating formation of crystals. These chemical changes are coupled with the presence of alkaline phosphatase activity up to the 13th day of gestation, after which they begin to fade rapidly [26]. This finding indicates that perhaps there are biochemical events taking place that make the gelatinous membrane favorable to crystallization during the critical period of otoconial formation. These biochemical changes in reverse may explain the deterring factor against otoconial formation in non-otoconia-forming structures of a similar nature in the inner ear (the tectorial membrane and cupula), as discussed by Veenhof [26]. His

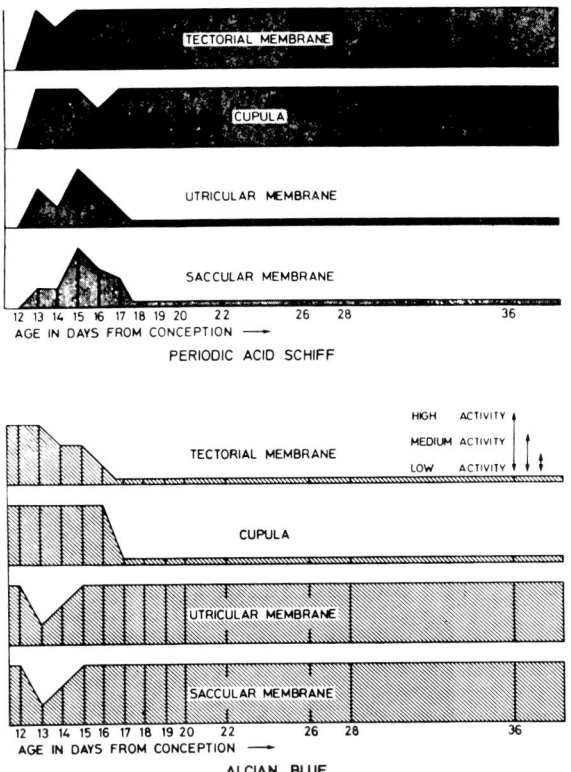

Fig. 4. Transient changes of PAS and Alcian blue staining characteristics in otoconial membranes, cupulae, and tectorial membranes during the gestational period of mice. (From Veenhof VB: "The Development of Statoconia in Mice." Amsterdam: North Holland, 1969, with permission.)

observations also indicate that there is no saturation of calcium in the tissue, although he could not determine whether a high concentration of calcium in the endolymph occurs before or during the crystallization period.

The "critical nucleation" concept of the initiation of crystal formation has been postulated [20, 26, 43]. According to this concept, preexisting heterogeneous nucleation initiates the growth of crystals. The nucleus in the crystal, described by a few investigators who used the light microscope [17, 44], has proved to be an organic substance [20] that may serve as a "nucleation point" from which an otoconium is formed (Fig. 5). The absence of obvious nuclei in some otoconia can be explained by the possibility that only "homogeneous nucleation" is responsible for formation of otoconia.

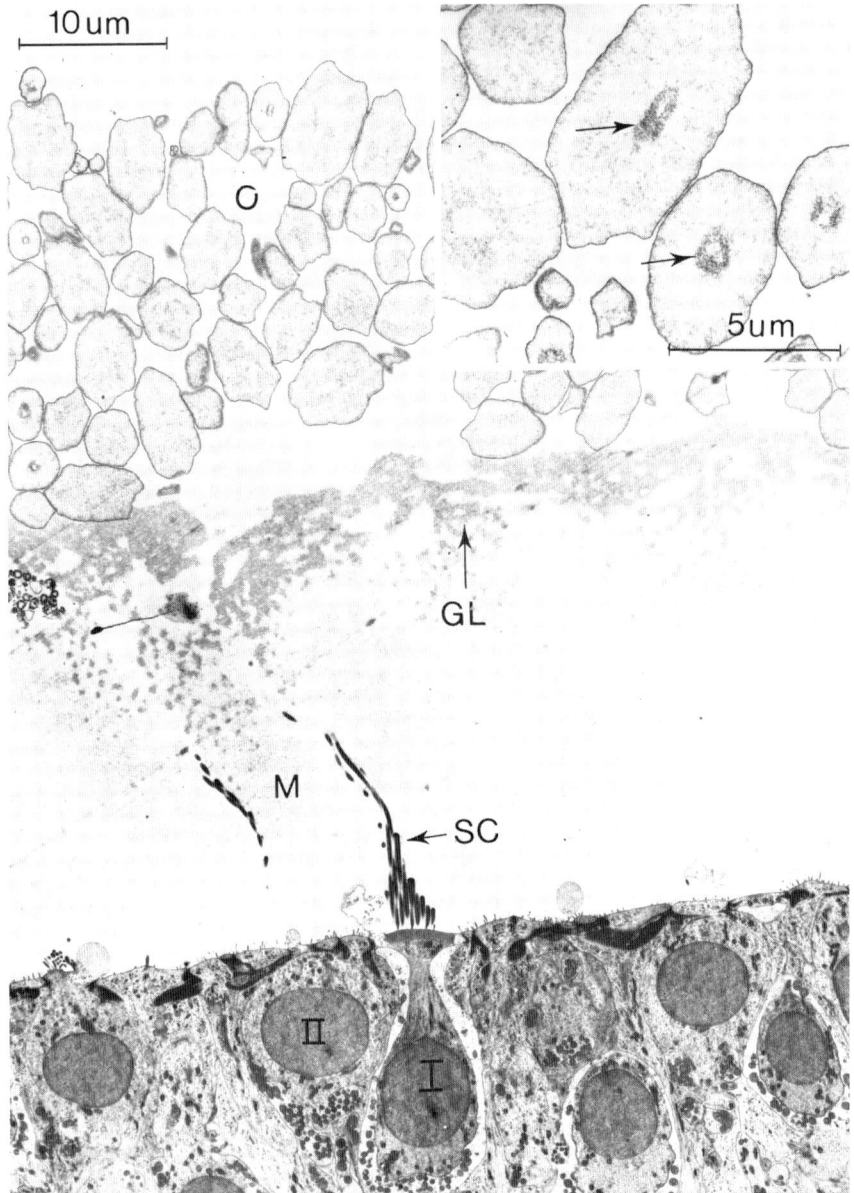

Fig. 5. A TEM photograph of the utricle of a squirrel monkey following EDTA decalcification. The otoconial membrane is formed of an otoconial layer (O), gelatinous layer (GL), and the subcupular meshwork (M). Type I and II sensory cells are also clearly noticeable. SC: sensory cilia. The insert is a close-up view of decalcified otoconia showing nuclei (arrows) formed by dense organic substances.

This process will take place in the presence of ionized calcium and carbonate ions present in the endolymph. The carbonate ions are easily produced from CO_2 by the catalytic activity of the enzyme carbonic anhydrase, which is abundantly present in the inner ear [45–47]. A negligible amount of radioisotope-labeled calcium (^{45}CA) was incorporated into the otoconia of young rats [48], of mice [26], and of gerbils [49]. In contrast to this, the fetal mouse has shown a high uptake of radioisotopic calcium by the otoconia during the gestational period (between day 13 and birth) [26, 46]. This finding strongly suggests that turnover of calcium in the adult is very slow and is negligible under normal conditions. However, it has been reported that when the otoconia are removed from the gravity receptors by high centrifugation, they grow back [50]. This finding has never been reported nor confirmed by recent experiments [51, 52]. (See also below under Mechanical Trauma.)

FATE OF OTOCONIA

Two mechanisms for the disappearance of otoconia can be considered: destruction in situ, or dissolution when they are displaced from the statoconial membrane. Ross et al [53] reported otoconia partly destroyed by surface pitting or, in advanced cases, excavation, presumably due to loss of calcium in situ. This mechanism is thought to be involved in the loss of otoconia in aged individuals. It is also conceivable that the loss of otoconia could be secondary to the loss of the glue-like gelatinous material that helps to hold the crystals together. Besides the thinning of the statoconial membrane by either loss of calcium or the shedding of crystals, modification of the shape and size of crystals due to fusion (aggregation) can occur, or total loss of otoconia can be caused by dislodgement of the entire statoconial membrane.

During the course of SEM study of the gravity receptors, numerous otoconia were observed [20] attached exclusively to the dark cell area of the utricle, which was evidence of decalcification as shown by the collapse of these otoconia (Fig. 6). This observation prompted the speculation that the dark cells may indeed be involved in the process of decalcification of the otoconia that are dislodged from the statoconial membrane. On this basis, it was suggested that perhaps the utricular dark cells are also involved in homeostasis of calcium in addition to their known function of maintenance of ionic environment in the endolymph in the pars superior. Because of the former function, these cells assume a protective role in checking dislodged crystals. However, this concept cannot be applied to the saccule, as the saccular wall is not known to contain dark cells.

Although the fate of the otoconia in the saccule remains unresolved, our recent observation has revealed that the stria vascularis, which is the organ analogous to the utricular dark cells in the pars inferior, is capable of dissolving otoconia that are in contact with it. This observation was also accidentally made in one animal

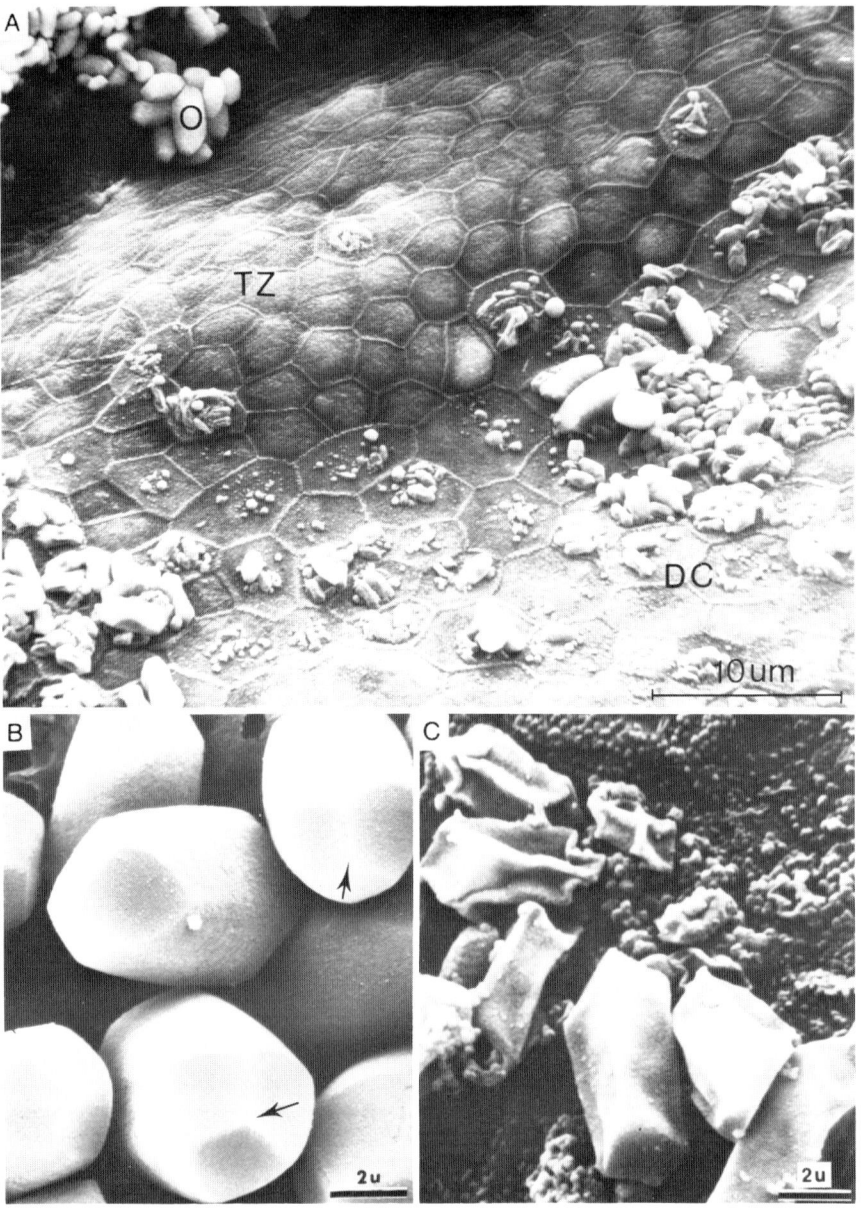

Fig. 6. A) SEM photograph of a guinea pig utricle shows normal otoconia (O) in the macular region and collapsed otoconia that are attached to the dark cells (DC). Cells of the transitional zone (TZ) are free of otoconia. B) Close-up view of normal otoconia. Arrows point to the pointed tips. C) Otoconia that are attached to the dark cells are collapsed, due to decalcification, indicating the presence of a large amount of organic substance. (From Lim DJ: Formation and fate of the otoconia. Scanning and transmission electron microscopy. Ann Otol Rhinol Laryngol 82:23, 1973, with permission.)

when we attempted to remove the saccular statoconial membrane under anesthesia using a fine pipette mounted on a micromanipulator; the otoconia must have flushed into the cochlear duct. It is not clear whether under natural conditions the dislodged otoconia in the saccule would go to the cochlear duct rather than migrating into the endolymphatic sac, following the presumed flow of endolymph. The theory of longitudinal flow postulates that the endolymph flows from the cochlear duct to the endolymphatic sac.

Finding otoconia in the cochlear duct in normal animals is extremely rare, although it occurs in some pathologic or experimental conditions. A large number of otoconia are formed in the cochlear duct of the offspring of normal mice when the mother has been oversupplemented with manganese during the gestational period [4]. Recently, Gussen [54] suggested that in cases of cochleosaccular degeneration in humans, the otoconia are found in the cochlear duct. She suggested that because the cochlea is located lower than the saccule in normal body position, the dislodged crystals or statoconial membrane have entered into the cochlear duct because of gravity. Johnsson and Hawkins [55] observed a large number of crystals in the apical coil of cochleae of patients with hydrops and congenital deafness and found that these crystals consist of apatite (on the basis of x-ray diffraction study) and are formed in situ (see below, under Hydrops). The role of the endolymphatic sac in the resorption of otoconia is virtually unknown at this point, and well-designed studies to test the function of the endolymphatic sac, stria vascularis, and dark cells are needed.

POSSIBLE CAUSES OF OTOCONIAL DEGENERATION (OR LOSS)

The clinical symptoms of subtle loss of otoconia are not well known. Even the massive loss often expected to accompany the degeneration of sensory cells is extremely difficult to diagnose. Schuknecht [56] first described a clinical symptom complex, cupulolithiasis, which he attributed to cupular deposits in the posterior ampulla. Later, Schuknecht [57] summarized the possible etiologic factors for this disorder, characterized by brief spells of paroxysmal vertigo in association with head movements. All of the conditions listed (spontaneous vestibular degenerative changes, labyrinthine concussion, otitis media, ear surgery, and occlusion of the anterior vestibular artery) could cause the dislodgement of otoconia or the statoconial membrane. He postulates that the calcareous deposits are dislodged otoconia or end products of degenerated otoconia. In addition to these conditions which may cause otoconial dislodgement or degeneration (or loss), there are several other conditions which can cause otoconial loss (Table 1).

Aging

Johnsson [58] and Johnsson and Hawkins [59] reported cases of severe loss of otoconia, mainly from the saccule, in temporal bones of humans of advanced age (over 60 years). Ross et al [53] described the pitting or serration of otoconial sur-

TABLE 1. Acquired Otoconial Degeneration and Malformation

1. Primary
   a) Aging
   b) Ototoxic drugs (eg kanamycin, neomycin, ethacrynic acid)
   c) Infection (eg labyrinthitis, otitis media)
2. Secondary
   a) Disruption of the blood supply (eg from the anterior vestibular artery)
   b) Mechanical damage (eg from linear acceleration, trauma to the head)
   c) Sensory degeneration (eg cochleosaccular)
   d) Intermixing of fluids of the inner ear (eg hydrops or rupture of the membrane)

faces and interpreted this to be the result of a loss of calcium in the process of degeneration. They also showed that degenerative change, or otoconial destruction, is more pronounced in the saccule than in the utricle and correlates with advancing age. Unlike the residual saccular otoconia, most of the remaining utricular otoconia had no visible evidence of degeneration even though there might be loss. They observed that the demineralization process affected the otoconia at the posterior tip of the organ most extensively and those most anterior in progressively diminishing degrees. The degeneration seems to begin by an attack on the body surfaces and on the line of intersection of the crystalline faces, which become pitted. The center of each otoconial crystal was penetrated early in the destructive process and eventually was hollowed out. Ultimately, the entire midportion of the otoconium was destroyed and disappeared without leaving any organic residue. Although these crystals appeared to be in the process of destruction, the crystallographic finding indicated that they still retained calcite crystalline formation. Ross et al also found evidence of degeneration in a 4-year-old child [53]. They also described the immature form of otoconium, which has a multifaceted appearance. They maintain that the individual otoconial crystal undergoes morphologic changes during life (immature, mature, and aged).

Ototoxic Drugs

It has been reported that a considerable reduction in the number of otoconia and increased incidence of malformed otoconia are found in ototoxicity by streptomycin [60, 61], ethacrynic acid [20], and neomycin [61]. While most of the drug-induced otoconial changes appear to be related to severe loss of otoconia, malformation of otoconia (formation of giant platelike otoconia) is also observed. In the former, Harada and Sugimoto [60] suggested that dislodging of otoconia and eventual dissolution by the vestibular dark cells are involved. In the latter, it is postulated that the abnormal (giant) otoconia are formed by dissolution and reaggregation by fusion of smaller otoconia (Fig. 7), which occur as a result of biochemical changes in the endolymph due to pharmacologic action of the drugs [20]. Vyslonzil

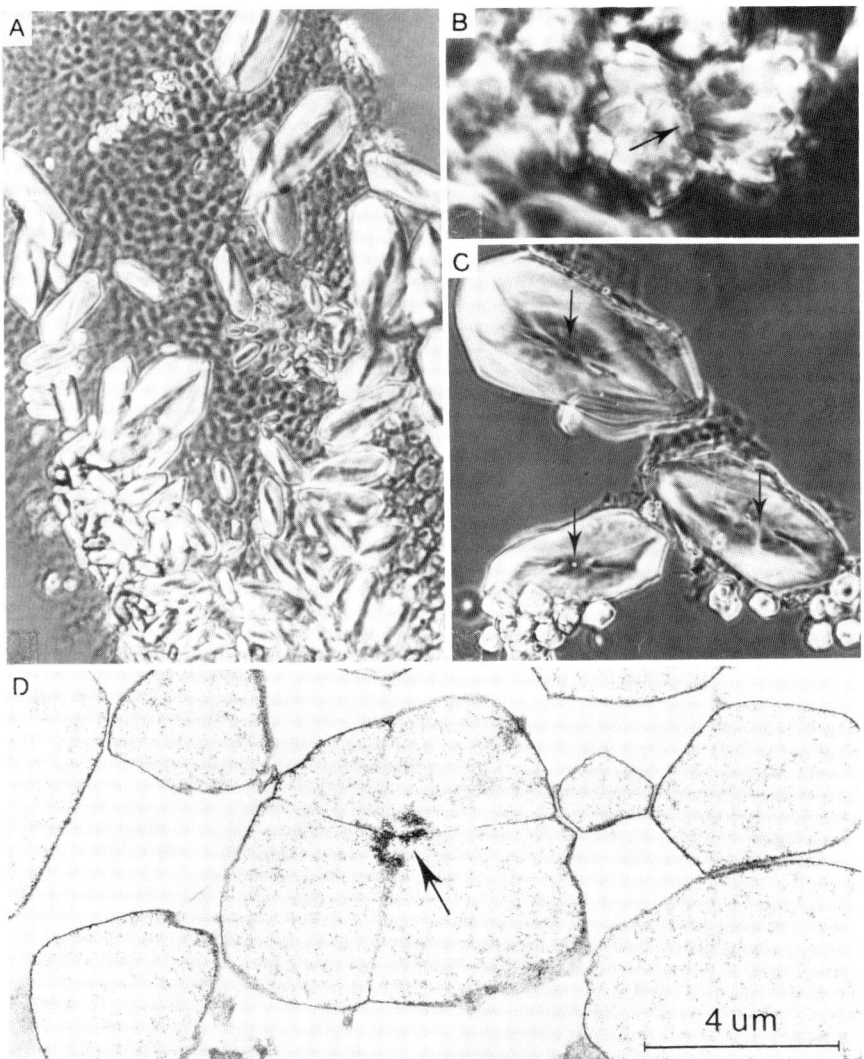

Fig. 7. A) A phase contrast microscopic picture of otoconia from guinea pig intoxicated with ethacrynic acid shows giant crystals intermixed with normal sized otoconia (× 120). B) The ethacrynic acid-induced giant crystal (butterfly formation) appears to be formed by aggregation of smaller crystals. An arrow indicates center portion (a narrowing) of the crystal (× 300). C) Ethacrynic acid-induced giant crystals also appear to contain nuclei (arrows). D) Evidence of fusion and nucleation (arrow) of small crystals to form a larger one is shown in this TEM micrograph.

[62] observed dislodged otoconia in the nondecalcified temporal bones of a human patient who had received a toxic dose of neomycin.

Infection

Viral or bacterial infection causing labyrinthitis involves total destruction of sensory organs, including the gravity receptors. The fate of otoconia in this case is not fully known. A high incidence of otitis media (26%) was also noted among patients suspected of having cupulolithiasis [63]. It is inferred that the dislodgement of the otoconial membrane as a result of labyrinthine reaction secondary to infection of the middle ear is a possible underlying cause of this correlation between the high incidence of otitis media and cupulolithiasis [57]. However, a recent study by Wright and Hubbard [64] on otoconial membranes of infants who had effusions from the middle ear failed to substantiate the notion that ears with effusion show a higher incidence of dislodgement of the otoconial membrane. When compared to the data from infants without effusion, the incidence of otoconial dislodgement was about equal in both groups. However, Wright and Hubbard found a higher incidence of giant crystals in the saccules of those patients who had otitis media. They also noted that dislodgement of the otoconial membrane occurred with greater frequency in older infants, suggesting that maturation of the otoconial membrane makes it more susceptible to displacement. If this is true, then one cannot rule out the possibility that the chance of displacement of the otoconial membrane is enhanced by otitis media in older individuals

Sensory Degeneration

The loss and dislodgement of the statoconial membrane as a result of cochleosaccular degeneration has been reported by Johnsson and Hawkins [59] and recently by Gussen [54]. In this type of degeneration, otoconial loss is confined mainly to the saccule [58, 59]. Gussen reported that the dislodged saccular otoconial mass could be found in the ductus reuniens and cochlear duct, inducing tissue reaction. The resultant occlusion of the ductus reuniens caused cochlear hydrops. She also suggested that the presence of these otoconia in the cochlear duct may cause damage to the delicate sensory cells, resulting in hearing loss.

Johnsson et al [65] described a human case of congenital deafness in which a large number of crystals were found in the apical coil of the cochlear duct. X-ray powder diffraction studies showed that the crystals consisted of apatite. Furthermore, in Dalmation dogs [55] they found minute crystals attached to the atrophied stria vascularis. X-ray diffraction study proved that some of the crystals apparently represented calcium phosphate. They suggested that in the cochlear duct these crystals are most likely produced locally and are not displaced otoconia [65]. In the absence of positive proof that the otoconia-like structures are indeed dislodged otoconia, the controversy about the origin of crystals in the cochlear duct remains unresolved.

Mechanical Trauma

Severe G-force from linear or angular acceleration or trauma to the head can cause displacement or loss of otoconia [51, 52, 66]. It can be either partial loss of some otoconia or total dislodgement of the statoconial membrane if the G-force or trauma is extreme. The fate of the dislodged otoconia is not known. Among patients with positional vertigo, 47% had longitudinal fractures of the temporal bone, and 21% had histories of injury to the head [67]. Schuknecht [57] has suggested that labyrinthine concussion may cause dislodgement of otoconia and may result in cupulolithiasis.

The question of possible regeneration of lost otoconia remains unresolved. Some authors report reappearance of otoconia, presumably by neogenesis, after removal of otoconia, in frogs, rabbits, guinea pigs [50], and in carp [68]. On the other hand, James [69] failed to observe any evidence of new generation of otoconia following their removal in rabbits.

Vascular Insufficiency

Experimentally induced disruption of the anterior vestibular artery and nerve caused degeneration of the macula utriculi, which included changes in the statoconial membrane [70]. It is most likely that the loss of otoconia represents a part of the total of degenerative changes of the macula.

Hydrops or Rupture of the Membrane

In 3 human specimens, Johnsson and Hawkins [55] observed otoconia made up of apatite rather than calcite: 2 cases had hydrops, and one had a collapsed saccular wall. One of these specimens was from a patient with congenital deafness and hydrops. In addition to abnormal otoconia, which were present in both the utricle and saccule, this ear had a calcification of all 3 cupulae, which consisted of apatite. Whether the abnormal crystals were altered otoconia or malformed otoconia, preformed by some genetic disorder or prior pathology, could not be determined.

Inner ear hydrops was also reported in fetal pallid mice. The pallid is a mutant which exhibits otoconial deficiency or malformation [71]. Whether there is a causal relationship between the transient hydrops and otoconial deficiency is not known; they may be unrelated events. Although the integrity of the otoconia when endolymph is mixed with perilymph is not known, saccular otoconial degeneration was observed in cats when the saccular wall was punctured experimentally [72]. It is also possible that otoconial degeneration in cases of hydrops is secondary to the intermixture of perilymph with endolymph.

CONGENITAL OTOCONIAL MALFORMATION AND DYSGENESIS

There are 2 groups of congenital otoconial pathology, one due to *environmental factors* during the critical period of gestation (during which the otoconia are formed) and the other due to *genetic factors* (Table 2).

TABLE 2. Congenital Otoconial Dysgenesis or Malformation

1. Environmental
    a) Mineral deficiency during gestation (eg Mn, Zn)
    b) Drugs during gestation (eg tetracycline, inhibitors of carbonic anhydrase)
    c) Viral infection during gestation (eg rubella)
    d) Weightlessness during gestation
2. Genetic
    a) Cochleosaccular dysgenesis (eg as in Dalmatian dog, albino cat, human)
    b) Dysgenesis (eg as in the pallid mouse, perhaps in human)
    c) Malformation (eg as in the tilted-head mouse)

Environmental Factors

Trace metals. It has been reported that deficiency of manganese or zinc in the diet of a pregnant mouse (thereby limiting the trace metals available to the fetus during the critical period of otoconial formation) affects the formation of otoconia [4, 9–11, 73]. It was found that the postural defects, particularly head tilting in guinea pigs, sheep, and many other laboratory animals, are associated with anomalous development of otoconia or deficiency of otoconia due to deficiency of trace metals in the diet. Although the exact mechanism by which these trace metals are involved in the formation of otoconia is highly speculative, it has been postulated that manganese is essential for the normal biosynthesis of sulfated mucopolysaccharide, which is an essential ingredient for the statoconial membrane, and that zinc is essential for the activity of the enzyme carbonic anhydrase, which provides carbonic acid and mobilizes calcium ions [5].

Drugs. Chelating agents, such as tetracycline and sulfanamide, and carbonic anhydrase inhibitors, such as dichlorophenamide, taken during the gestational period are known to cause otoconial dysgenesis [73, 74]. The exact mechanism by which otoconial dysgenesis is caused by these drugs is not known; however, it is postulated that chelating agents may interfere with trace metals, which may act as cofactors for enzymes, and inhibitors of carbonic anhydrase may interfere with carbonic anhydrase during the critical period of formation of crystals [5].

Viral infection. Viral infections, such as rubella, during the gestational period, are known to cause cochleosaccular dysgenesis when they occur during the time of the formation of the pars inferior [75, 76]. The exact pathology involving otoconial dysgenesis or degeneration of formed otoconia secondary to infection is not known.

Weightlessness. Vinnikov et al [77] reported absence and/or poor development of the otolith in a fish (*Branchyodanio rario*) when it was hatched in a weightless environment for 5–6 days. However, the sensory epithelium was well differentiated. When similar experiments were carried out for 16 days with a toad (*Xenopus laevis*) at the tail bud stage, abnormality of otoconia (glittering otoconia aggregated to form otolith) in the utricle and saccule and deficient otoconia in the lagena were observed, although the sensory epithelium was well differentiated. The authors ascribed these otoconial anomalies and otolithic deficiencies to general abnormalities of calcium exchange.

Genetic Factors

Cochleosaccular dysgenesis. Lack of otoconia in the saccule in association with dysgenesis of the cochlea and saccular maculae has been reported. A Scheibe type of congenital anomaly (cochleosaccular dysgenesis) in humans, dogs (Dalmation), mice (Shaker), mink (Hedlund), and cats (albino) is known to be due to genetic factors [57, 61, 78–80]. The absence of otoconia in some of these cases could be due to a failure of development (agenesis), but most likely is due to degenerative changes (or dysgenesis) involving the entire sensory organ that cause total dislodgement of the statoconial membrane.

Pallid Agenesis. The genetically mutant pallid mouse, which exhibits head cocking and inability to swim, is noted to have an otoconial deficiency (Figs. 8 and 9). In general, it is believed that this is the only consistent pathology involving its inner ear [3, 38, 81]. Severe deprivation of manganese or zinc in the diets of normal pregnant mice causes large numbers of the offspring to show ataxic and head-tilting behavior and otoconial deficiency, mimicking genetically mutant pallid mice. Inversely, the head-tilting behavior and otoconial deficiency in the pallid mouse can be prevented by supplementing the diet of the pregnant mouse with manganese or zinc, indicating that there is a causal relationship between the availability of trace metals and the deficiency of otoconia [11].

The relationship between pigmentation and genetically associated otoconial defects is of interest. Six mutant pigment genes in 4 species are now known to produce otoconial deficiency. All of these mutant pigment genes interfere with the development of melanocytes within the inner ear [5]. Manganese supplementation of pallid mice and pastel mink [4, 7] suggests that there may be a causal relationship between the presence of pigmented cells in the inner ear and the availability of manganese for otoconial development. This contention is strengthened by the finding that various pigmented tissues contain more manganese than tissues lacking melanocytes [82]. We have suggested [5] that the supplementing of pallid

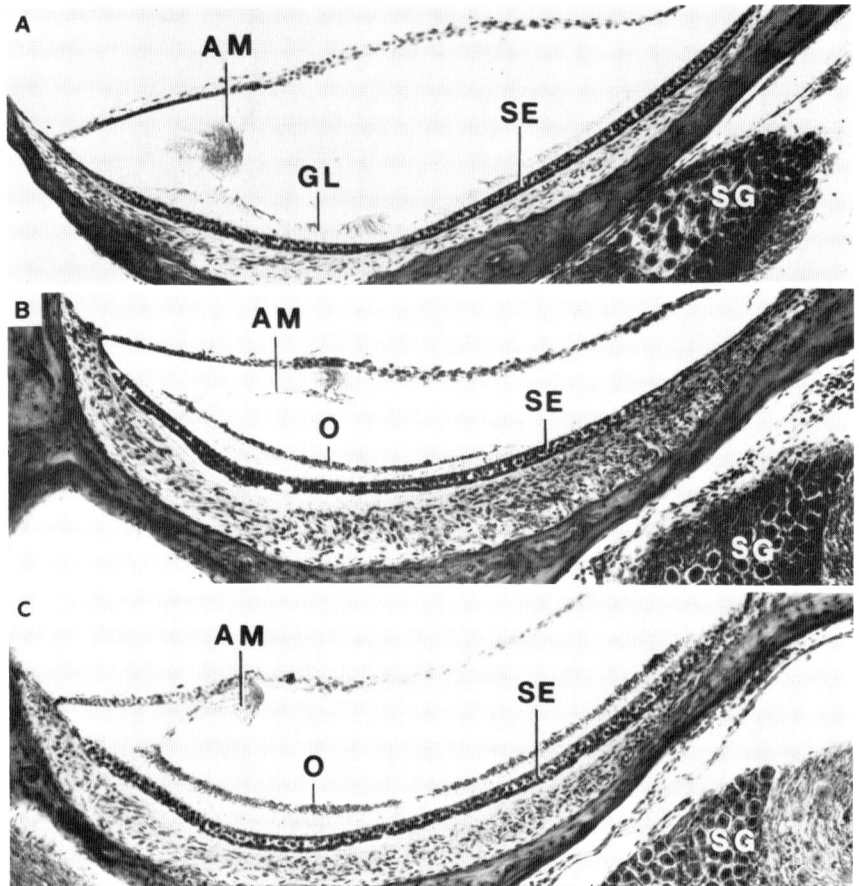

Fig. 8. A) Saccule of an untreated pallid mouse shows a well-developed gelatinous layer (GL), devoid of otoconia, but exhibiting an accessory membrane (AM), Scarpa ganglion (SG), and sensory epithelium (SE). (H & E, × 250). B) A saccule from a Mn-supplemented mouse shows numerous crystals in the otoconial membrane (O), plus well-developed accessory membrane (AM), sensory epithelium (SE), and Scarpa ganglion (SG). (H & E, × 250). C) A saccule from a normal control mouse shows well-developed otoconial membrane (O) and accessory membrane (AM). SG: Scarpa ganglion; SE: Sensory epithelium. (H & E, × 250). (Figs. 8 and 9 from Lim DJ, Erway LC: Influence of manganese on genetically defective otolith: A behavioral and morphological study. Ann Otol Rhinol Laryngol 83:565–581, 1974, with permission.)

mice with manganese may stimulate cells that synthesize melanin (as amelanotic melanocytes) present in the inner ears of pallid mice.

It is interesting to note that the enzymes involved in the synthesis of mucopolysaccharide in cartilage also require manganese [83]. Veenhof [26] suggested that

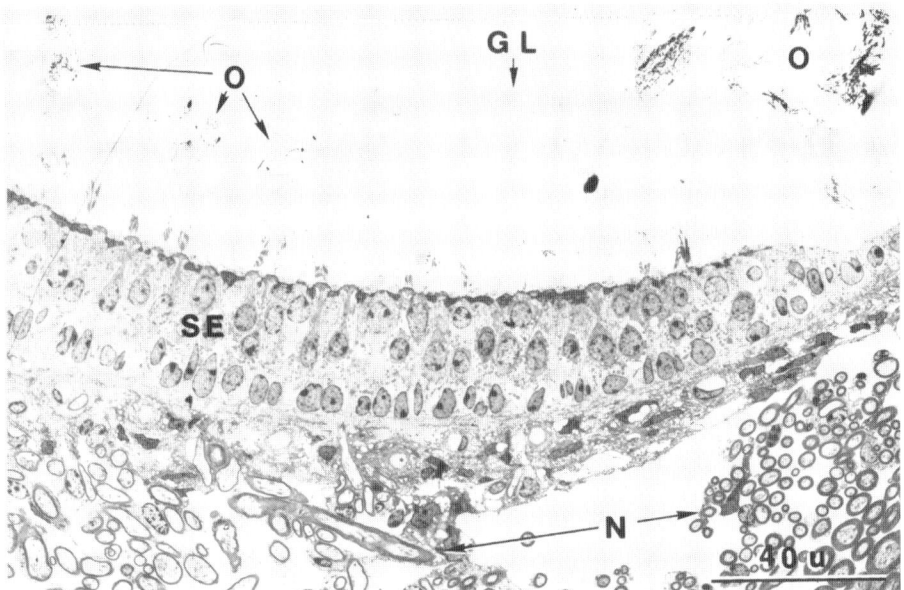

Fig. 9. Utricular otoconial membrane of an untreated pallid mouse shows several otoconia (O), well-developed gelatinous layer (GL), normal sensory epithelium (SE), and nerve fibers (N).

the PAS-positive substances (mucopolysaccharides) initiate crystallization in the membranes covering the maculae. The manganese-deficient and pallid mice, which lack otoconia, fail to incorporate labeled sulfate [84], suggesting that there might be subtle biochemical differences in the gelatinous layer of the statoconial membrane in those animals which fail to develop otoconia. Evidently, manganese is required only during the critical period of otoconial formation, as the effective period for supplementation of the diet with manganese ends on gestational day 15 in mice (the early part of the critical period). Unlike deficiency of manganese, deficiency of zinc affects statoconial formation as late as gestational day 16. Treatment with dichlorophenamide produces statoconial deficiency, and this effect may be mediated as late as gestational day 18. In the latter cases it was assumed that the statoconial deficiency is due to interference with activity of carbonic anhydrase; zinc is the cofactor for carbonic anhydrase; and dichlorophenamide inhibits activity of carbonic anhydrase.

Recently, Wright et al [85] reported a case of a possible pallid human in a 6-week-old victim of sudden infant death syndrome. By a technique for microdissection and surface preparation, the gravity receptors were examined by light and scanning electron microscopy, and a total deficiency of otoconia was found in the utricle and saccule on both sides. However, the gelatinous statoconial membrane, neuroepithelium and innervation were morphologically normal and strikingly resembled the gravity receptors of the pallid mouse [5]. Although skin pigmentation was reduced, this infant was not considered an albino, due to its dark eyes and black hair. There is no family or genetic history available. They concluded that this might be the first human pallid case, provided that the deficiency of otoconia is due to genetic factors.

Genetic malformation. The tilted-head mouse was discovered by Larsen [86] and is known to have an otoconial deformity as well as deficiency [4]. The pathol-

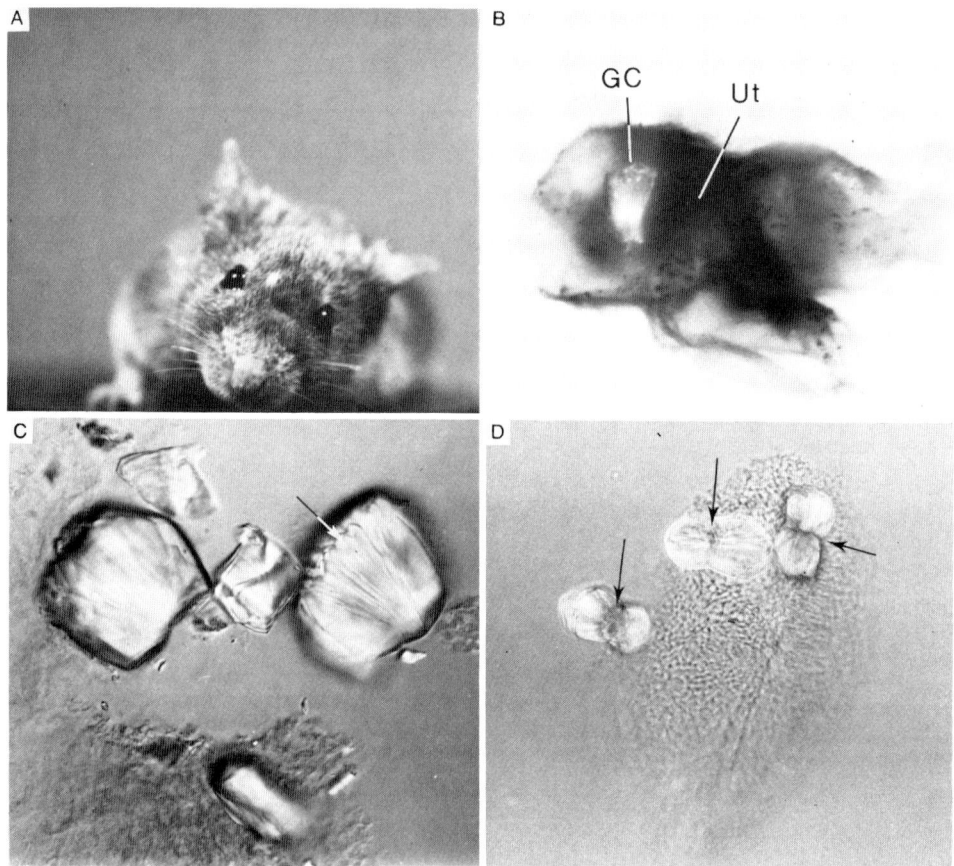

Fig. 10. A) Tilted-head mouse. B) Surface preparation of utricle (Ut) of tilted-head mouse, showing a giant crystal (GC) (× 50). C) Flower-petal-shaped giant crystals from tilted-head mouse. Arrow indicates lamellation (× 200). D) Bow-tie- or butterfly-shaped malformed giant otoconia with central narrowing (arrows). From a tilted-head mouse (× 125).

ogy mainly involves total deficiency of crystals or the formation of a giant crystal, which under the microscope resembles a butterfly or petals of a flower (Fig. 10). Abnormal crystals, when decalcified, show irregular distribution of organic substance in a large crystal and lamellation of the subunits of the crystal (Fig. 11). It is not clear whether the crystals are deformed from the start or are a reaggregation of smaller crystals. Electron micrographs suggest that in some cases they may be formed by fusion (Fig. 12). Some abnormal crystals resembling those of the tilted-

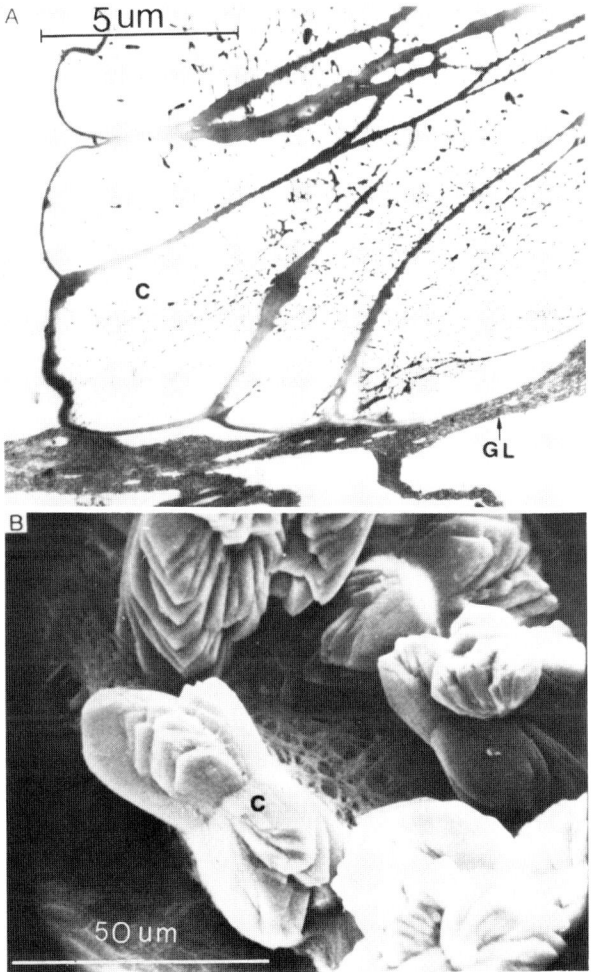

Fig. 11. A) Decalcified giant crystal (C) obtained from a tilted-head mouse shows lamellar arrangement of organic substance. GL: gelatinous layer. B) SEM view of malformed crystal (C) resembling bow tie.

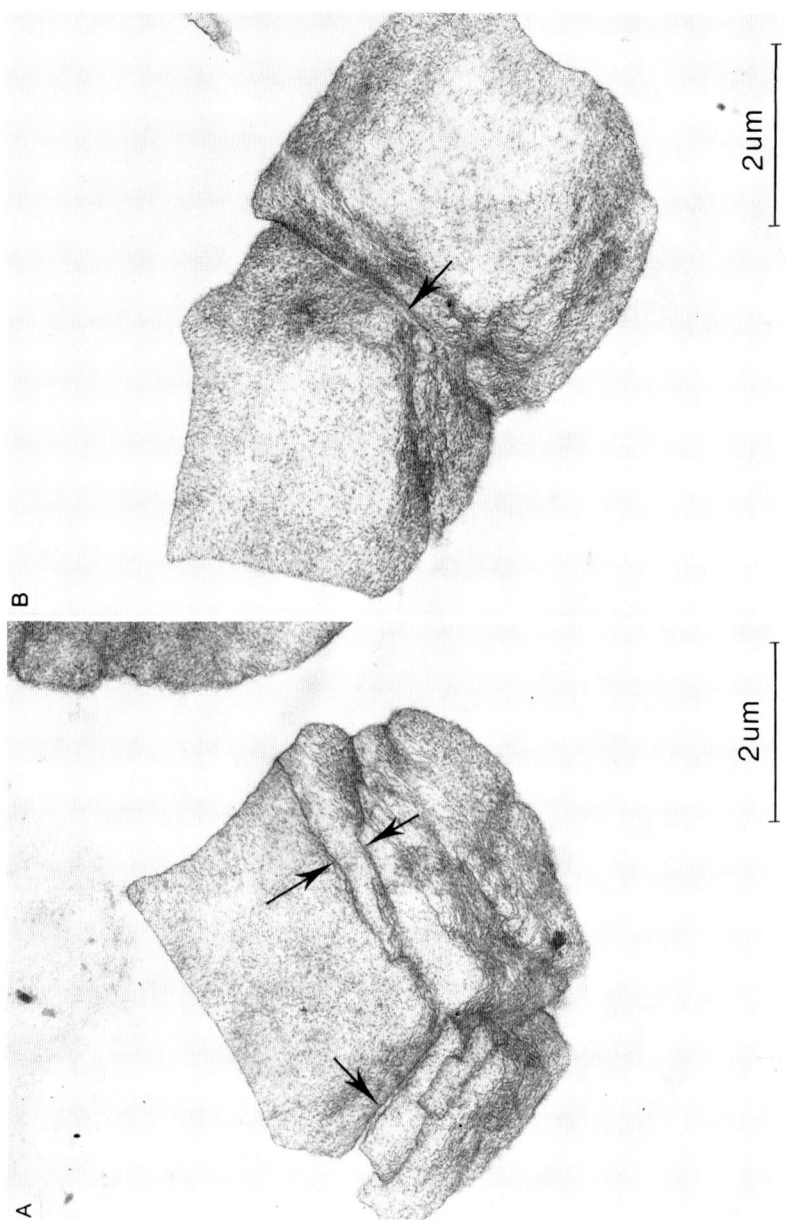

head mouse were also observed in guinea pigs treated with streptomycin [60] and in presumably normal humans [53].

Giant crystals with lamellar bodies are also found in pallid mice that develop some otoconia (Fig. 13). As shown in Figure 14, these giant crystals somewhat resemble hybrid cultured calcium carbonate, which can grow big at the expense of smaller crystals in the test tube [87], suggesting the complexity of the factors affecting formation of these crystals. As in the pallid mouse, the gelatinous layer of the statoconial membrane in the tilted-head mouse is well developed and appears to be normal, although biochemical information is not yet available. Unlike the pallid mouse, the tilted-head mouse is quite resistant to treatment by supplementation of its diet with manganese, suggesting that the biochemical mechanism involved in this genetic expression is different from that in the pallid mouse. Another mutant mouse exhibits congenital otoconial defects and progressive loss of otoconia during premature aging that are related to deficiencies of zinc or manganese or both [88]. These mutant mice produce zinc-deficient milk that is lethal to all sucklings.

The animals with otoconial anomalies reveal varying degrees of difficulty in swimming. Some are totally disoriented (underwater circlers); some are vertical swimmers, maintaining a vertical position and keeping their mouths and noses above the water line; some are normal and maintain a horizontal body position without any difficulty (Fig. 15) [6]. When the total area of sensory cells covered by crystals was determined by light microscopic and scanning electron microscopic observation, the areas covered or numbers of crystals present correlated well with the animals' swimming behavior in that the animals totally lacking otoconia in all gravity receptors invariably had underwater circling behavior; those with some crystals had vertical swimming behavior. When 30% or more of the gravitational sensory area in the saccule was covered by otoconia, the animal exhibited normal behavior in swimming [6]. Again, these data correlate well with those on air-righting reflex (Figs. 16 and 17). Furthermore, the eye movements elicited by rotation of these animals correlated with the anatomic data [12], presumably due to interaction between the gravity receptors and cristae.

Fig. 12. A) Early stage of formation of malformed crystal in tilted-head embryo shows lamellar condensation of organic substance (arrows), indicating the possibility of crystal fusion as a mechanism of malformation. EDTA decalcified. B) Same as A, but showing central condensation of organic substance by fusion of 2 small crystals. EDTA decalcified.

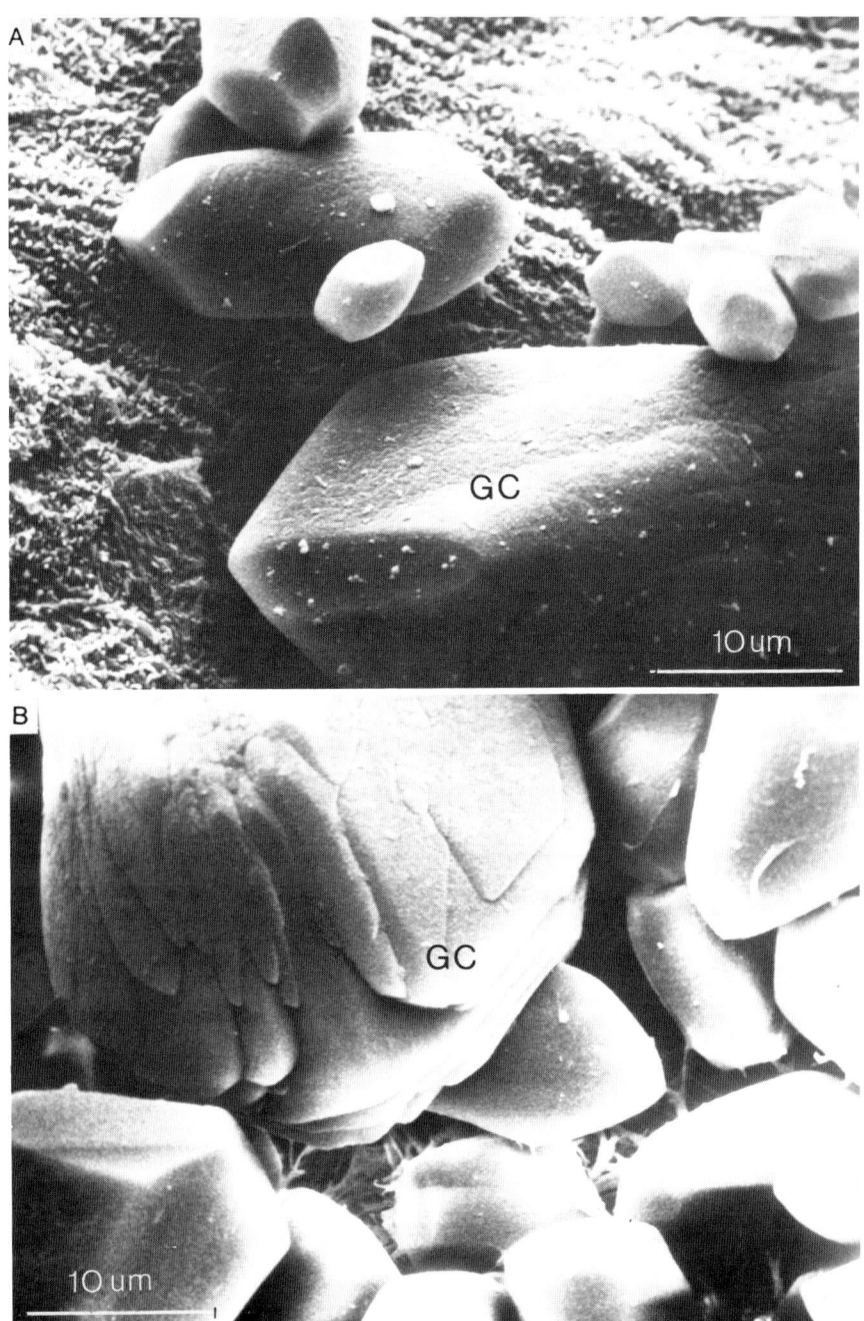

Fig. 13. A) A flat giant crystal (GC) seen in a pallid mouse. B) A lamellar crystal in a pallid mouse.

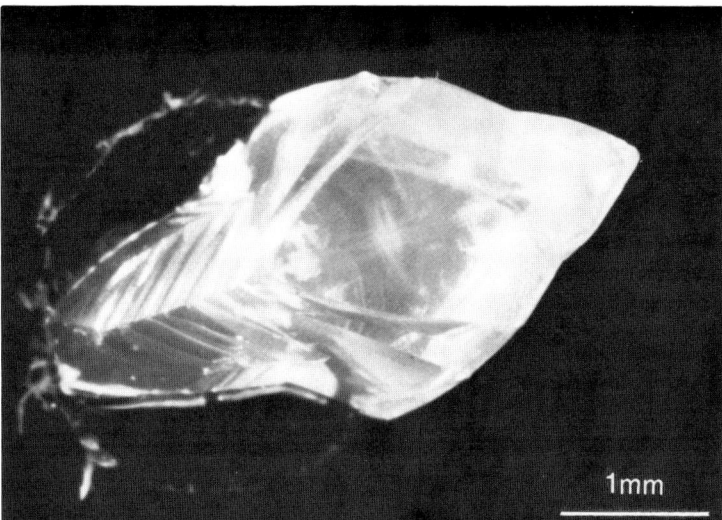

Fig. 14. A hybrid test tube-cultured calcium carbonate crystal shows rhombohedron arrangement and lamellation. The crystal was cultured in a test tube containing silica gel, calcium salt, and carbonate. It incorporates a large amount of gel in its body. The crystal was provided by Dr. H. K. Henisch of Pennsylvania State University.

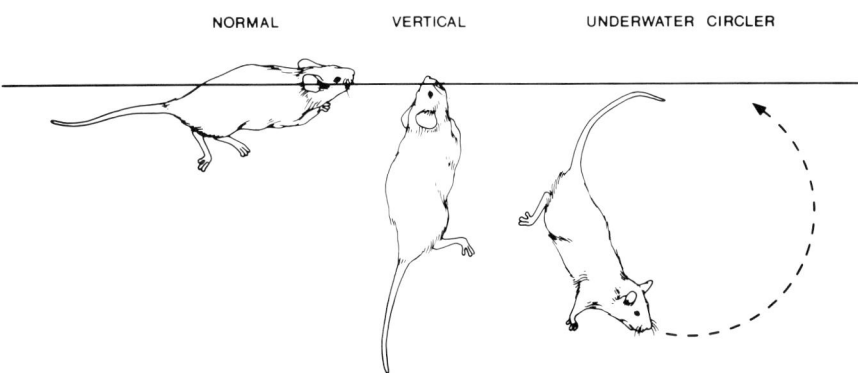

Fig. 15. Swimming behavior is classified as: –normal swimmer; –vertical swimmer; –underwater circler. (Figs. 15–17 from Lim DJ et al: Tilted-head mice with genetic otoconial anomaly. Behavioral and morphological correlates. In Hood JD (ed): "Vestibular Mechanisms in Health and Disease." London: Academic Press, 1978, pp 195–206, with permission.)

136 / Lim

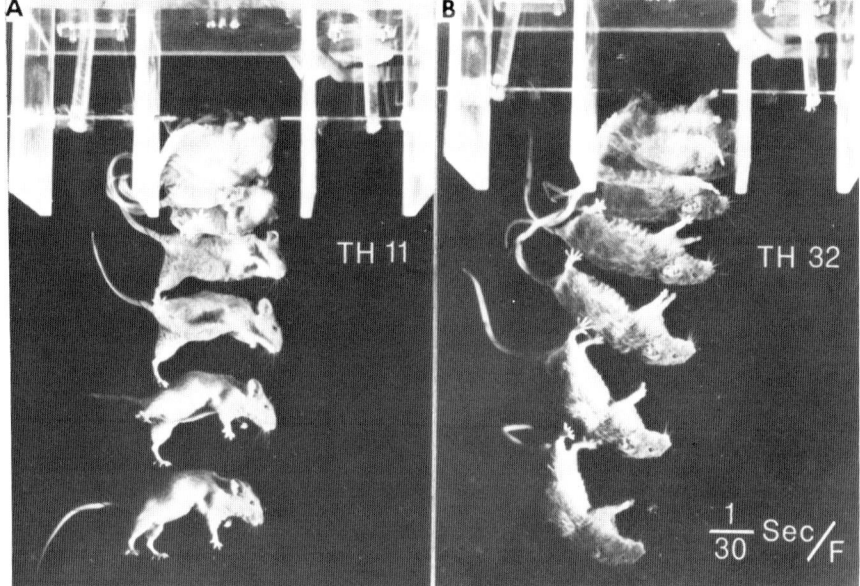

Fig. 16. A) This tilted-head animal righted at the 7th exposure (6/30 sec) (which is considered slower than normal), and is shown to have some otoconia in all gravity receptors. Timed strobe photograph. B) This tilted-head animal failed to right and is shown to have no otoconia in all gravity receptors.

CONCLUSION

Although traditionally the otoconia have been considered stable substances, recent studies indicate that otoconia are changeable and can rapidly undergo degeneration under various pathologic conditions. A marked loss of saccular otoconia in humans, correlating with advancing age, indicates that otoconial changes can also be considered part of the aging process of the body and suggests that the "statoconial deficiency syndrome" is common. The discovery of one human patient resembling the pallid mouse encourages us to look into the possibility that a genetic "statoconial deficiency syndrome" may exist in humans. To this end, we have to overcome the paramount difficulty of making the diagnosis that the human condition is due solely to otoconial deficiency. Clinical symptoms of gradual loss of otoconia in both ears may be subtle and require improved testing procedures. The conventional caloric test or Bárány chair test may be inadequate. Considering the large number of cases of genetic deafness associated with the saccule, a deliberate effort should be directed to the early identification of dysfunction of the gravity receptors.

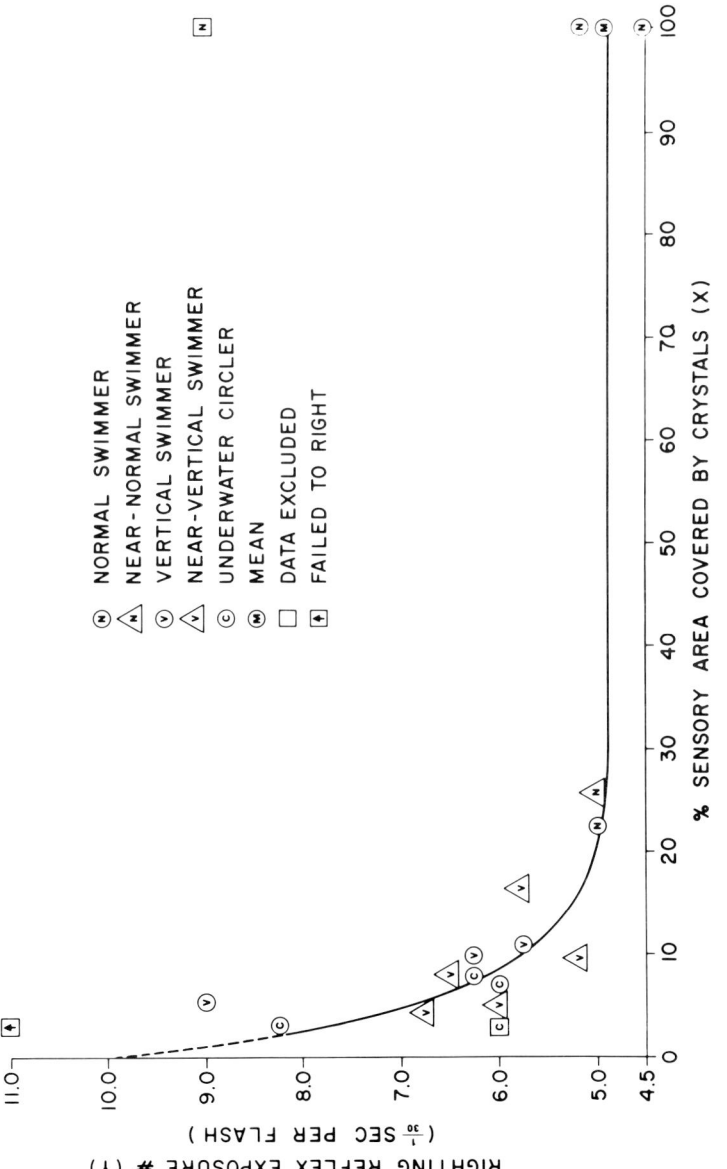

Fig. 17. Correlation between righting time and the averaged percentage of sensory area covered by crystals. The data for 3 animals are not included: 2 that deviated too much from the others, and the one that failed to right. The dotted line indicates the best fit curve extrapolated to its intercept even though we have no data for this area.

Webster and Webster [89] have shown that conductive hearing loss (experimentally induced) during the critical period of development of the brain can cause reduction in the size and number of some cells in the cochlear nuclei. A preliminary study [90] suggests that a significant reduction of numbers of cells in the posterior portion of the medial vestibular nuclei ipsilateral to the side with otoconial agenesis and a loss of neurons (30%) in the "Y" nucleus bilaterally occur in mice deficient in otoconia. A large-scale program of acquisition of temporal bones, combined with study of the brainstem, is needed to positively identify such a condition in well-documented human cases.

The discovery of mutant animals that either lack otoconia or possess abnormal otoconia provides a great opportunity for understanding the "statoconial deficiency syndrome." Furthermore, discovery that certain trace metals are involved in the morphogenesis and malformation of otoconia opens a new avenue for investigating the possible role of enzymatic dysfunction in these mutant genes. The prospect that genetic disorders involving tissue of the inner ear can be manipulated and corrected by trace elements is an exciting one, as we may be able to understand the exact biochemical disruptions caused by malfunctioning genes in the formation of otoconia.

ACKNOWLEDGMENTS

The author thanks Drs. Lars-G. Johnsson of the University of Michigan, Charles G. Wright of the University of Texas at Dallas, Lawrence C. Erway of the University of Cincinnati, and Ruth Gussen of UCLA for their kind cooperation in providing preprint manuscripts of their studies and critically reviewing the manuscript. The author also thanks Ilija Karanfilov, Joan Osborne, Linda Cox, Steven Lee McBride, Nancy Sally, and Katherine Adamson for their invaluable assistance in preparing the manuscript.

REFERENCES

1. Deol MS: Inherited diseases of the inner ear in the light of studies on the mouse. J Med Genet 5:137–155, 1968.
2. Erway LC: Otolith formation and trace elements: A theory of schizophrenic behavior. J Orthómolecular Psychiatry 4:16–26, 1975.
3. Lyon MF: Hereditary absence of otoliths in the house mouse. J Physiol 114:410–418, 1951.
4. Erway LC, Fraser AS, Hurley LS: Prevention of congenital otolith defects in pallid mice by manganese supplementation. Genetics 67:97–108, 1971.
5. Lim DJ, Erway LC: Influence of manganese on genetically defective otolith: A behavioral and morphological study. Ann Otol Rhinol Laryngol 83:565–581, 1974.
6. Lim DJ, Erway LC, Clark DL: Tilted-head mice with genetic otoconial anomaly. Behavioral and morphological correlates. In Hood JD (ed): "Vestibular Mechanisms in Health and Disease." London: Academic Press, 1978, pp 195–206.

7. Erway LC, Mitchell SE: Prevention of otolith defect in pastel mink by manganese supplementation. J Hered 64:111–119, 1973.
8. Erway LC, Hurley LS, Fraser A: Neurological defect: Manganese in phenocopy and prevention of a genetic abnormality of inner ear. Science 152:1766–1768, 1966.
9. Shrader RE, Everson GJ: Anomalous development of otoliths associated with postural defects in manganese-deficient guinea pigs. J Nutr 91:453–460, 1967.
10. Hurley LS: Approaches to the study of nutrition in mammalian development. Fed Proc 27:193–198, 1968.
11. Erway L, Hurley LS, Fraser AS: Congenital ataxia and otolith defects due to manganese deficiency in mice. J Nutr 100:643–654, 1970.
12. Coccia MR: "The Influence of the Otoliths on Semicircular Canal Induced Nystagmus." PhD dissertation, The Ohio State University, Columbus, Ohio, 1975.
13. Breschet G: Recherches anatomiques et physiologiques sur l'organe de l'audition des oiseaux. Paris, 1836 (as cited by Veenhof, [26]).
14. Kreiger E: De Otolithis. Thesis, Berlin, 1840.
15. Reibisch, Über die Eizahl bei Pleurobectes platessa und die Altersbestimmung dieser Form aus den Otolithen. Abt. Keil N.F. Bnd. 4, der Wissensch. Meeres Untersuchungen, 1899 (as cited by Veenhof, [26]).
16. Igarashi M, Kanda T: Fine structure of the otolithic membrane in the squirrel monkey. Acta Otolaryngol 68:43–52, 1969.
17. Lindeman HH: Studies on the morphology of the sensory regions of the vestibular apparatus. Adv Anat Embryol Cell Biol 42:1, 1969.
18. Marco J, Sanchez-Fernandez JMa, Rivera-Pomar JMa: Ultrastructure of the otoliths and otolithic membrane of the macula utriculi in the guinea pig. Acta Otolaryngol (Stockh) 71:1–8, 1971.
19. Sanchez-Fernandez JMa, Marco J, Rivera-Pomar JMa, Delgado RM: Electron diffraction studies on otolith organization in the macula utriculi of the guinea pig. Acta Otolaryngol (Stockh) 73:267–269, 1972.
20. Lim DJ: Formation and fate of the otoconia: Scanning and transmission electron microscopy. Ann Otol Rhinol Laryngol 82:23–36, 1973.
21. Lindeman HH: Anatomy of the otolith organs. Adv Otorhinolaryng 20:405–433, 1973.
22. Johnsson L-G, Hawkins JS Jr: Otolithic membranes of the saccule and utricle in man. Science 157:1454–1456, 1967.
23. Lim DJ: Fine morphology of the otoconial membrane and its relationship to the sensory epithelium. SEM/1979/III, pp 929–938.
24. Dohlman GF: The attachment of the cupulae, otolith and tectorial membranes to the sensory cell areas. Acta Otolaryngol (Stockh) 71:89–105, 1971.
25. Wislocki GB, Ladman AJ: Selective and histochemical staining of the otolithic membranes, cupulae and tectorial membrane of the inner ear. J Anat 78:3–12, 1955.
26. Veenhof VB: "The Development of Statoconia in Mice." Amsterdam: North-Holland, 1969.
27. Lim DJ: Unpublished data.
28. Carlström D, Engström H: The ultrastructure of statoconia. Acta Otolaryngol (Stockh) 45:14–18, 1955.
29. Hastings AB: Chemical analysis of otoliths and endolymphatic sac deposits in Amblystoma tigrinum. J Comp Neurol 61:295–296, 1935.
30. Lim DJ: The statoconia of the non-mammalian species. Brain Behav Evol 10:37–41, 1974.
31. Ades HW, Engström H: Form and innervation of the vestibular epithelia. "The Role of the Vestibular Organs in the Exploration of Space." NASA SP-77, Jan 20–22, 1965, pp 23–41.

32. Iurato S, de Petris S: Otolithic membranes and cupulae. In Iurato S (ed): "Submicroscopic Structure of the Inner Ear." Oxford: Pergamon Press, 1967, pp 210–218.
33. Trincker D: The transformation of mechanical stimulus into nervous excitation by the labyrinthine receptors. In Beament JWL (ed): "Biological Receptor Mechanisms." Cambridge: The University Press, 1962, pp 289–316.
34. Guardabassi A: L'organo endolinfatico degli Anfibi Anuri. Arch Ital Anat Embriol 57: 242–294, 1952.
35. Guardabassi A: Les sels de Ca du sac endolymphatique et les processus de calcification des os pendant le métamorphose normale et expérimentale chez les têtards de Bufo vulgaris, Rana dalmatina, Rana esculenta. Arch Anat Microsc Morphol Exp 42:143–167, 1953.
36. Stricker W: Die Otolithen und Cupulae terminalis im Gehörgan. Arch Mikr Anat Entw Gesch 103:259, 1928.
37. Belonoschkin B: Beitrag zur Frage der Natur und der Entstehung der Otolithen. Arch Ohrenheilk 128:208–224, 1931.
38. Lyon MF: The development of the otoliths of the mouse. J Embryol Exp Morphol 3: 213–229, 1955.
39. Geuze JJ: Observations on the function and the structure of the statocysts of Lymnaca stagnalis (L.). Neth J Zool 18:155–204, 1968.
40. Wiederhold ML: Personal communication.
41. Balsamo G, de Vincentiis M, Marmo F: The effect of tetracyclin on the processes of calcification of the otoliths in the developing chick embryo. J Embryol Exp Morphol 22: 327–332, 1969.
42. Vilstrup T: On the formation of the otoliths. Ann Otol Rhinol Laryngol 60:974–981, 1951.
43. Kolmer W: Gehörorgan. In Möllendorff W (ed): "Handbuch der mikroskopischen Anatomie des Menschen." Berlin: Springer-Verlag, 1927, pp 250–478.
44. Henle, quoted by Rudinger in Stricker's "Manual of Human and Comparative Histology," vol 3. London: New Sydenheim Soc, 1873, p 122.
45. Erulkar SD, Maren TH: Carbonic anhydrase and the inner ear. Nature 189:459–460, 1961.
46. Purichia NA: "Effects of Dichlorophenamide, Zinc, and Manganese on Otolith Development in Mice." PhD dissertation, University of Cincinnati, Cincinnati, Ohio, 1972.
47. Drescher DG: Purification of a carbonic anhydrase from the inner ear of the guinea pig. Proc Natl Acad Sci 27:892–896, 1977.
48. Bélanger LF: Development, structure and composition of the otolithic organs of the rat. In Sognnaes RF (ed): "Calcification in Biological Systems." American Association for the Advancement of Science, Washington, D.C., 1960, pp 151–162.
49. Preston RE, Johnsson L-G, Hill HJ, Schacht J: Incorporation of radioactive calcium into otolithic membranes and middle ear ossicles of the gerbil. Acta Otolaryngol (Stockh) 80: 269–275, 1975.
50. Werner CF: Die Differenzierung der Maculae im Labyrinth, insbesondere bei Säugetieren. A Anat 99:696–709, 1933.
51. Igarashi M, Nagaba M: Vestibular end organ damage in squirrel monkeys after exposure to intensive linear acceleration. "Third Symposium on the Role of the Vestibular Organs in Space Exploration." NASA SP-152, 1967, pp 63–81.
52. Parker DE, Covell WP, von Gierke HE: Exploration of vestibular damage in guinea pigs following mechanical stimulation. Acta Otolaryngol (Stockh) 239(Suppl):7, 1968.
53. Ross MD, Johnsson L-G, Peacor D, Allard LF: Observations on normal and degenerating human otoconia. Ann Otol Rhinol Laryngol 85:310–326, 1976.
54. Gussen R: Pathogenesis of cochleo-saccular degeneration with saccule otoconia displace-

ment into cochlea. Abstracts of the Research Forum, AAO and ARO, Las Vegas, 1978, p 38.
55. Johnsson L-G, Hawkins JE Jr: Hydrops and cupulolithiasis as seen in microdissections of human temporal bones. In Pulec JL (ed): "Meniere's Disease." Pacific Palisades, California: Palisades Publishing Co. (in press).
56. Schuknecht H: Cupulolithiasis. Arch Otolaryngol 90:755, 1969.
57. Schuknecht H: Cupulolithiasis. In "Pathology of the Ear." Cambridge, Mass: Harvard University Press, 1974, pp 465-473.
58. Johnsson L-G: Degenerative changes and anomalies of the vestibular system in man. Laryngoscope 81:1682-1694, 1971.
59. Johnsson L-G, Hawkins JE Jr: Sensory and neural degeneration with aging, as seen in microdissections of the human inner ear. Ann Otol Rhinol Laryngol 81:179-193, 1972.
60. Harada Y, Sugimoto Y: Metabolic disorder of otoconia after streptomycin intoxication. Acta Otolaryngol 84:65-71, 1977.
61. Johnsson L-G, Wright CG, Preston RE, Henry PJ: Streptomycin-induced defects of the otolithic membrane. Acta Otolaryngol (Stockh) (in press).
62. Vyslonzil E: Über eine umschriebene Ansammlung von Otokonien im hinteren häutigen Bogengang. Mschr Ohrenheilk 97:63, 1963.
63. Dix M, Hallpike C: The pathology, symptomatology and diagnosis of certain disorders of the vestibular system. Ann Otol Rhinol Laryngol 61:987, 1952.
64. Wright CG, Hubbard DB: Observations of otoconial membranes from human infants. Acta Otolaryngol (Stockh) 86:185-194, 1978.
65. Johnsson L-G, Hawkins JE Jr, Muraski AA, Preston RE: Vascular anatomy and pathology of the cochlea in Dalmatian dogs. In Darin de Lorenzo AJ (ed): "Vascular Disorders and Hearing Defects." Baltimore: University Park Press, 1973, pp 249-295.
66. Lim DJ, Stith JA, Stockwell CW, Oyama J: Observations on saccules of rats exposed to long-term hypergravity. Aerospace Med 45:705-710, 1974.
67. Barber H: Positional nystagmus: Testing and interpretation. Ann Otol Rhinol Laryngol 73:838, 1964.
68. von Frisch K: Über die Bedeutung des Sacculus und der Lagena für den Gehörsinn der Fische. Z Vergl Physiol 25:703, 1938.
69. James J: Some experiments on the function of the labyrinth. II. Pract Oto-Rhinol-Laryngol 24:348-350, 1962.
70. Schuknecht HF: The pathology of several disorders of the inner ear which cause vertigo. South Med J 57:1161-1167, 1964.
71. Lyon MF: The developmental origin of hereditary absence of otoliths in mice. J Embryol Exp Morphol 3:230-241, 1955.
72. Colman BH: Sacculotomy in cats. Conclusions from experimental fistula formation. J Laryngol Otol 82:1083-1094, 1968.
73. Purichia N, Erway LC: Effects of dichlorophenamide, zinc, and manganese on otolith development in mice. Dev Biol 27:395-405, 1972.
74. DeVincentiis M, Marmo F: Inhibition of the morphogenesis of the otoliths in the chick embryo in the presence of carbonic anhydrase inhibitors. Experientia 24:818-820, 1968.
75. Hemenway WG, Sando I, McChesney D: Temporal bone pathology following maternal rubella. Arch Klin Exp Ohr-Nas-Kehlk Heilk 193:287-300, 1969.
76. Lindsay JR: Profound childhood deafness: Inner ear pathology. Ann Otol Rhinol Laryngol 82(Suppl)5:1-121, 1973.
77. Vinnikov JA, Gazenko OG, Titova LK et al: Formation of vestibular apparatus in the weightless condition. Minerva Otorinolaringol 26:69-75, 1976.
78. Mikaelian D, Ruben RJ: Hearing degeneration in the Shaker-I mouse: Correlation of

physiological observation with behavioral response and with cochlear anatomy. Arch Otolaryngol 80:418, 1964.
79. Kikuchi K, Hilding DA: The defective organ of Corti in Shaker-I mice. Acta Otolaryngol (Stockh) 60:287–303, 1965.
80. Hilding DA, Sugiura A, Makai Y: Deaf white mink: Electron-microscopic study of the inner ear. Ann Otol Rhinol Laryngol 76:647–663, 1967.
81. Lyon MF: Absence of otoliths in the mouse: An effect of the pallid mutant. J Genet 51: 638–650, 1953.
82. Cotzias GC, Papavasiliou PS, Miller ST: Manganese and melanin. Nature 201:1228–1229, 1964.
83. Leach RM Jr, Muenster AM, Wein EM: Studies on the role of manganese in bone formation. II – Effect upon chondroitin sulfate synthesis in chick epiphyseal cartilage. Arch Biochem Biophys 133:22–28, 1969.
84. Shrader RE, Erway LC, Hurley LS: Mucopolysaccharide synthesis in the developing inner ear of manganese-deficient and pallid mutant mice. Teratology 8:257–266, 1973.
85. Wright CG, Hubgard DG, Graham JW: Absence of otoconia in a human infant. Ann Otol Rhinol Laryngol 86:779–783, 1979.
86. Larsen MM: Personal communication. Mouse News Letter 20:49, 1959.
87. Henisch HK: "Crystal Growth in Gels." University Park: The Pennsylvania State University Press, 1970.
88. Erway LC, Piletz JE, Ganschow RE: Lethal-milk mutant mice: Zinc deficiency and otolith defects. In Lim DJ (ed): "Abstracts of the Second Midwinter Research Meeting, Association for Research in Otolaryngology," 1979, p 24.
89. Webster DB, Webster M: Neonatal sound deprivation affects brain stem auditory nuclei. Arch Otolaryngol 103:392–396, 1977.
90. Clark GM, Douglas RJ, Erway LC, Wright CG, Hubbard DG: Vestibular nuclei: Neuronal loss in mice with otoconial agenesis and evidence of right-left asymmetry. Abstracts of Soc. of Neurosciences Satellite Symposium, "Vestibular Function and Morphology." Pittsburgh, 1978.

DISCUSSION

Dr. David Smith: Clinically, how can we assess an individual who has abnormal development of the saccule or other vestibular abnormalities which occurred in infancy or early childhood?

Dr. David Lim: This has been a real bottleneck as far as our research effort is concerned both in bringing this to the attention of the medical community and in designing tests to assess the problem.

Dr. Harold Schuknecht: A child with no vestibular function whatsoever seems to be a slightly unbalanced child who is a little bit less facile than his or her sibs. Sometimes the parents will notice this. However, the real disorders of vestibular function appear to come about when you have a viable vestibular system which becomes disordered so that you have aberrant function of the organ. A total loss is almost undetectable by the parent or the patient.

Dr. Isabelle Rapin: I beg to differ. Dr. Ruben and I have looked at a number of children with abnormal vestibular function and it appears that a portion, if not all of them, are slow to learn to hold their heads up, to sit, and to walk by themselves. Once they know how to do these things they do them exceedingly well, and if you want to detect this on clinical grounds the easiest test is to have them walk a balance bar. Also, these children would be a little clumsier than expected and become even more clumsy if another sensory organ for orientation is removed. Thus, a child without vestibular function when placed in the dark will have trouble going up stairs. A recent case was brought to my attention by a teacher who brought a child to me and stated that the child was neurologically impaired because she stumbled all the time in the movies. She observed that the child stumbled on the stairway in the Radio City Music Hall and we found out that there is very poor illumination there. Since we depend on our vestibular proprioceptive input and our visual input for coordination, if you remove one you can function well, but if you remove two of these inputs you can have serious problems with spatial orientation.

Dr. Robert Ruben: One point Dr. Rapin presented to me, which has been published (Clinical Pediatrics 13:922, 1974), and which I think has great importance is that motor signs are given by pediatricians for assessing the "development" of a child. One of the motor signs is the age when the child raises his head, walks, etc. Dr. Rapin has found that a number of children were delayed in this on the basis of vestibular dysfunction. Many of these children were considered to be brain damaged on the basis of their slowness in motor development. However, the slowness of motor development was due to lack of vestibular function.

Dr. David Smith: Dr. Rapin, how much of a time lag have you seen in the sitting and walking of children who had hypofunction of their vestibular apparatus?

Dr. Isabelle Rapin: I have seen it into the third year of life. However, it is not universally present because we have some children who walk within normal limits. We do not know whether this is within normal limits for a particular child. We had a family of children with Usher disease where one child walked at 14 months, and that was considered late compared to the other sibs. The second sib in that family who also had Usher syndrome did not walk until 18 months of age, which was clearly late.

Dr. Robert Gorlin: How accurate is an electronystagmogram for the infant?

Dr. Isabelle Rapin: As far as we know from Dr. Eviatar's report (Laryngoscope 89:1036, 1979), and our own reports, it is reasonably reliable. However, there are some pitfalls. For instance, we have found some children who had a positive electronystagmogram but this was probably caused by the effect of the irrigation, and was not repeatable. When doing caloric irrigation, one must also be careful that the water actually gets to the ear drum. Many times the ears are impacted with cerumen, or the stream of water only touches part of the canal wall.

Dr. Robert Ruben: For a number of years, we have used a control on all our caloric testing. Initially we do the caloric testing in the supine position and then reverse the child to the prone position. If the nystagmus is from a vestibular origin there should be reversal in the pattern of the nystagmus from supine to prone. If not, then we assume there is an artifact.

Dr. Walter Nance: Is any explanation of why these vestibular defects in mice lead to such dramatic movement, eg waltzing, turning around, etc? Is there an analog of that in man, or if not, why is man different?

Dr. Malkiot Deol: As far as it is known, this particular type of behavior is confined to rodents. However, it is unlikely that this particular malformation is confined *only* to rodents. It must occur at least in some of the related species, but the behavior does not. It could mean that in other species the compulsion to behave in this way is overcome by higher faculties. The reason for this type of behavior has been written about for the last 20 years, ever since I started working with the mouse. There are many lines of argument converging to one central concept, which is that the effects of these genes involve both the inner ear and the central nervous system. What is then observed is a behavioral effect on the central nervous system and not the inner ear, which also happens to be involved. It has been possible to produce the behavioral abnormality without damaging the inner ear. I have pursued this concept and work for more than the past two decades, but it appears not to have been noticed simply because it seemed so logical that the inner ear should be associated with the behavioral abnormality.

I also want to comment about some of the things which Dr. Lim described: the personal relationship between the absence of the otoconia and the abnormality of pigmentation. Pigmentation occurs in the utricle but not in the saccule of the mouse. The saccule usually does not even have a single melanocyte. The genes which were described affect pigmentation to some extent, but they also cause amelanotic melanocytes to occur in the utricle. However, we know there are similar melanocytes in albino animals where the otoconia are normal. There are also a number of spotting genes that totally eliminate both amelanotic and melanotic melanocytes, and these have otoconia which are not affected. So much for the relationship with pigmentation.

Secondly, I would like to discuss the absence of the otoconia and the manganese and zinc deficiency. The deficiency occurs not in the organism concerned, but in the mother. Thus, we are probably talking about the teratologic effect of manganese and zinc deficiency. In other words, it has to be present in the mother during gestation. It is true that the manganese deficiency would lead to an absence of otoconia but does not affect pigmentation. If the manganese is added to the pregnant mother, the offspring will have otoconia, but they will still be deficient in pigment.

Another aspect is the possible origin of the otoconia. There is a mutant mouse called Dancer, in which the macula of the saccule is always present but the macula of the utricle is always absent. However, the membrane upon which the macula should sit is present. In some of these animals the macula and saccule are confluent and connected by a wide channel. Thus, all the substances that are available in one chamber are available to the other. Yet in spite of this, we find that in the macula of the saccule there are almost normal otoconia while in the macula of the utricle there is not a single granule.

This suggests that the formation of the otoconia is in some way dependent upon the macula. Whether it is with the neural epithelial cells activated or whether this is done by the supporting cells is unknown. However, the presence of the macula is essential to the formation of the otoconia, as illustrated in the Dancer mutant. The absence of otoconia is really an indication of the abnormality of the macula itself. Thus, if the macula is abnormal, the abnormalities of balance are not necessarily due to the absence of the otoconia, but to the function of the neural epithelium itself.

Finally, I would like to discuss the relationship between the absence of the otoconia and the behavioral abnormalities which have been noted in many of the mice. The animals who have normal otoconia should behave normally, but they do not. These animals are hyperactive and tend to circle. They have other neurologic symptoms. I would hypothesize that the manganese deficiency in some unknown manner affects the central nervous system on the one hand, and goes to make up the otoconia on the other. There is a link between these observations; that these symptoms can be controlled genetically proves three things concerning the manganese: that the manganese affects pigment, that the manganese affects otoconia, and that the manganese also affects the central nervous system. This may be done by independent pathways. In other words, this is a pleiotropic effect and, if we knew more about what happens, we could know in what ways they are connected.

Dr. David Lim: In connection with Dr. Deol's comments, I feel that there is another possibility to explain the continued circling behavior. The information that has been found by the Websters, that in sensory deprivation there is a change in the anatomy of the central cochlear nuclei, may be applicable to the absence of sensory input from the otoconia-deficient mice. If the mice are deprived of macular input, this might cause permanent changes within the central nervous system which could lead to the aberrant vestibular function. Concerning the relationship of pigmentation and manganese, I feel that there are many steps in the morphogenic pathway of the otoconia. At any one of these points there could be an abnormality.

Dr. Isabelle Rapin: I would like to make one other comment concerning vestibular disease in infants. Dr. Ruben and I have seen some children in whom it is possible that there is involvement of the gravity receptors, as we have seen these children crawl with their heads hanging down. This symptomatology would be quite hard to imagine on the basis of abnormality of the semicircular canal.

Dr. David Lim: I would like to complement you for suspecting that there may be some patients with gravity receptor dysfunction. Some of them may have been thought to have been psychologically disturbed or severely retarded.

Dr. Charles Berlin: Sometimes children with abnormal vestibular reactions like this are misdiagnosed as being autistic. We have seen one child who was diagnosed as retarded and autistic based on his slow language development, slow walking, and aberrant balance behavior. The child was subsequently found to have a congenital fistula of the round window. The round window fistula was closed and the aberrant motor development ceased.

Dr. David Smith: I have always been bothered by the term "sensorineural deafness." I feel it would be important to localize the source of the deafness in a more precise manner in terms of cochlear or central nervous system. I would appreciate some practical thoughts concerning this, also including the use of tomography.

Dr. Charles Berlin: It has recently become possible, even in one-day-old infants, to obtain measurements of whether or not the auditory system is responsive. The simplest technique which is being used is to record electrical potentials from the scalp with the use of a computer average and a preamplifier. We are able to record whether or not the subject has a reasonable auditory system. One can record hair cell activity, synchronous discharge of the 8th nerve, synchronous discharge of the 2nd order neurons, and of the 3rd, 4th, and 5th order neurons and sometimes 6th order neurons. With the use of other equipment (electroacoustic impedance bridge), one can also make determinations concerning the function of the middle ear.

Dr. Isabelle Rapin: I would like to make some further comments concerning the term sensorineural. By and large, we are really still talking about cochlear problems when this term is used. In the literature there are a number of cases in which people have spoken about "central deafness" or "auditory perceptual problems." I feel many of these cases have been children with peripheral problems who have been mislabeled. I think, however, as we become more sophisticated we should be able to make diagnoses in cases which have true central auditory pathology.

Dr. LaVonne Bergstrom: I would like to answer Dr. Smith's question concerning tomography. Actually, one does not have to do tomography with the examination of the infant. One can take a routine x ray which will give you significant information. Some of these examples are to be found in my paper (this symposium).

Dr. Robert Ruben: Our experiences are congruent with Dr. Bergstrom's. Approximately, up to a year to a year and a half routine x rays will give excellent pictures of the bony labyrinth.

The Morphogenesis of the Middle and External Ear*

Thomas R. Van De Water, PhD, Paul F.A. Maderson, DSc, and Tina F. Jaskoll, PhD

INTRODUCTION

Van De Water and Ruben's review [1] of otic morphogenesis is concluded by reiterating Yntema's contention [2] that the inner ear could be considered independently of the middle and external ear. While this is true in certain respects, and indeed provides the rationale for so treating otic morphogenesis in the present symposium, it must be emphasized that there is as yet insufficient information to be certain of the developmental interrelationships among them. The middle ear and external ear are complex anatomic regions which receive contributions from ectoderm, endoderm, mesoderm, and neural crest during development. This melange of potentially interacting tissues not only makes these regions difficult to approach experimentally, but probably also explains to a large extent why even the history of descriptive analyses of development of the ear has lagged so far behind that of most other, more delineated, systems of the vertebrate body (see page 8 of Reference 3).

---

*This research was supported in part by grants from the NIH #NS-08365 (T.R. VDW.) and NS-13924 (P.F.A.M.), the Deafness Research Foundation (T.R. VDW.) and C.U.N.Y. "PSC-BHE" nos. 11629 and 12267 (P.F.A.M.).

If data on the normal morphogenesis of any system are to be used to explain the etiology of congenital defects therein, a complete modern anatomic description is a sine qua non. Where appropriate detail is lacking, it must be provided before experiments can be planned. In certain cases, and this is especially true of the middle ear, we must also be aware that problems in the interpretation of experimental data could arise if the evolutionary relationships of the animal models used are inadequately understood. Since the time of writing and eventual publication of Van De Water and Ruben's review [1], several disciplines have contributed data which, while considerably enhancing our knowledge of morphology of the middle and external ear, have also spotlighted the theoretic and practical problems which exist in designing and executing appropriate experiments concerning possible developmental mechanisms therein. We will a) review germane current evolutionary interpretations of interrelationships among lower tetrapods, b) review advances in our knowledge of the morphology of otic development, c) review the results of past and recent experimental studies on development, and d) attempt to relate the available data to our current knowledge of cell and tissue interactions in development. We will attempt to show how these data contribute to our understanding of developmental anomalies.

THE EVOLUTION OF THE MIDDLE AND EXTERNAL EAR

Henson [4] has provided an excellent detailed account of the comparative anatomy of the middle ear, dealing en passant with certain comments concerning the external ear. To facilitate the presentation and analysis of currently available developmental data, it is necessary to reiterate certain issues discussed at length by Henson [4]. As a prelude however, a brief review of our current understanding of tetrapod evolutionary relationships is required to provide a background for a recently presented thesis concerning evolution of the middle ear.

Figure 1 shows a greatly simplified scheme of our understanding of tetrapod evolution (for more detailed accounts see Olsen [5] and Romer and Parsons [6]). In the mid-Devonian period (about 370 million years ago) an unknown rhipidistian fish gave rise to the first amphibian. Since this creature is unknown except by inference, we refer to a "basic amphibian stock." From this stock, 2 distinct lineages arose: one giving rise to the modern amphibia, the other to the reptiles. From the "stem reptiles" (Cotylosaurs) arose the turtles (Chelonia), the tuatara, lizards and snakes (Lepidosaurs), the Archosaurs (whose descendants included the "dinosaurs," crocodiles, and eventually the birds), and, on a totally different lineage, the "mammal-like reptiles" (Therapsids) which, as their name implies, were the ancestors of modern mammals. As noted on the figure, most of the important intermediate forms are extinct (being known only as fossils). As Henson [4] has detailed, among extant tetrapods, only frogs, turtles, the tuatara, most lizards, crocodiles, and also birds and mammals have functioning middle

Morphogenesis of Middle and External Ear / 149

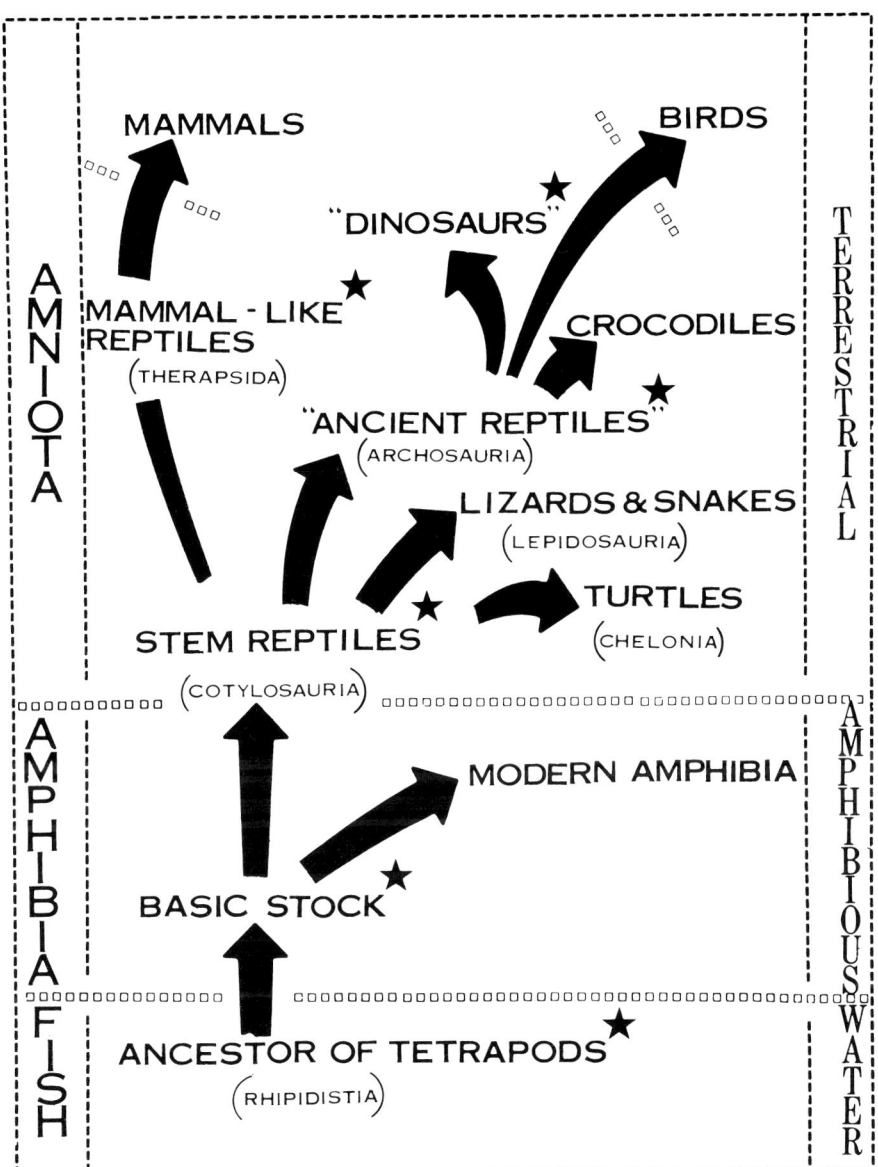

Fig. 1. Schematic and simplified phylogeny of the tetrapod vertebrates. The left-hand vertical column indicates the major taxonomic level, while the right hand vertical column indicates the environments primarily occupied by the groups concerned. Lines made of open squares represent transitions from one vertebrate class to another. Those groups indicated by stars are extinct and are known only as fossils, or by inference from other fossils. For detailed accounts, see Olson [5] and Romer and Parsons [6].

ears (ie serving to transmit airborne sound vibrations to the inner ear). Lack of availability of appropriate embryonic series, let alone live embryos for experimental purposes, is a problem which must be added to the general intellectual problem of the patterns of evolution of the soft parts in these diverse forms.

Figure 2 presents highly schematic representations of the basic anatomy of the middle and external ear which we observe and/or infer during the 370 million years of evolution which we have just briefly reviewed. The units of the characteristic mammalian ossicular chain — stapes, incus, and malleus (Fig. 3) — have long been accepted by paleontologists and comparative anatomists as having been derived respectively from the hyomandibular, quadrate, and articular skeletal elements of our piscine ancestors. Henson [4] has provided a fully documented discussion of this contention, including comments on the structural and functional aspects of the "middle ear" of certain extant fish. These latter data are not germane to the present study, and will not be mentioned further. The jaws of most fish are not firmly attached to the neurocranium, and in most cases they are suspended therefrom by the hyomandibular component of the hyoid (2nd branchial) arch which articulates proximally with the otic capsule. The point of attachment of the fish hyomandibular to the jaws is close to the articulation (suspensorium) which consists of the quadrate (the most posterior component of the pterygoquadrate bar, the embryonic primordium of the upper jaw), and the articular (the most posterior component of the Meckel cartilage, the embryonic primordium of the lower jaw). These facts have 2 significant corollaries. First, the mammalian ossicular chain which functions to transmit vibrations from the tympanum to the fenestra ovalis consists of elements whose function was histori-

---

Fig. 2. A highly schematic representation of middle and external ear morphology during the course of tetrapod phylogeny. Many of the processes on the rhipidistian hyomandibular and the columella of the tetrapods have been omitted for simplicity. Patterns of stippling represent homologies accepted by paleontologists and comparative anatomists. A — articular bone; ADJ — skin adjacent to tympanum and/or mammalian pinna; CA — columella auris; EAM — external auditory meatus; EC — extracolumella (the variety of processes involved in this structure may not be homologous among amniotes [see text]); FEC — frog extracolumella, which according to Lombard and Bolt [11] is almost certainly not homologous with the amniote structure(s); ?FO — fenestra ovalis of uncertain form in many early tetrapods; FT — frog tympanum, again probably not homologous with that of amniotes [11]; HYM — rhipidistian hyomandibular bone; I — incus; M — malleus; OC — otic capsule; OP — operculum, a dermal bone putatively occupying the position of the primitive tetrapod tympanum in rhipidistian fishes; OPP — opercular process of rhipidistian hyomandibular thought to be homologous with the distal end of the tetrapod columella [6]; P — pinna of mammalian ear; PF — pars flaccida of mammalian tympanum (Shrapnell membrane); ?PRT — presumptive tetrapod tympanum, structure completely unknown, location subject of much debate [4, 5]; PT — pars tensa of mammalian tympanum; Q — quadrate bone; ST — mammalian stapes.

cally quite different — they were all associated with jaw suspension. Second, since mammals are the only tetrapods with 3 ear ossicles, we must examine the data concerning how and why this situation arose, as well as the question of whether the single columella auris in other tetrapods evolved once or several times.

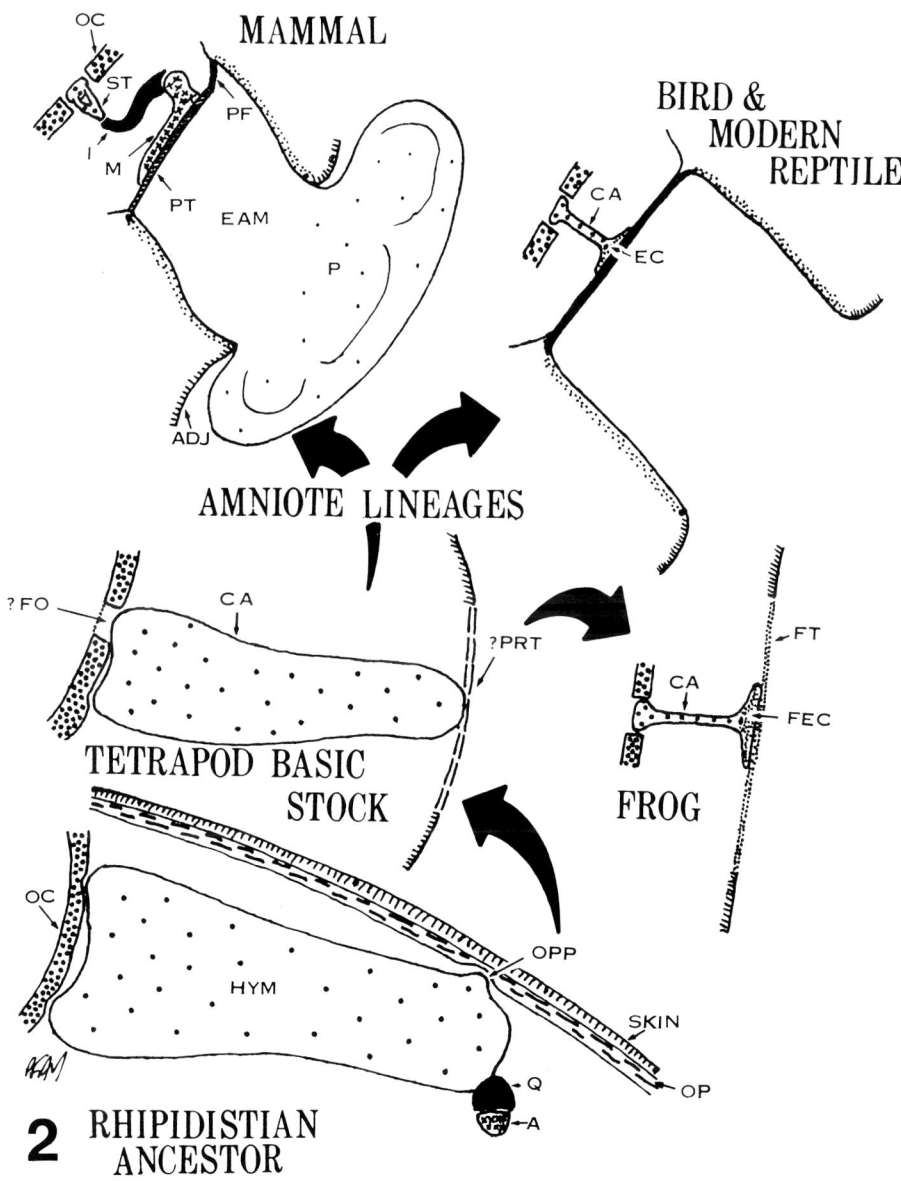

The importance of the second corollary cited above concerns our choice of experimental animals for investigations of otic morphogenesis. While the actual cellular mechanisms involved in developmental processes in all vertebrate embryos are indubitably similar [7], this does not necessarily imply that the sequence of interactions among components of a complex system are identical in all tetrapods. Such an inference is valid only if the available evidence indicates genetic homology between the components under consideration. Recent studies have raised some interesting problems in this context, which can now be discussed.

While Thomson [8] provided an excellent account of the transition from the suspensory fish hyomandibular to a potentially vibration-transmitting columella auris, many students before and since have been reasonably concerned by the relatively massive size of the homologous unit (where known) in most Paleozoic and Mesozoic tetrapod fossils. Henson [4] has documented much of the discussion of whether such a relatively massive unit could function in transmission of sound. It now seems clear that that transition from a massive (?continuing auxiliary suspensory) unit to a more delicate unit with an "ossicular function" occurred several times during reptilian evolution, and occurred particularly late in that lineage leading to mammals [9]. Many detailed studies by Crompton, Hopson and their students (for references, see [10]) have indicated that while the long-assumed homologies of the reptilian quadrate and articular with the mammalian incus and malleus, respectively, are substantiable on paleontologic grounds, the transition from a suspensory to an ossicular function was definitely a two-step process. Initially these elements were replaced in the suspensorium by the squamosal and dentary (the temporomandibular joint) to improve the masticatory apparatus. Thus, only secondarily could the quadrate and articular have become part of the characteristic mammalian ossicular chain. The fossil record cannot provide any information on the how or why of the sequence of incorporation, but some plausible speculations can be derived from developmental data. However, we shall probably never know the time at which the "mammalian auditory mechanism" arose in the sense we recognize it in extant forms. In many nonmammalian species there is an "extra–stapes" which actually inserts on the tympanic membrane [4]. The extra-stapes poses an outstanding revolutionary problem since its adult morphology suggests a polyphyletic origin. This issue could be resolved by appropriate detailed developmental anatomic studies, and is relevant to the "clinical-medical-anatomic" interpretation of the embryonic origin of the mammalian middle ear ossicles. Lombard and Bolt [11] have presented a most persuasive argument concerning the evolution of the tetrapod ear which is of great importance to our understanding of the developmental processes therein. They argue that the tympanic ear, as seen in modern tetrapods, is of diphyletic origin, while that of amniotes seems to have arisen from a common ground plan, that seen in modern amphibia is the result of independent evolution.

This conclusion implies that the results of experimental studies on amphibians [1, 2, 12] may have provided data somewhat or totally irrelevant to the problems of the developmental dynamics of amniotes.

A final comment in this section concerns the tympanum and the "external ear." First, given the arguments of Lombard and Bolt [11], the superficially-placed tympanum of modern amphibia (and perhaps fossil forms [4]) not only lacks anything which might be termed an external auditory meatus, but indeed the tympanum itself may not be homologous with that of other tetrapods. Second, the tympanum of modern nonmammalian amniotes, while almost certainly homologous, may be variously superficially situated (Fig. 4), or may lie in a shallow (Fig. 5) or deep "meatus" (Fig. 6). The only major difference seen in mammals is the presence of a definitive pinna which is of widely diverse form. Therefore, the external tympanic epithelium and the meatus — to whatever degree the latter is present — represent examples of the many other localized regional specializations of the integument [13], and thus present significant developmental problems. The evolutionary relationship between the mammalian tympanum and that of other amniotes has been the subject of debate for nearly a century. Shute [14] reviews the history of the problem and credits Westoll [15] with first suggesting that the pars flaccida (the Shrapnell membrane) is the vestigial homolog of the original reptilian tympanum, while the pars tensa — the "functional mammalian tympanum" — is therefore probably a neomorph. If this argument is true, it suggests an interesting possible answer to one of the most vexing questions of otic evolution. Presuming the mammal-like reptilian (or even early mammalian) ear had some vibratory receptive function, in any sequence of intermediate steps wherein the quadrate and articular rudiments, released from their suspensory function, *gradually* encroached upon the tympanum, they would have had a "dampening effect" on tympanic vibration. As such, their presence would have been functionally disadvantageous, and presumably "natural selection" would have removed them entirely. On the other hand, if their incorporation into the ossicular chain involved the appearance of a new tympanic membrane (?under their joint inductive influences during early embryogenesis), the stapes could have become incorporated into such a chain, perhaps with an "extra-stapes" still activating the original tympanum until the pars tensa (*sensu stricto*) became functional Such an hypothesis can never be verified directly, but improved knowledge of the role of the ossicular anlagen in ectodermal differentiation to form a tympanum would provide some direct support. Furthermore, it should be noted that apart from a single sentence concerning the Shrapnell membrane on page 305 of reference 16, no *comparative* study of the amniote tympanum has been conducted since the work of Filogamo [17], who concentrated mainly on the distribution of elastic fibers therein. More information is urgently needed in this context, especially on epithelial and mesenchymal cell organization.

THE ANATOMY OF DEVELOPMENT OF THE TETRAPOD MIDDLE EAR

Interpretation of experimental results in contemporary developmental biology necessitates detailed knowledge of cell and tissue differentiation. In this section we review the current status of middle ear development, emphasizing those cytologic data which have recently become available and focusing attention on significant gaps in current knowledge.

Amphibia

All previous reviews [1, 2, 4] of information concerning the development of the anuran middle ear have been based almost solely on studies where only the cartilaginous elements were analyzed, and there is a great need for detailed cytologic investigations of that period when the columella establishes contact with the definitive tympanum which appears during metamorphosis (Wasserzug, personal communication). A number of previous experimental studies on possible neural contributions to the otic region are reviewed by Toerien [12]. While his conclusion that the columella is completely absent from animals whose neural crest has been removed seems conclusive evidence of a branchial arch origin of this ossicle, the fact that the rest of the ear, including the tympanum, is quite normal under such circumstances is rather surprising. Toerien [12] also reports that if the otocyst is removed, the columella is present but has a misshapen footplate. These data together imply that the interactions among capsule, columella, and tympanum in these animals are significantly different from those seen in amniotes. Since Lombard and Bolt [11] believe that the anuran tympanic ear evolved independently of that of amniotes, further developmental investigations may be warranted for their intrinsic interest, but at present, the relevance of any of these results to mammalian congenital ear abnormalities seems dubious.

Amniotes

The general knowledge of amniote middle ear development through the late 1920s was summarized by Goodrich [18]. Romanoff [19] deals with later literature concerning the avian middle ear, and Anson [20] and Stephens [21] each

---

Fig. 3. Dissection of the left ear of a human cadaver, photographed looking down the external auditory meatus (large arrow) after removal of the tympanum to reveal the ossicular chain. The approximate region which would have been covered by the pars tensa of the tympanum is represented by a roughtly ovoid region of large stipple; that occupied by the pars flaccida is similarly indicated by fine stipple. The ossicles and their component parts are labeled as follows: MM — manubrium of the malleus; M — body of malleus; I — incus; IS — incostapedial articulation; CS — crus of stapes.

Fig. 4. Photograph of the left side of the head of the lizard, *Iguana iguana* (the green iguana), to demonstrate a species with a fairly superficially placed tympanum (TM). The insertion of the extracolumellar processes (ECP) may be seen through the dorsal portion of the tympanum.

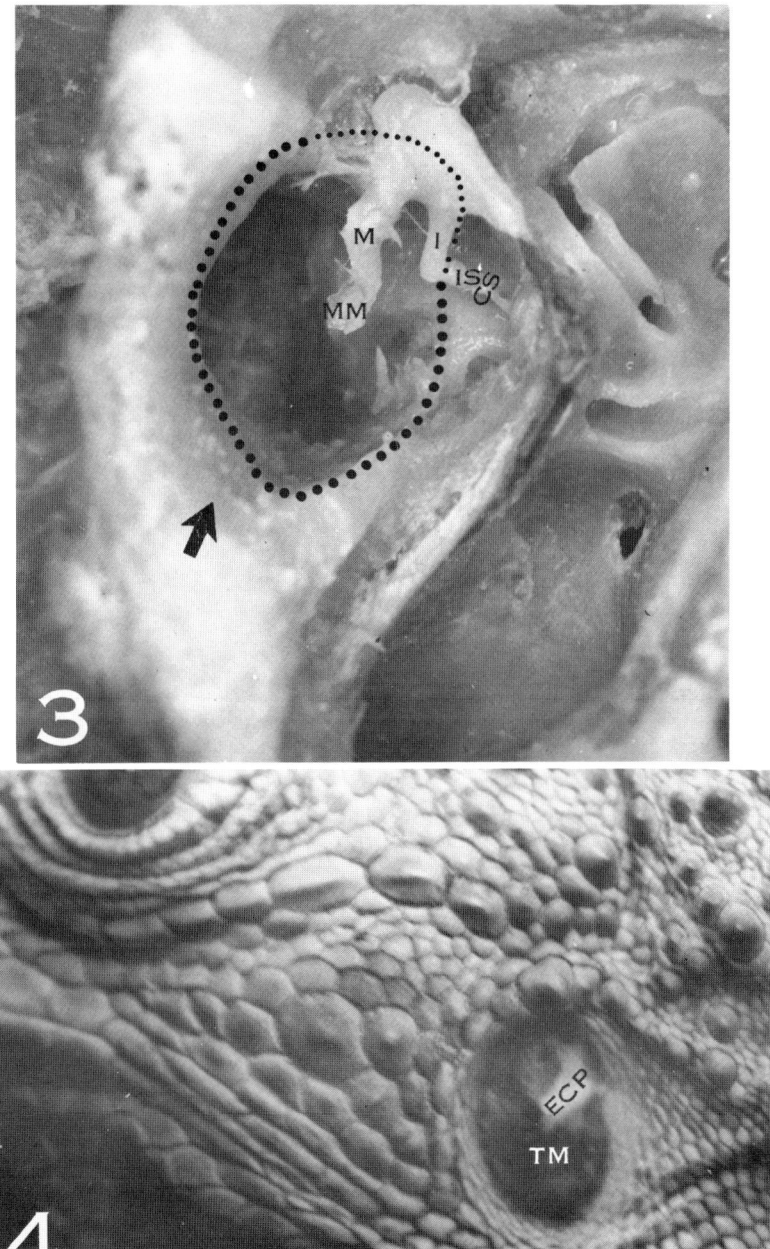

provided new data, while reviewing older information concerning the mammalian condition. However, until recently, the available data did not permit a detailed evaluation of problems concerning the mechanism of expansion of the hyoid pouch (tubotympanic sulcus), problems in cytologic observations pertaining to patterns of chondrification of ossicle(s), tympanic differentiation, etc.

Figure 7 provides a schematic representation of middle and external ear differentiation in an amniote. While derived primarily from a study of a timed sequence of chick embryos [22], it also illustrates mammalian (Figs. 8 and 10), and lizard (Fig. 9) otic differentiation (Jaskoll [23]; Van De Water and Maderson, unpublished data). The first indication of middle and external ear differentiation is the lateral outgrowth of the hyoid pouch ventral to the otocyst, in the general direction of an ectodermal invagination (the primordium of the external auditory meatus). By the time the otic capsule consists of early chondroblasts, similar cells representing the primordia of the ossicle(s) may be seen (Fig. 7A). As chondrification of the ossicle(s) proceeds, the external auditory meatus becomes significantly deeper, and the tubotympanic sulcus begins to send 2 or more pouches growing dorsad around the ossicle(s); these may now be termed middle ear cavities (Fig. 7B). In reptiles (Maderson, unpublished data) and in birds [22], the epithelial lining of the middle ear cavity is more or less flat, but in mammals it is highly convoluted [23]. As the expansion of the cavities continues dorsad, they eventually meet dorsal to the ossicle(s), which bridge the space between the fenestra ovalis and the presumptive tympanum (Figs. 7C, 7D, and 9).

In birds there is a complex interaction between the proximal cells of the primary columellar shaft involving the dedifferentiation of previously chondrified cells to produce the annular ligament [22]. Such a process is not so apparent in the mouse embryo [23] nor in reptile embryos (Maderson, unpublished data). This observation has considerable import with respect to the problem of the "contribution" of capsule cells to the stapedial footplate and will be discussed further below. In birds [22] and lizards (Maderson, unpublished data), the definitive tympanic cavity, and therefore the tympanum itself, is completed at the time of hatching or birth, but in the mouse the endodermal epithelium of the tympanic cavity does not "compress" the residual tympanic mesenchyme until 16 days postpartum [23]. There is a significant external auditory meatus in birds (Fig. 6) whose epithelium has the same characteristics and keratinizes at the same time

---

Fig. 5. Photograph of the right side of the head of *Crocodylus acutus*. The tympanum, lying at the bottom of a fairly well-defined "external auditory meatus," is indicated by an arrow.

Fig. 6. Photograph of the left side of the head of *Gallus domesticus*. In an intact bird, the external opening of the auditory meatus may be seen only if the feathers are parted. Here, the skin, much subcutaneous connective tissue, and some muscle have been removed from the regions indicated by X, to reveal the deep-lying tympanum (T). The extracolumellar processes may be seen just as white marks on the posterior aspect of the tympanum to the right of the symbol. The large arrow indicates the direction of the meatus in an intact bird.

Morphogenesis of Middle and External Ear / 157

as, apterous regions of the body [22]. Similarly, the lizard meatus remains patent throughout embryonic life, and although it remains nonscaled, its epidermis enters the characteristic shedding cycle [24] at the same time as the rest of the embryo (Maderson, unpublished data).

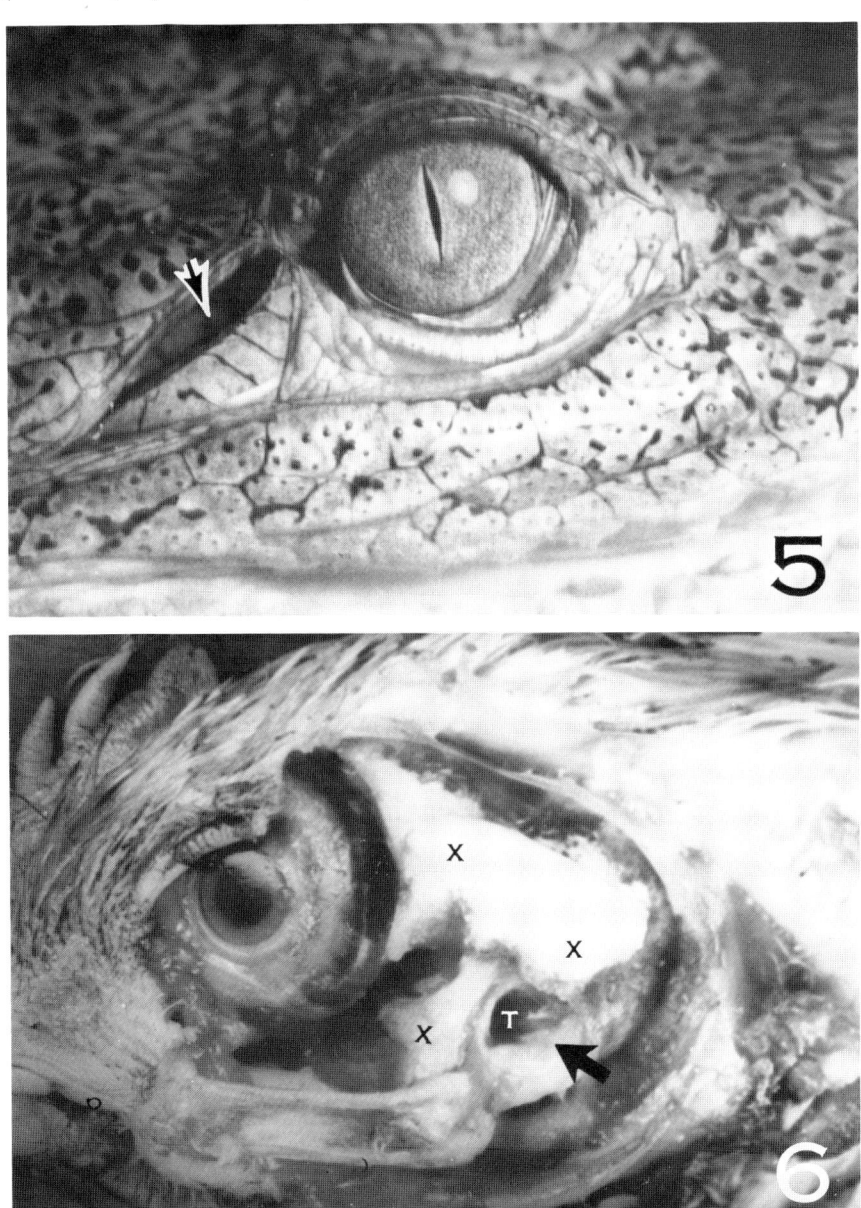

In the mammalian embryo, the external auditory meatus has a complex history. At 13 days gestational age in the mouse (Fig. 11A), it is a simple depression on the lateral aspect of the head, and the histology of the epithelium is exactly the same as that of the rest of the body surface — a simple cuboidal germinal epithelium overlaid by a single layer of flattened peridermal cells. By 15 days (Figs. 11B and 8), the simple depression begins to be covered over by the downward growth of the presumptive dorsal pinna. In the ventromedial margin appears the primordium of the so-called "meatal plate" which has been described previously as an "invagination" of ectodermal cells. Such an interpretation does not appear to be correct. Close examination of the invagination reveals that it is merely 2 closely apposed epidermal surfaces, which are often still separated most laterally. The close apposition is probably brought about by the rapid growth of mesenchymal cells representing the presumptive cartilages of the pinnae. This interpretation is confirmed by close examination of the plate and the external pinnal epidermis at day 19 (Figs. 10, 11C, and 12). By this time, the external pinnal epidermis has a multilayered periderm, and a single layer of presumptive cornifying cells, while the meatal plate still appears as a closely apposed pair of younger epidermal epithelia. By 9 days postparturition, the central peridermal cells of the deep meatal plate (Fig. 13) are filled with conspicuous keratohyalin granules, while distally, the meatus is reopening as its cells become cornified (Fig. 14), although its outer surface is still covered by a multilayered periderm. Further details of pinnal development have been provided previously [1].

Fig. 7. A schematic representation of the development of the amniote middle and external ear. While based mainly on a study of chick embryonic development [22], it essentially resembles the major stages of development in all amniotes. A) The tubotympanic sulcus (TTS), an extension of the hyoid pouch — is growing dorsolaterally from the pharynx (PH) beneath the otic capsule (OC), in the general direction of an ectodermal depression, the anlage of the external auditory meatus (EAM). At this time, mesenchymal condensations representing the anlage(n) of the ossicle(s) (O) may be seen surrounded by mesenchyme (M). B) The single columella (reptiles and birds), or the ossicular chain (mammals) (O) — now runs through the mesenchyme from a fenestra ovalis close to the lagena of the cochlea (L) to the presumptive tympanic region (TM). The tubotympanic sulcus has grown dorsally directed pouches anterior and posterior to the ossicle(s) which represent the first indications of the developing middle ear cavity (MEC). The external auditory meatus may have reached its maximal degree of relative depth at this time, or further depression may occur later in development, especially in mammals and birds. C) As the middle ear cavities continue their dorsad growth and enlargement, the footplate (FP) of the columella (mammalian stapes) becomes suspended by a presumptive annular ligament (AL) within the fenestra ovalis. In birds [22] and reptiles (Maderson, in preparation, see below, Fig 9), the continued lateral expansion of the middle ear cavities is beginning to compress the mesenchyme against the ectoderm of the presumptive tympanum. In mammals, the development of the meatal plate may delay this event until much later in embryonic development, or even postnatally [23]. D) As the mesenchyme is removed [22], the endodermal epithelium of the middle ear cavity encroaches upon the ossicle(s). In mammals, joint differentiation between the ossicles would be well advanced at such a time, and ossification would have begun in any amniote embryo. Other abbreviations are:-HB- hindbrain; IEC - inner ear cavity; N - notochord; SQ - squamosal.

Morphogenesis of Middle and External Ear / 159

The fate of the mesenchyme which originally occupied the region of the tympanic cavity has been a source of contention for some years [1], with the associated problem of the germ layer origin of the epithelium lining the mature tympanic cavity. This issue has been discussed at length elsewhere [22, 23], and we may now be reasonably certain of 2 facts. First, the entire epithelial lining of the tympanic cavity is of endodermal origin, and the putative discontinuities described by previous workers were certainly histologic artifacts. Second, since it appears that the cavity expands by simple growth of the epithelium, the fate of the mes-

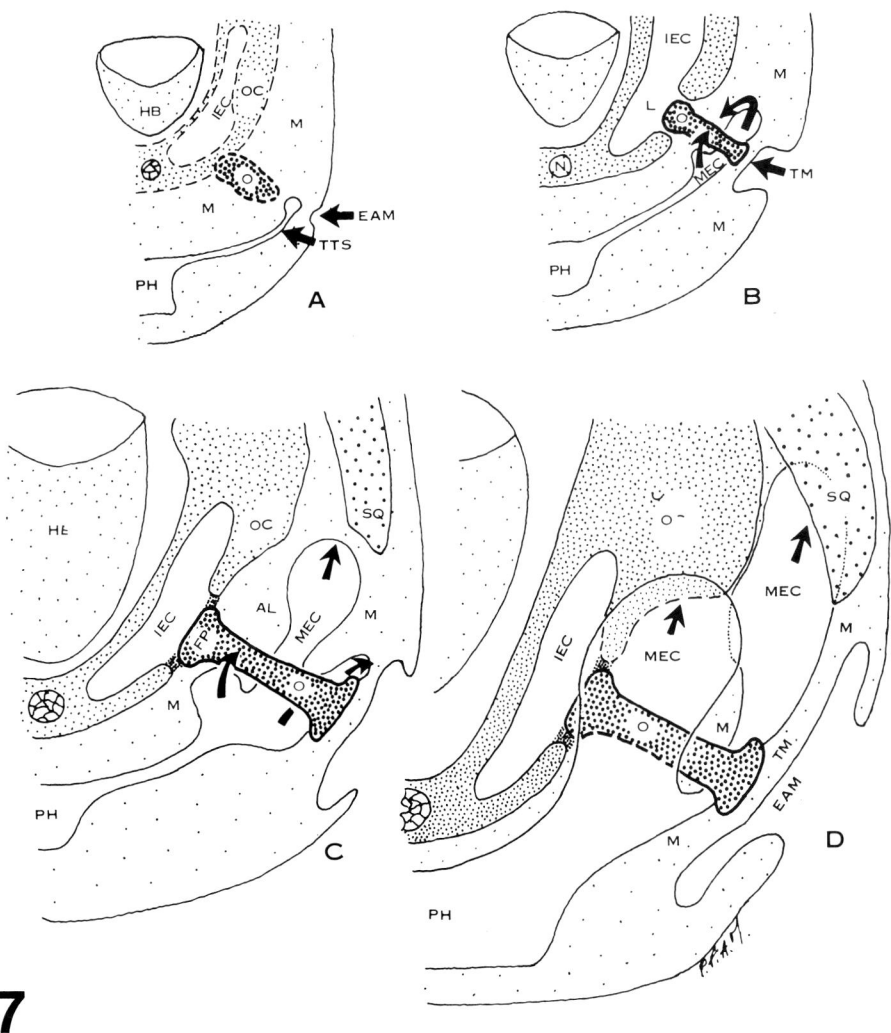

enchyme is significant. Jaskoll and Maderson [22] have shown that it appears to be a minor site of hemopoiesis in birds: the mesenchyme differentiates, either as blood cells or as vascular endothelia which drain into the nearby jugular vein; cell death is either absent or of minor importance. A similar situation probably exists in lizard embryos (Maderson, preliminary observations). By contrast, no evidence of sinus vascularization or hemopoiesis is apparent in mammals, and cell death predominates [22, 23]. A summary comparing the major histogenic events in the differentiation of the middle ear of chick and mouse is shown in Table 1.

EXPERIMENTAL CONTRIBUTIONS TO OUR UNDERSTANDING OF MORPHOGENESIS OF THE MIDDLE AND EXTERNAL EAR

Until recently, very few experimental studies of the development of the middle and external ear per se were available. However, advances in our knowledge of the anatomy of development of the regions discussed above permit an analysis and interpretation of data derived from studies not specifically addressed thereto. The diversity of these specific and nonspecific approaches leads us to present the available facts here in an operational sequence, and discuss their significance in the last section of this review.

NEURAL CREST CONTRIBUTIONS TO THE MIDDLE AND EXTERNAL EAR

Since the classic summary of this fascinating embryonic cell population by Hörstadius [25], there has been a virtual exponential increase of interest in its developmental capacities. This has been due mainly to the fact that where earlier workers were confined almost exclusively to evaluation of the effects of unilateral extirpation, or even mere morphologic description, a battery of new techniques has come available. The use of implants of radioactively labeled grafts, and, more

---

Fig. 8. Transverse section through the otic region of a 15-day mouse embryo showing the depression that will become the external auditory meatus (EAM) whose dorsal margin is beginning to show the first indications of pinnal development. In the ventromedial margin at X, the first indication of the meatal "invagination" may be seen; further along the series from which this section was taken, this invagination still clearly posesses a patent lumen. Note that the histology of the epidermis over the entire region is essentially the same. The tubotympanic sulcus (TTS) is also shown.

Fig. 9. Transverse section through the otic region of an embryonic *Lacerta vivipara* whose general degree of development resembles that of a Hamburger-Hamilton chick stage 35–36. The tympanum (TM) is already well defined at the base of a shallow meatus, but the middle ear cavity (MEC) has not yet completely compressed the tympanic mesenchyme. The columella (C) bridges the space between the fenestra ovalis where the footplate (FP) is suspended by the annular ligament (arrows). The cochlear (COCH) and vestibular (VEST) portions of the inner ear are also shown, surrounded by capsular cartilage (OC).

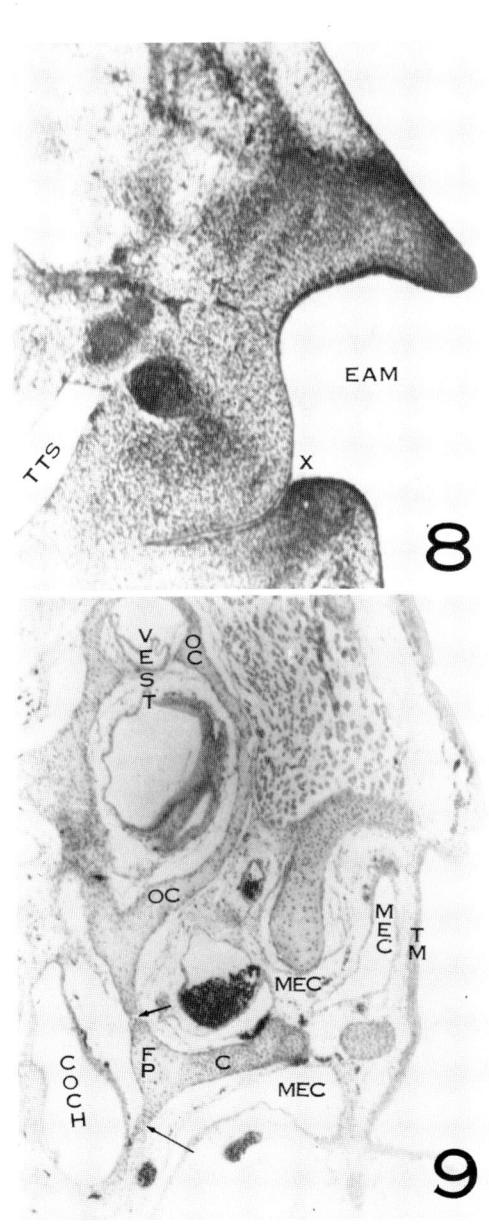

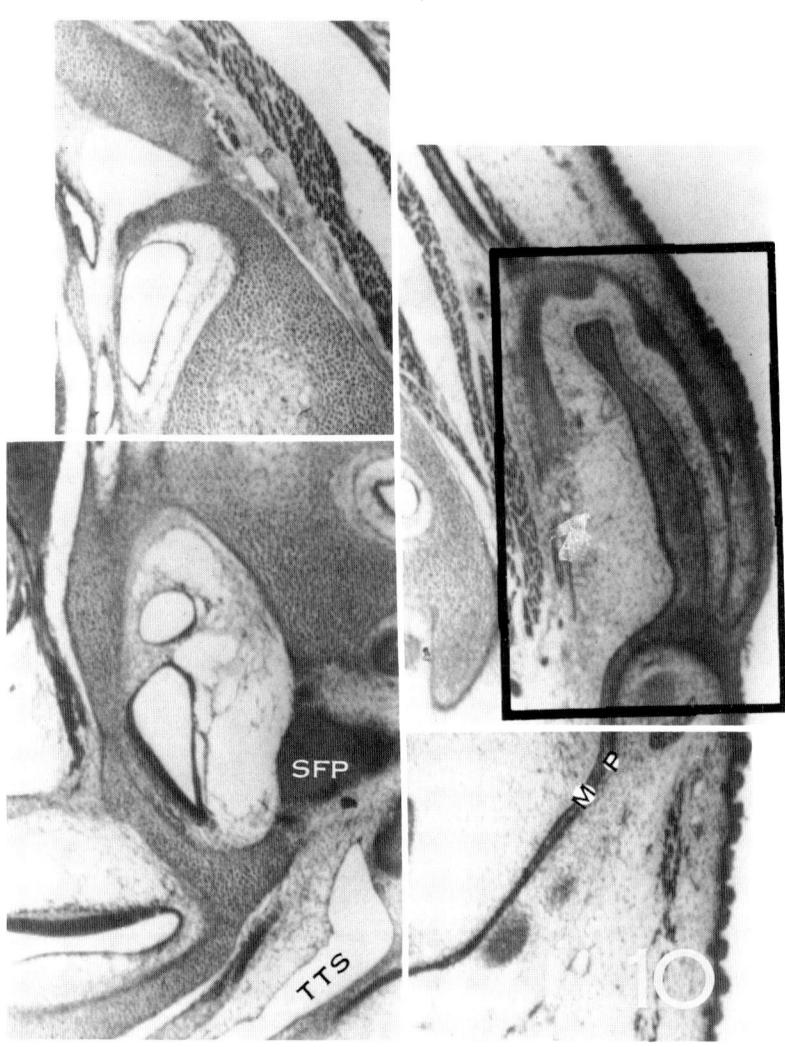

Fig. 10. Section through the otic region of a 19-day-old mouse embryo showing maximal development of the meatal plate. The region outlined by a rectangle is shown in greater detail in Fig. 12. The meatal plate (MP) runs far ventrally, but the tubotympanic sulcus (TTS) has scarcely begun its pattern of dorsolateral growth to form either an inner ear cavity or a tympanum. Thus the ossicles, represented here only by the footplate of the stapes (SFP), are still surrounded by mesenchyme (M).

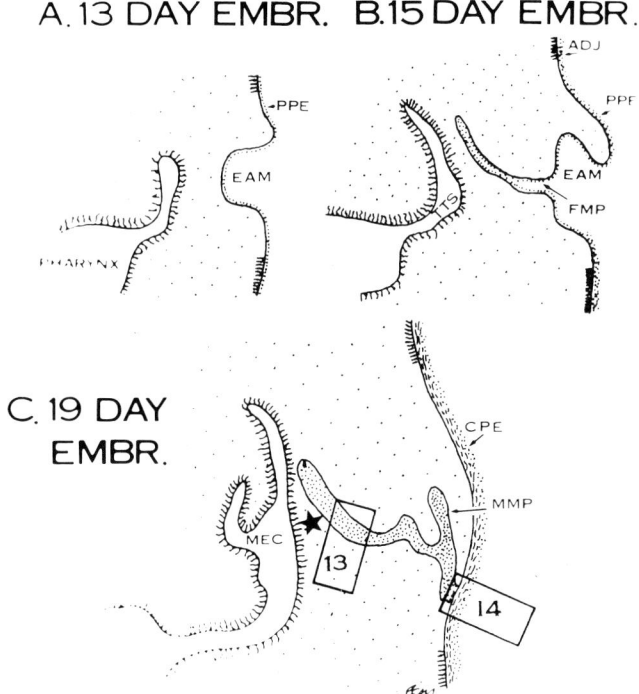

Fig. 11. Diagrammatic representation of the development of the external auditory meatus and meatal plate in A) 13-day-old, B) 15-day-old, and C) 19-day-old mouse embryos. Initially the epidermal histology of the adjacent, nonotic skin (ADJ) is the same as that lining the external auditory meatus (EAM) and over the presumptive pinnal tissues (PPE). By the 15th day, the tubotympanic sulcus (TTS) has grown somewhat dorsad from the pharynx, and its endodermal lining approaches the presumptive meatal plate (FMP) in some sections. The lumen of the latter may still be patent distally, but its epidermis, like that of the meatus, bears only a single layer of superficial peridermal cells, while that of the pinna (PPE) and the adjacent skin now has several layers of peridermal cells. By 19 days, the lumen of the external meatus and the enlarged meatal plate (MMP) have become completely occluded. The epidermis of the pinna and the adjacent skin shows the first signs of cornification beneath the multi-layered periderm, while the meatal plate itself seems to be merely a simple plate, but is in fact 2 younger epidermes lying en face. The star indicates the approximate location of the presumptive tympanic tissues. The rectangles numbered 13 and 14 indicate the locations of the subsequent Figs. 13 and 14 below.

recently, reciprocal transplantation of chick and quail neural crest cells, has permitted the tracing of neural crest contributions through hatching, which was previously impossible. The individual contributions of Chibon, Drews, Johnston, Le Douarin, Le Lievre, Noden and Weston, using these techniques, and a considerable body of other data from other workers concerning the neural crest as studied by electron microscopy, histochemistry, biochemistry, and cell culture are too numerous to list here, but the interested reader will find full documentation in several recent papers [26–29].

Noden [26] provides a complete table of the known contributions of neural crest cells to various parts of the avian head and body. Of particular interest in the present context are the origins of the Meckel cartilage and the quadrate (1st arch derivatives), and of the columella (a 2nd arch derivative). While Jaskoll and Maderson (page 184 [22]) report a personal communication from Le Lievre to the effect that the otic capsule contains some neural crest cells, Noden (page 300 [27]) states that the otic complex is of mesodermal origin. The phrase "otic complex" refers to the capsular region excluding the columella (Noden, personal communication). Noden [26] repeatedly emphasizes that the ultimate fate of neural crest cells is dependent upon the final environment in which they find themselves when their migration is completed. Nowhere is this environmental dependence better demonstrated than in Kollar's report [30] that explants of early mouse maxillary or mandibular rudiments grown in vitro fail to develop teeth, unless pieces of 5th ganglion are included in the culture. Apparently the penetrations of nerve axons into the jaw primordia are the final thrust that migrated neural crest cells need to transform them into preodontoblasts that in turn induce ameloblast differentiation in the overlying ectoderm. The penetration of nerve axons into this region at this critical time has been confirmed in vivo [31]. Available data suggest that the skeletogenic capacities of vertebrate cranial neural crest may be vestiges of a once pan-body capacity [32]. While some skeletal structures are definitely of pure crest origin, Noden (page 301 [27]) discusses the chimeric origin of a number of posterior cranial elements, indicating an interaction with other mesodermal cells. As Hörstadius (pages 8–9 [25]) indicates, designation of the neural crest to the mesoderm is not a new concept but one which arose from a series of morphologic studies by Miss Platt in the 1890s. Her terms "ecto-

---

Fig. 12. A high-power micrograph of the region indicated in Fig. 10 showing the details of the dorsal part of the meatal plate (MMP) as compared to the pinnal epidermis (PPE). The latter is now multilayered and the very first indications of cornification are apparent. Note the dense mesenchymal aggregations representing the future pinnal cartilages (PC).

Fig. 13. The histology of the deep meatal plate in a 7-day-postpartum mouse. The peridermal cells of the core are filled with basophilic keratohyalin granules.

Fig. 14. The histology of the distal, superficial meatal plate of a 7-day-postpartum mouse. The multilayered periderm (P) may be seen overlying the cornified tissues (C). Note the presence of keratohyalin granules presaging cornification in the meatal plate cells to the left of the photograph. Many hair follicles may be seen (H).

Morphogenesis of Middle and External Ear / 165

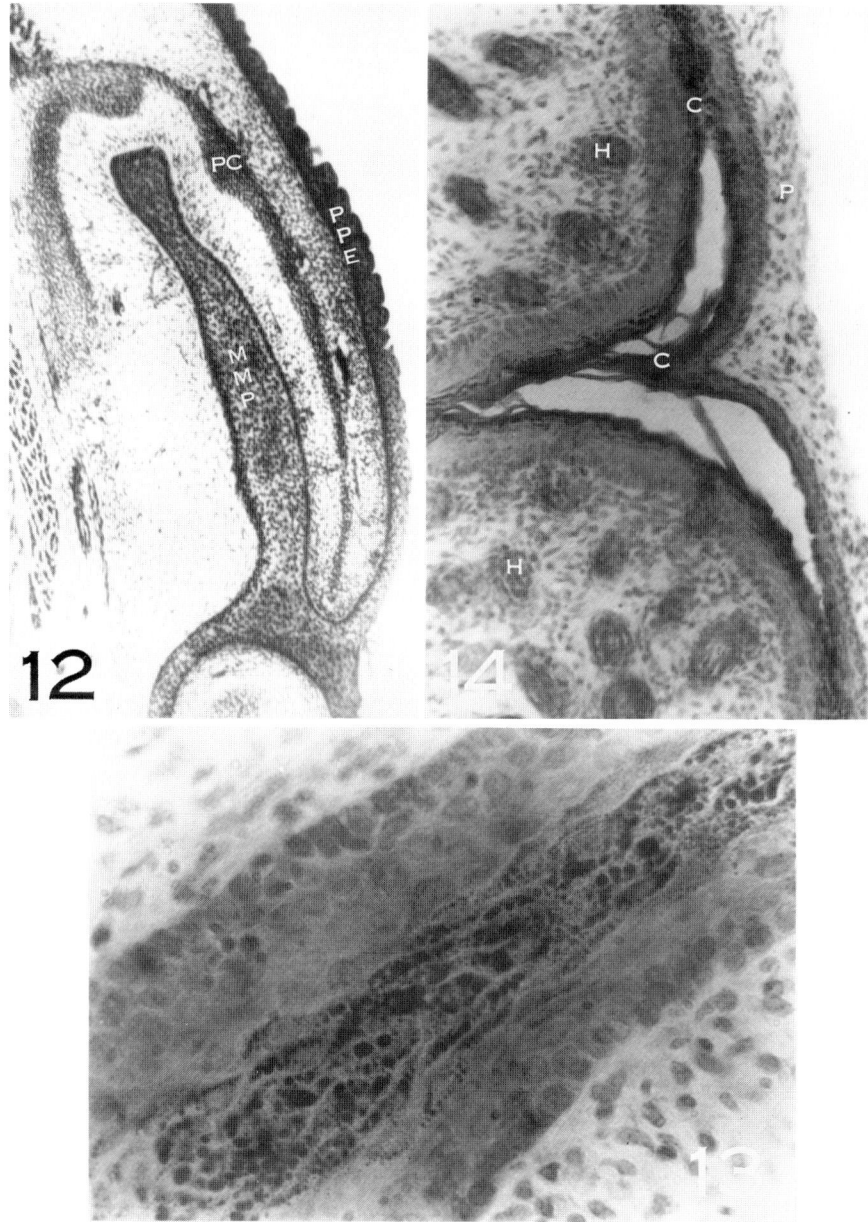

TABLE 1. A Comparison of the Development of the Middle Ear in the Chick and Mouse

	Chick/HH Stages*	Mouse/Days/Gestation
Ossicle(s) condensation	25	11
Ossicle chondrification	32–34	14
Footplate "fusion" with otic capsule	32–34	15**
Footplate suspended by annular ligament cells	35	15–16
Annular ligament differentiation	38	18–22 (1 day postnate)
Ossicle(s) ossification	41	25 (4 days postnate)
Middle ear cavity surrounds ossicle(s)	38	16 days postnate
Tympanic membrane differentiation		
a) inner aspect	37–38	14–16 (postnate)
b) outer aspect	40–41	2–16*** (postnate)
Keratinization	41	6 (postnate)

*The stage that a character is first observed will be given except in cases where it continues over a period of time.
**The footplate is never completely continuous with the otic capsule.
***The appearance of the ectodermal epithelium changes little from days 2–16 postnate.
(Taken from Jaskoll [23])

mesoderm" (ie neural crest) and "endomesoderm" (ie mesoderm in the more usual sense) might be usefully reinstated, since they greatly facilitate discussion of tissue interactions in complex regions such as the middle ear.

THE MORPHOGENESIS OF THE MIDDLE AND EXTERNAL EAR STUDIED BY EXTIRPATION PROCEDURES

Reagan [33] cauterized the otocyst in young chick embryos and observed that a columella was formed which lacked a footplate. As Jaskoll and Maderson [22] indicate, this experimental result not only caused considerable debate among evolutionists, but for many years was the basis for textbook statements to the effect that the stapedial footplate is of capsular origin. Simons [34–37] has repeated and confirmed Reagan's experiment [33] using more sophisticated techniques; but Toerien [38] reported only slight deformities of the medial end of the columella of the turtle in the absence of an otic capsule following excision of the early otocyst. Toerien (page 270 [38]) summarizes a variety of extirpation experiments on turtles as follows: "The experimental evidence supports the more recent views obtained from a study of normal series of chelonians *that the footplate is not developed as a separate entity from capsular cartilage*" (italics added). As indicated above, preliminary study of lizard columellar development seems to substantiate Toerien's conclusion [38], so that Jaskoll and Maderson's description [22] of the complex series of chondrocytic interactions in development of the chick footplate may be peculiar to this class of vertebrates. It is hoped that ongoing studies of reptilian columellar development will resolve this problem. Regrettably, 2 recent reports by Frank and Smit [39, 40] concerning the crocodile and the ostrich, respectively, are illustrated only by line drawings and no cytologic descriptions are given.

While we are most anxious not to initiate a semantic argument concerning a distinction between "capsular cells *contributing* to the stapedial footplate" and "capsular cells *interacting* with the stapedial shaft cells to form a footplate," the issue is of great importance in interpreting certain experimental data. Spirit and Van De Water (unpublished data) have analyzed the effects of the removal of varying amounts of the early chick otic cup. While their endeavors were directed primarily towards an understanding of the regulative capacities of the remaining tissues, their results clearly indicate that as long as *some* sensory tissue develops, there always will be found an otic capsule (albeit sometimes of abnormal shape and size), and a fenestra ovalis with a normal footplate suspended therein will develop. Figure 15 shows a section of the middle ear of a Hamburger-Hamilton stage 36 embryo recovered after operation at HH stage 12, with only a minute region of lagena present, and yet the middle and external ear morphology is virtually identical to a normal embryo (compare Fig. 15 to Fig. 9 in Jaskoll and Maderson [22]).

MIDDLE AND EXTERNAL EAR MORPHOGENESIS STUDIED BY EXPLANTATION PROCEDURES

As recent reviews [1, 41] have indicated, most studies involving the explantation of embryonic otic rudiments into situations in vitro have been predicated toward study of differentiation of the inner ear. However, some of these studies have provided incidental information of interest here. Figure 16 shows a living mouse inner ear, explanted on the 13th day of gestation and grown for 9 days in vitro. A stapedial footplate is clearly visible, and an excellent photograph of a similar situation in reference [42] shows that the footplate is fused to the capsule and that the annular ligament is absent. These studies might be taken as indicating that in fact the capsule is *responsible* for the stapedial footplate, but it must be borne in mind that thus far no one has managed to clean adherent mesenchyme from otocyst explants (see Discussion [41]). This mesenchyme might contain either endomesoderm or neural crest cells, or both. The fusion of the footplate to the capsule in such studies in vitro has also been observed by Van De Water (unpublished data) and is of interest because a similar result has been obtained in quite different experiments discussed below. Van De Water (unpublished data) has explanted mouse otocysts surrounded by larger quantities of mesenchyme, even including some ectoderm. In some circumstances, an apparent ossicular chain forms. Further experiments of this type are planned in the near future.

MORPHOGENESIS OF THE MIDDLE AND EXTERNAL EAR STUDIED IN CHORIOALLANTOIC GRAFTS

Bradley [43] showed that rudiments of chick limb grown on chick chorioallantoic membranes (CAM) produced more complete differentiation of skeletal tissues and joints than techniques in vitro. Jaskoll and Maderson [22] described "joint differentiation" as manifested in the development of the annular ligament suspending the footplate as a major feature of avian middle ear development, and have evaluated "joint differentiation" of middle ear anlagen that were explanted to chick chorioallantoic membranes [44]. In 110 recovered grafts of entire otic regions derived from donor embryos, Hamburger-Hamilton stages 15–29, 96 showed recognizable middle ear structures. A columella was readily identifiable in 75 grafts, and 9 were indistinguishable from normal specimens, although some abnormalities of the external meatus were observed. The other grafts showed various degrees of columellar abnormality which could be characterized in 3 types according to a schedule compiled by Jaskoll, Maderson and Weiner [45]. These types will be defined briefly here for subsequent reference: Type I – footplate either completely or partially fused with the otic capsule (Fig. 17); Type II – columella not fused with capsule, but separated from it by mesenchymal cells, both capsule and columella being surrounded by differentiated perichondria; Type III – abnormal columella, including a wide range of deformities such as lack of processes, extreme small size, or even absence. These types of abnormalities are precisely those which have been obtained by the use of various teratogens, but CAM grafting – and probably, in vitro techniques – have certain inherent problems for the study of the development of a structure as complex as the middle and external ear. When the otic rudiment is removed (including the otocyst), the embryo is extremely small, and there is no way of controlling which other presumptive tissue and organ areas are included. Thus, in some cases keratinizing epithelia continuous with epithelia of obvious digestive tract characteristics, or even feathers adjacent to the columella, were sometimes seen, and Figure 17 includes a structure identified as a tongue. The inevitable exposure of such a

---

Fig. 15. Section through the otic region of a chick embryo sacrificed on the 14th day (Stage 36) of incubation following extirpation of a large portion of the otic cup at Hamburger-Hamilton stage 12. Although the cochlea is represented by only a small piece of neural tissue (COCH), the columella (C) is perfectly normal in appearance with a footplate (FP) suspended in a fenestra ovalis, and an extracolumella (EC) inserting onto a well-developed tympanum (TM). The middle ear cavity (MEC) and the external auditory meatus (EAM) are quite normal in appearance.

Fig. 16. A living mouse inner ear in vitro, removed as an otocyst from a 13-gestational-days-old embryo, photographed after 9 days. Two ampullae (A) of 2 of the semicircular canals are indicated; the cochlear duct (COCH) has a normal configuration, and a stapedial footplate (SFP) may be seen.

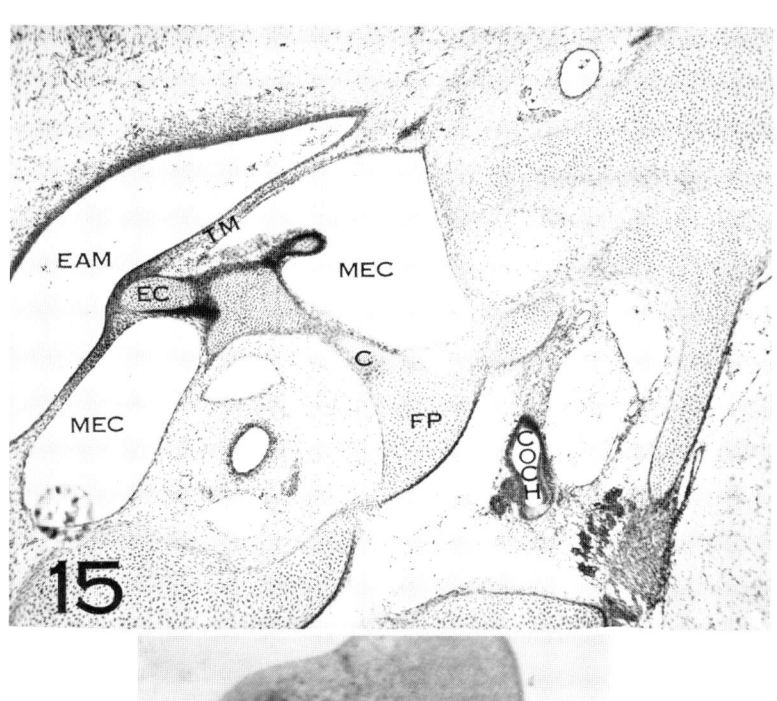

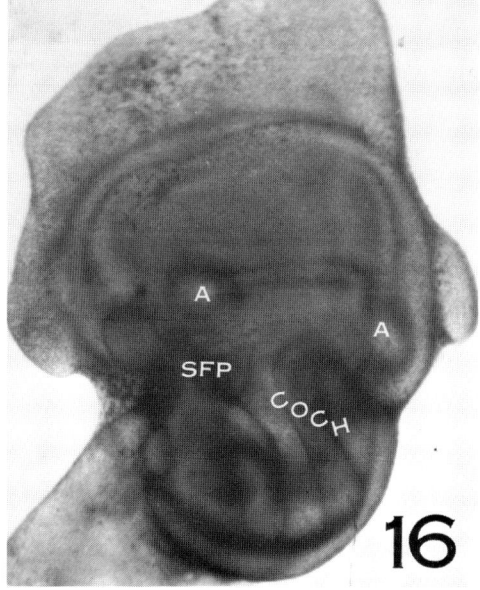

melange of endodermal and ectodermal epithelia, endomesoderm, and ectomesoderm is such that controlled experiments will probably prove impossible to perform on a repeatable basis. For this reason, extirpation experiments (as above) and drug interference in vivo would seem to be more promising.

MORPHOGENESIS OF MIDDLE AND EXTERNAL EAR STUDIED BY TERATOGENIC INTERFERENCE

Teratology — involving either simple description or experimental production of abnormal morphogenesis — was for many decades a rather minor, even dull, side branch of embryology. However, the thalidomide tragedy of the 1960s gave considerable impetus not only to more rigorous testing of drugs developed for potential therapeutic use but also to the use of drugs as investigative tools. Deliberate production of abnormalities in embryos of known normalcy by application of drugs or by exposure of the developing organism to damaging environmental conditions, and a comparison of the abnormal morphogenesis with the normal state, has often made it possible to identify key events in organogenesis which are not detectable by other techniques [46–48]. It is most important to bear in mind that in very few cases do we know very much about the actual cellular mechanisms which are disrupted by these agents. However, if we can identify drugs or environmental conditions which regularly produce specific defects, then at least we can establish a firm basis for the ultimate identification of the appropriate transcriptional, translational, or posttranslational event(s) which is/are the cause(s) of the developmental lesion. Obviously this is a long step away from the initial investigation. The ideal is the production of a phenocopy which can be compared with a known mutant.

There have been several hundred publications describing craniofacial malformations produced by teratogens, for example Shah [49]. However, with the exception of Morriss' production [50] of a condition resembling Treacher Collins syndrome by feeding pregnant rats excess vitamin A, and Scherschlicht's [51, 52] noting columellar defects in chick embryos following administration of triethylamine melamine, little is known of the effects of teratogens on development of the middle and external ear. It should be noted, however, that most authors simply do not mention these regions in their reports, so that there is no way of knowing whether or not effects were produced therein. A reexamination of much stored slide material in this context could produce extraordinarily valuable contributions to our knowledge of otic morphogenesis.

Jaskoll [23] has conducted investigations of the effects of several different teratogens on development in ovo of chick middle ear. A full account of the results produced by hadacidin [45] (Fig. 18), and a preliminary account concerning beta-aminoproprionitrile, beta-2-thienylalanine, 5-fluorouracil, triethylamine melamine and pilocarpine [53] are available. The results of these investigations may be summarized as follows. Although no morphologic signs of middle ear differentiation are apparent until Hamburger-Hamilton stages 25–26, abnormalities can only be produced when the drugs are applied at earlier stages. All drugs which produce columellar abnormalities produce very high mortalities (50–90%). Three basic types of abnormality are produced (see above), their frequency being approximately associated with the time of application of the drug. In many cases, extreme craniofacial abnormalities were observed without any detectable effect on the columella.

These data have been interpreted [23, 45, 53] as follows: cephalic neural crest derivatives are so rarely absent in surviving embryos that it would appear that if teratogens do adversely affect early neural crest metabolism, and therefore the primary determination of its derivatives, they are probably lethal. In those embryos which survive, the columellar defects may be explained in terms of interference with the complex series of interactions between its anlage and that of the otic capsule, which lead to the formation of the footplate, the fenestra ovalis, and the annular ligament [22]. Minor effects on other columellar processes, and on its size or exact shape, as well as those seen in other cranial neural crest derivatives (frontonasal and lower jaw abnormalities) are explicable in terms of effects on later cell proliferation and morphogenesis rather than on primary determination. These conclusions have implications in the context of the etiology of congenital defects of the ear.

CONTRIBUTIONS TO OUR KNOWLEDGE OF MORPHOGENESIS OF THE MIDDLE AND EXTERNAL EAR BY STUDY OF MUTANT PHENOTYPES

In a 1977 review, Deol [54] states that well over 50 genes affecting development of the inner ear in the mouse are known; other mammalian species have also been described in this context. However, with very few exceptions, data on the middle and external ear in these mutants are totally lacking, and indeed lack of reference thereto renders it impossible to state whether these regions are normal in these mutants, or simply have not been described. We are for the most part dependent on inferences which may be drawn from descriptive clinical studies [46, 55], where, of course, there is no way of knowing whether the conditions have a genetic base or whether they are the result of environmental effects in utero.

Van De Water and Ruben [1], and Ruben [56] have reported on the homozygous Kreisler mouse. This mutant shows extreme variability in the degree of development of the inner ear, and in those cases where the greatest deficiencies are observed (see Fig. 5B [1] and Fig. 13 [56]), the effects on the capsular cartilages and ossicles show certain similarities to those produced by partial extirpation of the avian otic cup (Spirit and Van De Water, unpublished data).

Two clinical case reports describing malformation of the ossicular chain [57] and fixation of the stapes within the region of the fenestra ovalis [58], associated respectively with Treacher Collins syndrome and renal abnormalities, and with symphalangism and syndactylia, are of interest for 2 reasons. First, they both illustrate the fact that even in cases of extreme anatomic deficiency of the middle ear, the ossicles are never absent, only malformed (see above). Second, they are both examples of the curious association of deficiencies in 2 or more quite distinct organ systems. There are bounteous opportunities for evaluation of not only possible deficiencies in middle and external ear in mutant mammalian strains known to possess defects of the inner ear, but also for consideration of possible deficiencies in other organ systems.

DISCUSSION AND CONCLUSION

The Current Status of Our Understanding of Tissue Interactions

Recently there has been a resurgence of interest in the phenomenon of "embryonic induction," that apparently ubiquitous activity wherein embryonic cell populations exchange information, thus promoting and/or maintaining patterns of specific differentiation. Although first suggested in the 1st decade of this century by studies of vertebrate eye development, the concept of embryonic induction was formalized following the experiments by Spemann and Mangold [59] on amphibian gastrulation and neurulation. These experiments, demonstrating the effect exerted on the presumptive neural plate by the underlying chordamesoderm, rank among the great classics of biologic research, and derived studies have exercised the imagination and ingenuity of dozens of workers for the last 50 years [60]. The history of this 50-year search for the identity and mode of action of the elusive "primary inducing agent" essentially reflects the general trends in biologic research during that period. Beginning with studies of general cellular activity as reflected by patterns of oxidative metabolism along gradients, passing into a period of increasing refinement of biochemical study, and then involving the construction of models based on the latest information from molecular biology, the continuing search has raised many interesting questions. Hundreds,

---

Fig. 17. A section through a CAM graft of a chick otic region removed from a donor of Hamburger-Hamilton Stage 17, 10 days earlier. The columella (C) shows the characteristic shape, and the footplate (FP) is suspended within the fenestra ovalis by the annular ligament (arrows). A middle ear cavity (MEC) with an endodermal epithelium (E) surrounds the columella. The extracolumella (EC) inserts into the mesenchyme adjacent to the endodermal epithelium, but note the absence of an ectodermal epithelium on the "tympanic membrane." Structure X has all the histologic characteristics of a normal tongue. Otic capsule is marked (OC).

Fig. 18. A section through the columella of a chick embryo injected with 2.0 mg Hadacidin at Hamburger-Hamilton Stage 18 and recovered 7 days later (HH Stage 34). The columella (C) inserts into the tympanic membrane (TM). The footplate (FP) is partially fused with the otic capsule (OC). Note the absence of the dorsal portion of annular ligament (arrow), although the footplate is clearly separate from the otic capsule. Regions are marked: IE– inner ear, P – perichondrium.

if not thousands, of publications have "spun off" from this inquiry into primary embryonic induction, and amply demonstrate that inductive events characterize not only all phases of embryonic development, but are also the basis for the maintenance of the differentiated adult state [61–65].

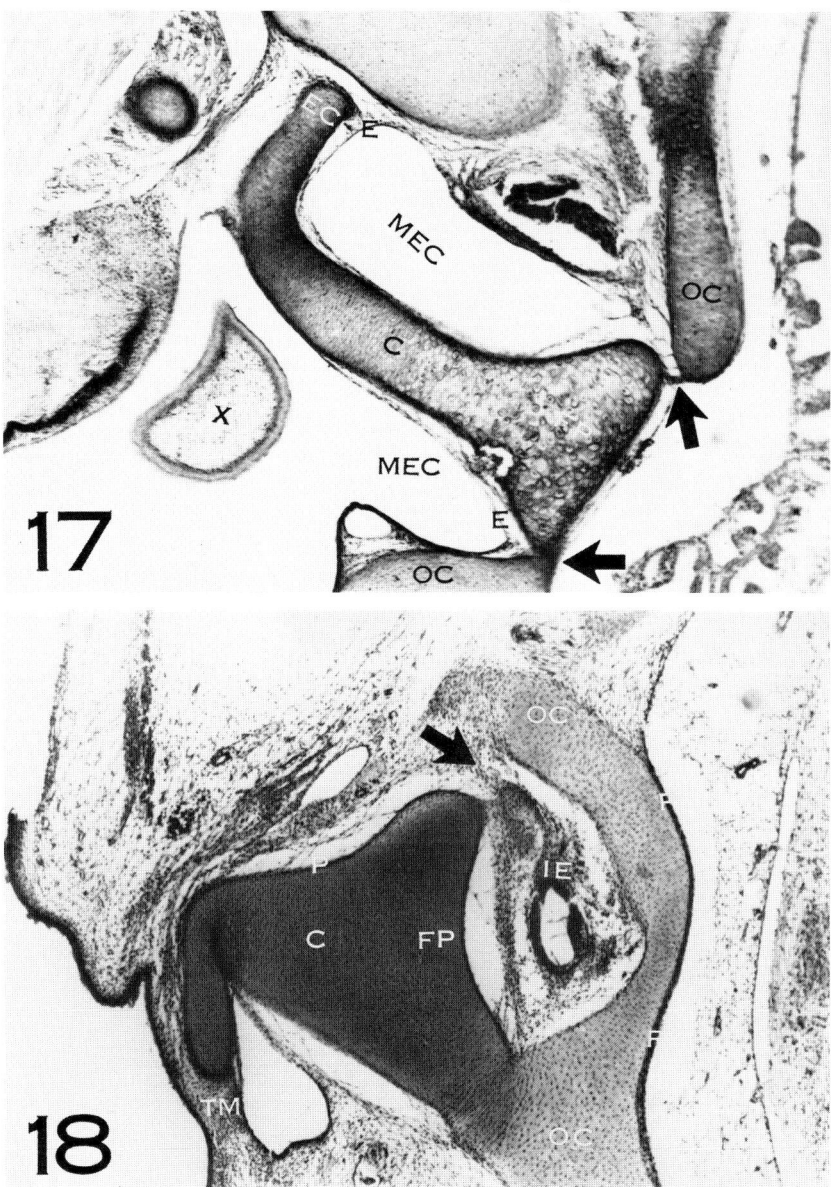

Study of a great variety of problems has led us to understand that there are common factors to any and all developmental programs [7]. While there may be some validity in Meier and Hay's [66] thoughtful comments to the effect that the nature of the *controlling mechanisms* in different "inductive interactions" may be so varied that we are approaching a time when the concept has become unmanageably broad, we may be certain of the following. When we approach the study of a given system, we now know exactly the sort of data we need in order to evaluate the critical events in its development. Further, we can appreciate that without a solid background of knowledge of the cellular interactions involved in normal embryogenesis and later homeostasis, attempts to understand the etiology of congenital abnormalities will be fruitless.

The steps involved in the understanding of embryonic development and adult homeostasis of any biologic system are all the same. First, we need detailed information on normal differentiation — especially the distribution of certain extracellular materials [7], patterns of cell division, movement (perhaps even death), and final cytodifferentiation. Such descriptive information may be obtained by the use of a variety of techniques — light and electron microscopy, histochemistry, biochemistry, etc; it is important to assess the degree of sophistication that is necessary to answer specific questions at specific points in an investigation. Such studies permit the identification of key events in development and thus facilitate the interpretation of experimental interferences. The second step is the identification of mutant phenotypes which must then be described to a comparable degree of completeness with respect to their ontogeny. A point will be found wherein the organogenesis of a given mutant system shows a recognizable difference from that seen in the normal system; we may infer that it is around this period of time when the mutant allele exerts its effect. The third step involves experimentation. An attempt must be made to produce a phenocopy of a mutant condition by exposing a normal genome to a known external variable. Using the term "phenocopy" in the very broad sense, this may be effected by manipulation of tissues by extirpation, transplantation, or drug treatment. Such a sequence of investigative steps has been used to singular advantage in our understanding of the normal morphogenesis of skin and limb [3, 7, 13, 67]. While it cannot be claimed that we have as yet reached the stage where dermatologists or orthopedic specialists can utilize such data as part of their everyday clinical activities, we can say that either plausible explanations of presented symptoms or a basis for the planning of appropriate experiments for testing of drugs for therapeutic use has been reached.

Clinical Implications and Problems for Future Research

In the light of all these data, it is obvious that our ignorance of the morphogenesis of the middle and external ear far exceeds our knowledge, but we may glean some small items of useful information from what we do know. Severe developmental anomalies such as otocephaly [68, 69], Treacher Collins syndrome [70], Robin syndrome [71], 1st and 2nd branchial arch syndrome [72], and congenital deafness resulting from ossicular defects [73], are all associated with anatomic structures and regions which are known to receive contributions from neural crest. Indeed, it has been suggested that otocephaly and other craniofacial abnormalities may be associated with a deficiency in this embryonic tissue [74, 75]. In the light of the data reviewed here concerning the actions of teratogens on development of the middle ear, we wish to express the general view that the neural crest is so important to vertebrate head development that any genetic lesion or major teratogenic factor which influences primary neural crest function would certainly be lethal. Such would not therefore ever manifest as a clinical problem since the fetus would almost certainly be spontaneously aborted. Thus, to the extent that these malformations might be due to deficiencies of subsequent morphogenesis of tissues derived from neural crest, we will remain dependent upon advances in reconstructive surgery to ameliorate them. Squamous metaplasia of the epithelium of the middle ear, either as a congenital condition or following chronic otitis media, *might* be due to alterations in normal epithelial-mesenchymal interactions [76, 77], but experimental investigations are needed to substantiate such contentions. It is *possible* that if, indeed, defects in mesenchymal metabolism are involved in such conditions, drugs might be found which would restore their normalcy, but appropriate tests cannot be considered until we have direct experimental evidence of the normal mechanisms of epithelial maintenance.

In the first section of this paper, we emphasized the very special problem attendant upon experimental investigations of the middle and external ear in light of recent views concerning evolutionary relationships of the modern amphibia. There is a more subtle related problem which is illustrated in Figure 19. As has been emphasized (at least implicitly), students of paleontology and comparative anatomy are quite convinced that the mammalian stapes, incus, and malleus are respectively the homologs of the nonmammalian columella (fish hyomandibular), quadrate, and articular (Fig. 19A). However, many clinicians and medical anatomists would argue [1] that portions of the incus and malleus derive from the 1st (mandibular) arch, while the stapes, part of the incus, and the manubrium of the malleus derive from the 2nd (hyoid) arch (Fig. 19B). Figure 19C, based primarily on Noden's review [26] concerning experimental studies on the avian neural crest, would imply that all components of the mammalian ossicles are of neural crest origin. If and when it becomes possible to manipulate mammalian embryos throughout the appropriate stages of morphogenesis, perhaps this impasse could be resolved. We should bear in mind, however, that once such experiments become possible, those of us, experimental biologists and clinicians alike, who share a common fascination for the processes whereby the human body is formed, will be so busy pursuing our own particular system of choice and its attendant prob-

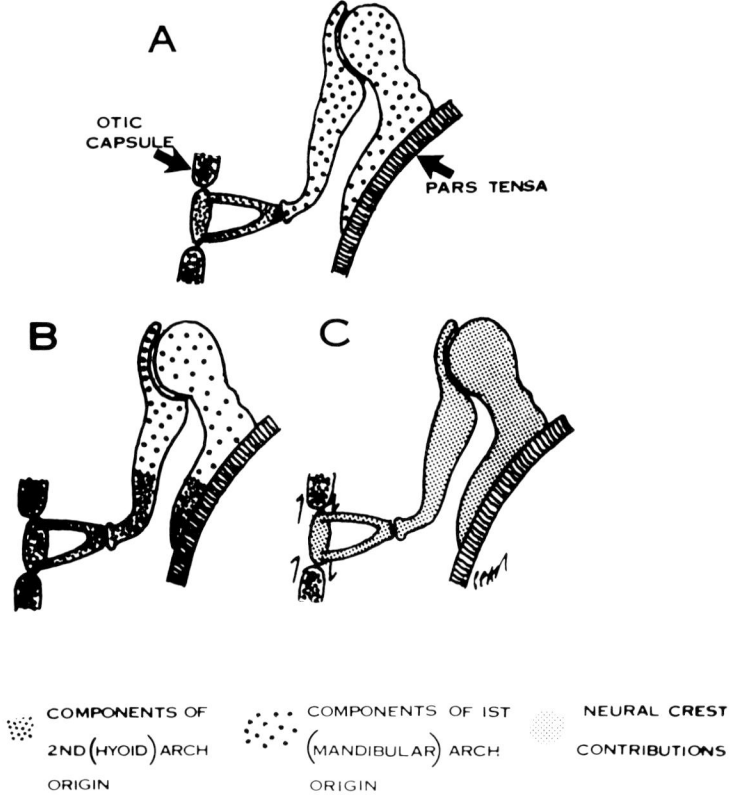

Fig. 19. Diagrammatic representation of 3 different interpretations regarding the homologies and embryonic branchial arch origins of the mammalian ear ossicles.

lems that not only will previously existing paradoxes be forgotten, but we might all become too involved to attend meetings and symposia and continue cross-pollenization at them.

ACKNOWLEDGMENTS

The authors thank Ms. Una Maderson for typing the manuscript.

REFERENCES

1. Van De Water TR, Ruben RJ: Organogenesis of the ear. In Himcliffe R, Harrison D (eds): "Scientific Foundations of Otolaryngology." London and Chicago: W Heinemann Year Book, 1976, pp 173–184.

2. Yntema CL: Ear and nose. In Willier BA, Weiss PA, Hamburger V (eds): "Analysis of Development." Philadelphia: WB Saunders, 1955, pp 415–428.
3. Flaxman BA, Maderson PFA: Growth and differentiation of skin. J Invest Dermatol 67:8–14, 1976.
4. Henson OW: Comparative anatomy of the middle ear. In Keidel WD, Neff WD (eds): "Handbook of Sensory Physiology: Auditory System." Berlin and New York: Springer-Verlag, 1974, vol 5, part 1, pp 40–110.
5. Olson EC: "Vertebrate Palaeozoology." New York and London: Wiley-Interscience, 1971.
6. Romer AS, Parsons TS: "The Vertebrate Body." Philadelphia: WB Saunders, 1977.
7. Maderson PFA: Embryonic tissue interaction as the basis for morphological change in evolution. Am Zool 15:315–327, 1975.
8. Thomson KS: The evolution of the tetrapod middle ear in the rhipidistian-amphibian transition. Am Zool 6:379–397, 1966.
9. Allin EF: Evolution of the mammalian middle ear. J Morphol 147:403–438, 1975.
10. Crompton AW, Parker P: Evolution of the mammalian masticatory apparatus. Am Sci 66:192–201, 1978.
11. Lombard RE, Bolt JR: Evolution of the tetrapod ear: An analysis and reinterpretation. Biol J Linn Soc 11:19–76, 1978.
12. Toerien MJ: Experimental studies on the origin of the cartilage of the auditory capsule and columella in Ambystoma. J Embryol Exp Morphol 11:459–473, 1963.
13. Sengel P: "Morphogenesis of Skin." Cambridge: Cambridge University Press, 1976.
14. Shute CCD: The evolution of the mammalian eardrum and tympanic cavity. J Anat 90:261–281, 1956.
15. Westoll TS: The mammalian middle ear. Nature 154:114–115, 1945.
16. Johnson FR, McMinn RMH, Atfield GN: Ultrastructural and biochemical observations on the tympanic membrane. J Anat 103:297–310, 1968.
17. Filogamo G: Réchèrche sur la structure de la membrane du tympan chez les differents vertébrés. Acta Anat (Basel) 7:248–272, 1949.
18. Goodrich ES: "Studies on the Structure and Development of the Vertebrates." New York: MacMillan, Dover Reprint Edition (1958), 1930.
19. Romanoff AL: "The Avian Embryo." New York: MacMillan, 1960.
20. Anson BJ: Development of the auditory ossicles. Laryngoscope 248:561–569, 1947.
21. Stephens CB: Development of the middle and inner ear in the Golden Hamster (Mesocricetus auratus). Acta Otolaryngol (Suppl) (Stockn) 74:296, 1972.
22. Jaskoll TF, Maderson PFA: A histological study of the development of the avian middle ear and tympanum. Anat Rec 190:177–200, 1978.
23. Jaskoll TF: "The Microscopic Anatomy and Dynamics of Avian and Mammalian Middle Ear Development." Unpublished PhD Thesis, City University of New York, 1978.
24. Maderson PFA: The embryonic development of the squamate integument. Acta Zool 46:275–295, 1965.
25. Hörstadius S: "The Neural Crest." Oxford: Oxford University Press, 1950.
26. Noden DW: Interactions directing the migration and cytodifferentiation of avian neural crest cells. In Garrod DL (ed): "The Specificity of Embryological Interactions." London: Chapman and Hall, 1978.
27. Noden DW: The control of avian cephalic neural crest cytodifferentiation. I. Skeletal and connective tissues. Dev Biol 67:296–312, 1978.
28. Noden DW: The control of avian cephalic neural crest cytodifferentiation. II. Neural tissues. Dev Biol 67:313–329, 1978.

29. Johnston MC, Noden DW, Hazelton RR, Coulombre JL, Coulombre AJ: Origins of avian ocular and periocular tissues. Exp Eye Res 29:27–43, 1979.
30. Kollar EJ: The use of organ cultures of embryonic tooth germs for teratological studies in tests of teratogenicity in vitro. In Ebert JD, Marois M (eds): "Tests of Teratogenicity in Vitro." New York: North-Holland Publishing Co, 1976, pp 303–334.
31. Kollar EJ, Lumsden AGS: Tooth morphogenesis: The role of innervation during induction and pattern formation. J Biol Buccale 7:49–60, 1979.
32. Maderson PFA: On the early evolutionary history of the neural crest. Am Zool 18:586, 1978.
33. Reagan FP: The role of the auditory sensory epithelium in the formation of the stapedial plate. J Exp Zool 23:85–108, 1917.
34. Simons EV: The effects of experimental unilateral anotia on skull development in the chick embryo. I. Introduction, techniques and preliminary results. Acta Morphol Neerl Scand 12:331–344, 1974.
35. Simons EV: The effects of experimental unilateral anotia on skull development in the chick embryo. II. Essentials of the development of the chondrocranium in normal embryos of 7–20 days of incubation. Acta Morphol Neerl Scand 13:287–304, 1975.
36. Simons EV: The effects of experimental unilateral anotia on skull development in the chick embryo. III. Chondrocranial development in anotic embryos of 7–20 days of incubation. Acta Morphol Neerl Scand 14:61–78, 1976.
37. Simons EV: The effects of experimental unilateral anotia on skull development in the chick embryo. IV. Development of the bony skull in embryos of 9–20 days of incubation. Acta Morphol Neerl Scand 15:75–87, 1977.
38. Toerien MJ: Experimental studies on the columella-capsular interrelationship in the turtle Chelydra serpentina. J Embryol Exp Morphol 14:265–272, 1965.
39. Frank GH, Smit AL: The early ontogeny of the columella auris of Crocodilus niloticus and its bearing on problems concerning the upper end of the reptilian hyoid arch. Zool Africana 9:59–88, 1974.
40. Frank GH, Smit AL: The morphogenesis of the avian columella auris with special reference to *Struthio camelus.* Zool Africana 11:159–182, 1976.
41. Van De Water TR, Li CW, Ruben RJ, Shea CA: Ontogenic aspects of mammalian inner ear development. This volume.
42. Friedmann I, Hodges MG, Riddle PN: Organ culture of the mammalian and avian embryo otocyst. Ann Oto Rhinol Laryngol 86:371–380, 1977.
43. Bradley SJ: An analysis of self-differentiation of chick limb buds in chorioallantoic grafts. J Anat 107:479–490, 1970.
44. Jaskoll TF, Maderson PFA: The differentiation of the avian middle ear on chick chorioallantoic membrane. J Morphol (Submitted for publication).
45. Jaskoll TF, Maderson PFA, Weiner BE: The differentiation of the columella in avian embryos treated with hadacidin with some observations on other skeletal abnormalities. Teratology 18:321–332, 1978.
46. Warkany J: "Congenital Malformations: Notes and Comments." Chicago: Year Book Medical Publishers, 1971.
47. Neubert D, Merker HJ (eds): "New Approaches to the Evaluation of Abnormal Embryonic Development." Stuttgart: Thieme-Edition, Publishing Sciences Group, Inc, 1975.
48. Ebert JD, Marois M (eds): "Tests of Teratogenicity in Vitro." New York: North-Holland Publishing Co, 1976.
49. Shah RM: Effect of prenatal administration of hadacidin, a cancer therapeutic agent, on the development of hamster fetuses. J Embryol Exp Morhphol 39:203–220, 1977.

50. Morriss GM: Abnormal cell migration as a possible factor in the genesis of Vitamin A induced cranio-facial abnormalities. Supra #47, pp 678–687.
51. Scherschlicht R: Malformations in the head of the chick after treatment with TEM during organogenesis. I. Skeleton, musculature, brain and cranial nerves. Wilh Roux Arch 173:83–106, 1973.
52. Scherschlicht R: Malformations of the head of the chick after treatment with TEM during organogenesis. II. Sensory organs and upper beak. Wilh Roux Arch 177:241–245, 1975.
53. Jaskoll TF, Maderson PFA: The effects of teratogens on avian columella development. Anat Rec 190:432, 1978.
54. Deol MS: Deficiencies of the inner ear in the mouse and their origin. In "Mecanismes de la Rudimentation des Organes chez les Embryons de Vertébrés. Actes du Colloque International #266," CNRS. Paris, 163–171, 1977.
55. Rapin I, Ruben RJ: Patterns of anomalies in children with malformed ears. Laryngoscope 87:1469–1502, 1976.
56. Ruben RJ: Developmental and cell kinetics of the Kreisler (kr/kr) mouse. Laryngoscope 83:1440–1468, 1973.
57. Ruben RJ, Toriyama M, Dische MR, Bransilver B, Daley JF: External and middle ear malformations associated with mandibulofacial dysostosis and renal abnormalities: A case report. Ann Otol Rhinol Laryngol 78:605–624, 1969.
58. Vase P, Prytz S, Pederson PS: Congenital stapes fixation, symphalangism and syndactylia. Acta Otolaryngol 80:394–398, 1975.
59. Spemann H, Mangold H: Über Induktion von Embryonalan durch Implantation Artfrender Organisatoren. Arch Mikros Anat Entwicksmech 100:599–638, 1924.
60. Toivonen S, Tarin D, Saxen L: The transmission of morphogenetic signals from amphibian mesoderm to ectoderm in primary induction. Differentiation 5:49–55, 1976.
61. Ursprung H (ed): "The Stability of the Differentiated State." New York: Springer-Verlag, 1968.
62. Fleischmajer R, Billingham RE (eds): "Epithelial-Mesenchymal Interactions." Baltimore: Williams and Wilkins, 1968.
63. Goldspink G (ed): "Differentiation and Growth of Cells in Vertebrate Tissues." New York: Halstead, 1974.
64. Lash J, Whittaker JR (eds): "Concepts of Development." Stamford: Sinauer Assoc Inc, 1974.
65. Wessels NK: "Tissue Interactions and Development." Menlo Park, CA: WA Benjamin, Inc, 1977.
66. Meier S, Hay ED: Stimulation of corneal differentiation by interaction between cell surface and extracellular matrix. I. Morphometric analysis of transfilter induction. J Cell Biol 66:275–291, 1975.
67. Goetinck PF: Genetic aspects of skin and limb development. Curr Top Dev Biol 1:253–284, 1966.
68. Klein D: Genetic factors and classification of craniofacial abnormalities derived from a perturbation of the first and second branchial arch. In Longacre JJ (ed): "Cranio-Facial Anomalies: Pathogenesis and Repair." Philadelphia: JB Lippincott, 1968, pp 31–42.
69. Wright S, Wagner K: Types of subnormal development of the head from inbred strains of guinea pigs and their bearing on the classification and interpretation of vertebrate monsters. Am J Anat 54:383–447, 1934
70. Holborow CA: Deafness and the Treacher Collins syndrome. J Laryngoscope 75:978–984, 1961.
71. McKenzie J: The first arch syndrome and associated anomalies. Supra #68, pp 135–195.

72. Longacre JJ: The surgical management of first and second branchial arch syndrome. Supra #68, pp 243–256.
73. Hough JVD: Congenital malformations of the middle ear. Arch Otolaryngol 78:335–343, 1963.
74. Johnston MC: The neural crest in abnormalities of the face and brain. In Bergsma D (ed): "Morphogenesis and Malformations of the Face and Brain." Alan R. Liss for the March of Dimes Birth Defects Foundation, BD:OAS XI(7):1–18, 1975.
75. Johnston MC, Pratt RM: The neural crest in normal and abnormal craniofacial development. In Slavkin H, Greulich R (eds): "Extracellular Matrix Influences in Gene Expression." New York: Academic Press, 1975, pp 773–777.
76. Lim DJ, Shimada R, Yoder M: Distribution of mucus-secreting cells in normal middle ear mucosa. Arch Otolaryngol 98:2–10, 1973.
77. Hentzer E: Ultrastructure of the middle ear mucosa. Ann Otol Rhinol Laryngol 85(Suppl 5a): 30–36, 1976.

Pathoembryology of the Middle Ear

Joseph B. Nadol, Jr., MD

Surgical exploration of the middle ear over the last 3 decades has documented a variety of malformations that may result in a conductive hearing loss [1]. These anomalies may be limited to the middle ear or comprise part of a regional or systemic syndrome. Among the known causes of malformations of the middle ear are genetic defects, demonstrating mendelian or multifactorial inheritance or chromosomal abnormalities, and nongenetic factors, such as thalidomide.

The theoretic possibilities for etiologies of nongenetic congenital malformations of the middle ear are limited only by the imagination, but analysis of these sporadic anomalies is unlikely to lead to a better understanding of underlying developmental defects, unless a specific etiology is recognized. It is for this reason that the study of malformations induced by thalidomide is valuable, since the induced developmental defects are phenocopies of disorders also caused by genetic defects. Furthermore, they may be reproduced and studied in the experimental animal. Nevertheless, study of human malformations that are caused by genetic defects, particularly single gene defects, is more likely to elucidate underlying mechanisms of dysmorphogenesis. The objective of such study is the determination of specific defects, such as an enzyme deficiency, upon which a rational plan for diagnosis and/or treatment of a disorder could be developed [2]. Unfortunately, in contrast to inborn errors of metabolism in which specific enzymatic defects are recognized, the study of human malformations has progressed only to the point of recognition of a genetic basis in some disorders, and the formation of hypotheses concerning the probable systems responsible for the defects.

In the area of malformations of the middle ear, although there is a plethora of case reports documenting anomalies both of genetic origin and of unknown cause, there has been little effort to classify the known genetic syndromes that produce a conductive hearing loss in a way that suggests underlying developmental defects, even in a general way [3].

TABLE 1. Summary of Classification of Genetic Syndromes That Cause a Conductive Hearing Loss

Progressive hearing loss

1. Bone dysplasias
2. Abnormalities of connective tissue
3. Abnormal metabolism of mucopolysaccharides
4. Unknown underlying developmental defect

Nonprogressive hearing loss

1. Dysostoses, abnormalities of cartilage, bone, or connective tissue
2. Mesodermal defects
3. Regional (localized) defects
4. Chromosomal abnormalities
5. Unknown underlying developmental defect

Progression of hearing loss unknown

1. Bone dysplasias, dysostoses
2. Unknown underlying developmental defect

There are over 50 syndromes that include a conductive hearing loss and in which the mode of genetic inheritance is reasonably certain. What follows is a preliminary attempt at classification of these syndromes and a discussion of representative examples. During this organizational process, several limitations were recognized. First, the assignment of a genetic basis is tentative in some cases. Second, the data concerning the type of defect of the middle ear are often incomplete or based on single case reports. Third, a great deal of the anatomic data is based on surgical exploration rather than postmortem histopathology. Hence, the data must be biased toward those malformations of the middle ear that cause a conductive hearing loss. Discovery of other defects, such as an anomalous course of the facial nerve, malposition of the great vessels, and lesser malformations of the ossicular chain and its ligaments and tendons, often depends on the presence of a coincident conductive hearing loss. Furthermore, contraindications to exploratory surgery, such as anomalies of the eustachian tube, or coincident severe mental retardation or sensorineural hearing loss, will further bias the data. With these limitations in mind, the following classification is offered.

CLASSIFICATION OF GENETIC SYNDROMES THAT CAUSE A CONDUCTIVE HEARING LOSS

Table 1 summarizes the broad categories of classification. The syndromes were separated first into 2 groups, based on whether or not a progressive hearing loss had been reported in each case. This resulted in automatic segregation of broad classes of defects. For example, the bone dysplasias, as would be expected, seemed to fall exclusively into the category of progressive conductive hearing loss, while all localized or regional congenital defects, such as Robin or Treacher Collins syndromes, fell into the nonprogressive group.

The next step was the tentative assignment of a proposed underlying defect, or at least a unifying concept that provided a "least common denominator" for the various systemic defects represented in each syndrome. In other words, an attempt was made to explain the pleiotropic effect of a single gene defect on the basis of a single underlying developmental defect. It must be realized that these assignments are only hypothetic. Furthermore, in many cases only a very general area of the likely underlying defect could be assigned. Thus, a category such as "mesodermal defect" is vast and is several steps removed from the desired goal of assigning a specific enzymatic defect. A synopsis of each of the syndromes with the known clinical data and a tentative assignment of an underlying defect in each case is presented in Table 2.

PROGRESSIVE CONDUCTIVE HEARING LOSS

Bone dysplasias. The most specific group of genetic disorders that cause a progressive conductive disorder is that categorized as "bone dysplasias," in which there is faulty growth and modeling of bone. In the disorders in which data are available, the conductive hearing loss is due to fixation of all 3 ossicles, with the exception of otosclerosis which represents a localized dysplasia of the otic capsule. Cranial nerve palsies and sensorineural hearing loss are common in this group, presumably due to coincident narrowing of neural foramina by bony overgrowth. In addition, toxic substances may be released from the involved otic capsule resulting in primary degeneration of the organ of Corti. The histopathologic features of bone dysplasias are illustrated by 2 cases, the first of Albers-Schönberg disease, and the second of sclerosteosis.

Case 1. Albers-Schönberg disease was diagnosed at birth. The child was blind and mentally retarded and died at 15 months of age of bronchopneumonia. Histologic examination of the temporal bone illustrated the increased density and thickness of bone that is characteristic of this disease (Fig. 1). The stapes was thickened, and the pathology was similar to that observed in long bones. There was persistence and heavy calcification of cartilage, suggesting an abnormality of endochondral ossification or its remodeling.

TABLE 2. Synopsis of Clinical Characteristics of Genetic Syndromes That Cause a Conductive Hearing Loss

Syndrome	Middle ear malformations	Associated Malformations Local	Associated Malformations Systemic	Inheritance[a]	Underlying developmental defect
		Progressive — 1. Bone dysplasias			
Otosclerosis [4]	Fixation of stapedial footplate	?Sensorineural hearing loss	None	AD	Limited bone dysplasia
Paget disease of bone (osteitis deformans) [5–8]	Ankylosis of ossicles	Sensorineural hearing loss	Generalized skeletal changes	AD	Bone dysplasia
Hereditary hyperphosphatasia (juvenile Paget disease; hyperostosis corticalis juvenilis deformans) [9–11]	ND	Enlargement of head	Thickening of bones	AR	Bone dysplasia
Hyperostosis corticalis generalisata (van Buchem disease) [12, 13]	—	Facial paralysis, cranial nerve palsies, sensorineural hearing loss, thickening of skull and mandible	Increased density of ribs, clavicles, diaphyses of long bones	AR	Bone dysplasia
Albers-Schönberg disease (recessive osteopetrosis) [14]	All ossicles composed of abnormal bone	Facial paralysis, sensorineural hearing loss	Increased density of all bones	AR	Bone dysplasia

[a]AD: autosomal dominant; AR: autosomal recessive; X: X-linked; CHR: chromosomal abnormality; ND: not described.

Sclerosteosis [15]	Fixation of ossicles, closure of round window	Sensorineural hearing loss, hypertelorism, midfacial hypoplasia, cranial nerve paralysis	Generalized osteosclerosis	AR	Bone dysplasia
Dominant craniometaphyseal dysplasia [16–18]	Fixation of malleus and incus in epitympanum	Hypertelorism, progressive sensorineural hearing loss, progressive facial paralysis	Progressive hyperostosis of cranial and facial bones, splaying of metaphyseal ends of long bones	AD	Bone dysplasia
Recessive craniometaphyseal dysplasia [19]	Fixation of ossicles in epitympanum	Hypertelorism, cranial nerve abnormalities (II, VII, VIII)	Metaphyseal widening of long bones	AR	Bone dysplasia
Frontometaphyseal dysplasia [3, 20]	Fixed malleus and incus (one case)	Enlarged supraorbital ridge, hypoplasia of angle of mandible	Muscle wasting, flexion, deformities of fingers, increased density in diaphyseal region of long bones, generalized skeletal changes (progressive)	AD *or* X	Bone dysplasia
Cleidocranial dysplasia [3, 21–23]	Incudomalleal fusion and ankylosis in epitympanum, congenital fixation of the stapedial footplate	Narrowed external canals	Hypoplastic clavicles, wormian bones	AD	Bone dysplasia
Achondroplasia [3]	Fusion of ossicular chain at multiple sites	Malformation of entire cochlear capsule	Generalized retardation of cartilaginous growth	AD	Bone dysplasia

(continued next page)

TABLE 2 (Continued)

Syndrome	Middle ear malformations	Associated Malformations		Inheritance	Underlying developmental defect
		Local	Systemic		
		Progressive — 2. Abnormalities of connective tissue			
Osteogenesis imperfecta [24–26]	Fixation of stapedial footplate	Facial dysplasia, sensorineural hearing loss	Blue sclerae, brittle bones, loose ligaments, dentinal defects	AD	Disorder of connective tissue
Keratoconus, blue sclerae, loose ligaments, conductive deafness [27, 28]	Fixation of stapedial footplate	None	Blue sclerae, keratoconus, progressive visual impairment, hyperextensible joints, scoliosis, spondylolistiasis	AR	Disorder of connective tissue
Multiple synostoses and conductive deafness (symphalangism-brachydactyly syndrome) [29]	Ankylosis of stapes, malformed stapes and incus	None	Progressive proximal symphalangism, carpal and tarsal coalition, hypoplasia of nails	AD	Disorder of connective tissue
Progressive lipodystrophy of the face and arms, multiple bone cysts, and conductive deafness [30]	—	None	Lipodystrophy of face and arms, bone cysts	AR	Disorder of connective tissue
Kniest syndrome [31]	—	Cleft palate	Short limbs, clubfeet, stiff joints, myopia, retinal detachment	AD	Disorder of connective tissue

Progressive – 3. Mucopolysaccharide metabolism				
Mucopolysaccharidoses (Hurler and Hunter) [32–34]	Absence of incudo-malleal joint, exostoses in tympanic cavity, absence or obliteration of oval and round windows, mesenchyme in middle ear	None	Skeletal abnormalities, mental retardation, decreased mobility of joints	AR (Hurler and Hunter)	Metabolism of mucopolysaccharides
Progressive – 4. Unknown underlying developmental defect				
Progressive external ophthalmoplegia, retinal pigmentary degeneration, cardiac conductive defects, and mixed hearing loss [35]	—	Facial weakness, vestibular hypofunction	Cardiac conductive defects, cerebellar ataxia, corticospinal tractal signs, ptosis, progressive external ophthalmoplegia, retinal pigmentary degeneration, bulbar weakness, proximal limb girdle myopathy	?	?
Nonprogressive – 1. Dysostoses, disorders of cartilage, bone, connective tissue				
Dyschondrosteosis (Madelung deformity, Leri-Weill disease) [36]	Vestigial incus, absent malleus, deformed stapes, fixation of footplate	Narrow external canals	Mesomelic dwarfism, deformity of distal radius and ulna and proximal carpal bones	AD	Systemic dysostosis
Metaphyseal dysostosis, mental retardation, and conductive deafness [37]	—	None	Short stature, metaphyseal changes in long bones	AR	Dysostosis

(continued next page)

TABLE 2 (Continued)

Syndrome	Middle ear malformations	Associated malformations		Inheritance	Underlying developmental defect
		Local	Systemic		
Dominant symphalangism and conductive deafness [38]	Fixation of footplate	None	Symphalangism (absence of proximal interphalangeal joints), coalition of carpal and tarsal bone	AD	Bone/joint
Joint fusions, mitral insufficiency, and conductive hearing loss [39]	Fixation of footplate	None	Joint fusions (carpus, tarsus, and cervical vertebrae), mitral insufficiency	AD	Cartilage/bone
Carpal and tarsal abnormalities, cleft palate, oligodontia, and fixation of stapes [40, 41]	Fixation of footplate	Cleft palate, oligodontia	Carpal and tarsal abnormalities	AR	Connective tissue, cartilage/bone
Calcification of cartilages, brachytelephalangy, multiple peripheral pulmonary stenoses, and mixed deafness [42]	—	Sensorineural hearing loss	Brachytelephalangy, calcification of cartilages, multiple peripheral pulmonary stenoses	AR	Cartilaginous disorder
Knuckle pads, leukonychia, and mixed hearing loss [43]	Malformation of ossicular chain	Sensorineural loss, vestibular hypofunction	Knuckle pads, leukonychia	AD	Connective tissue

Nonprogressive – 2. Mesodermal defects

Microtia, hypertelorism, facial clefting, and conductive hearing loss [44]	Hypoplasia of incus and stapes, fusion of ossicles	Microcephaly, facial clefting, hypertelorism, malformed auricles, absent external auditory canal	AR	Mesodermal
Renal, genital anomalies and anomalies of the middle ear [45]	Malformed incus and fixation of malleus and incus in attic, absent incus	Narrow external auditory meatus		
		Mental retardation, ectopic kidneys, congenital heart disease, hypoplasia of thenar eminence	AR	Mesodermal
		Renal hypoplasia, internal genital malformations, vaginal atresia	AR	Mesodermal
Hypoplasia of upper limbs, cardiac arrhythmias, malformed pinnae, and unilateral conductive deafness [46]	Absence of stapes and oval window	Malformed pinnae		
		Hypoplasia of upper limbs, sinus arrhythmia	AD	Mesodermal
Orofaciodigital II syndrome (Mohr syndrome) [47, 48]	Shortened incus, fixation of stapedial footplate	Cleft tongue, cleft lip and palate, lobulated nodular tongue, broad nasal root, hypoplasia of body of mandible and zygoma, microtia, atresia of external canal		
		Polydactyly, syndactyly, microcephaly, muscular hypotonia, brachydactyly	AR	Mesodermal

Nonprogressive – 3. Regional defect

X-linked mixed hearing loss with congenital fixation of the stapedial footplate and perilymphatic gusher [49]	Fixation of stapedial footplate	Perilymphatic gusher, sensorineural hearing loss, vestibular hypofunction	None	X	Regional abnormality

(continued next page)

TABLE 2 (Continued)

Syndrome	Middle ear malformations	Associated malformations		Inheritance	Underlying developmental defect
		Local	Systemic		
Dominant hereditary conductive deafness through lack of incudostapedial junction [50, 51]	Abnormal incudostapedial joint	Hypertrophic auricular lobules, pinnal abnormalities	None	AD	Regional defect
Atresia of the external auditory canal and conductive deafness [52]	Incus and malleus deformed, stapes and tympanic membrane missing	Atresia of bony canal	None	AD	Limited regional abnormality
Lop ears, micrognathia, and conductive deafness [53]	Footplate fixed, anomalous posterior crus, rudimentary stapedial muscle and tendon	Narrow external auditory canal, lop ears, micrognathia	None	?	Regional malformation
Malformations of the ear, cervical fistulas or nodules, and mixed hearing loss, or branchial cleft anomalies, cup-shaped ears and deafness [54, 55]	Stapedial fixation, shortened lenticular process, malformed incus and stapedial fixation, rudimentary ossicles, small malleus and incus, fusion of incus and stapes, absence of oval window	Auricular deformity, preauricular pits or appendage, atresia of external canal, Mondini deformity, cervical fistulas, facial paralysis	Renal dysplasia	AD	Regional abnormality (except renal dysplasia)

				Regional abnormality
Treacher Collins syndrome, Franceschetti-Klein syndrome (mandibulofacial dysostosis) [56, 57]	Malleus fixed, fusion of malformed malleus and incus, absence of stapes and oval window, absent stapedial tendon, deformed incus and stapes, absent incus, ankylosis of stapedial footplate, bony bridge from stapes to facial canal, absence of middle ear, monopodal stapes and thinned incus	Hypoplasia of zygomas, coloboma of lower eyelids with lack of cilia medial to colobomas, mandibular hypoplasia, malformed pinnae, malformed or atretic external canal	None	AD
Crouzon syndrome (craniofacial dysostosis) [58]	Deformity of ossicles, stapedial fixation, ankylosis of malleus, ankylosis of incus	Atresia of external auditory canal, midfacial hypoplasia, hypertelorism, absence of tympanic membrane	Premature craniosynostosis	AD	Regional bone dysostosis
Robin syndrome [59]	Stapedial suprastructure and footplate thickened	Deformity of bony labyrinth, scala communis	Micrognathia, glossoptosis, cleft palate	Multifactorial?	Regional defect
Goldenhar syndrome (oculo-auriculovertebral dysplasia, OAV syndrome) [3, 60]	Incudomalleal fusion and fixation to epitympanum, stapedial malformations, fixation of the footplate, absence of oval window, absence of stapes	Anomalies of the facial nerve, atresia of external canal, auricular abnormalities, hemifacial microsomia	Coloboma of eyelids	Multifactorial?	Regional defect

(continued next page)

TABLE 2 (Continued)

Syndromes	Middle ear malformations	Associated malformations		Inheritance	Underlying developmental defect
		Local	Systemic		
		Nonprogressive — 4. Chromosomal abnormalities			
Turner syndrome [3]	Malformations of stapedial suprastructure, congenital fixation of footplate, absence of stapedial tendon	Sensorineural hearing loss, low-set elongated pinnae, cup-shaped thick lobules	Gonadal dysgenesis short stature, osteoporosis, cutaneous nevi, pterygium colli, cubitus valgus	CHR (XO)	—
Trisomy 13 [3]	Deformed stapedial suprastructure, absence of incudostapedial joint, absence of stapedial muscle and tendon	Abnormalities of modiolus	Microcephaly, mental retardation, multiple anomalies of the eye, cleft lip and palate, cardiac anomalies, abnormal palm prints	CHR	—
Trisomy 18 and deafness [61, 62]	Abnormal ossicles, abnormal course of facial nerve	Atresia of external auditory canal, malformed pinnae, micrognathia, defects in inner ear	Hypertonia, mental retardation, talipes, short sternum, cardiac abnormalities	CHR	—
Trisomy 21 and mixed deafness (Down syndrome) [63]		Sensorineural hearing loss, small rounded ears with prominent antihelix	Mental retardation, short stature, cardiac malformations, loose ligaments	CHR	—
Chromosome 18, long arm deletion (18q-) syndrome and deafness [64]	Fused and malformed ossicles	Stenosis or atresia of external auditory canal, midfacial hypoplasia, hypertelorism	Short stature, psychomotor retardation, muscular hypotonia, congenital heart disease	CHR	—

Nonprogressive – 5. Unknown underlying developmental defect

Syndrome	Middle ear findings	Other findings	Inheritance	?
Otofaciocervical syndrome [65]	—	Preauricular pits, high-arched palate, small mandible, large conchae	Lateral cervical fistulas, dermatoglyphic abnormalities, weakness of cervical muscles, retarded development of carpal bones	AD	?
Klippel-Feil anomalad and abducens paralysis with retracted bulb and sensorineural or conductive deafness (Wildervanck syndrome or cervicooculoacoustic dysplasia) [66]	Abnormal ossicles, absent oval window	Cleft palate, sensorineural hearing loss, preauricular tags, malformation or atresia of external canal, abnormal semicircular canals, dysplasia of bony labyrinth	Fusion of cervical vertebrae, mental retardation, abducens paralysis, spina bifida	Multifactorial	?
Cup-shaped ears, mixed hearing loss, and the lacrimo-auriculodentodigital syndrome [67]	—	Cup-shaped ears, sensorineural hearing loss	Hypoplasia of lacrimal puncta, digital abnormalities, small teeth	AD	?
Malformed low-set ears and conductive hearing loss [68]	Malformation of the malleus, missing incus and stapes	Malformed auricles, low-set external canals without atresia	Mental retardation, cardiac murmur, hypogonadism	AR	?
Cryptophthalmia syndrome and mixed deafness [69]	Malformed ossicles?	Atresia of outer half of ear canal, cryptophthalmia, coloboma of nasal alae, laryngeal stenosis	Syndactyly (fingers and toes), urogenital abnormalities, spina bifida occulta	AR	?

(continued next page)

TABLE 2 (Continued)

Syndrome	Middle ear malformations	Associated malformations		Inheritance	Underlying developmental defect
		Local	Systemic		
DiGeorge syndrome [70]	Absent ossicles, absent oval window	Atresia of external auditory canal, auricular defects, Mondini defect, scala communis, horizontal canal absent, hypoplasia of facial and auditory vestibular nerves	Thymic aplasia, aplasia of parathyroid	?	?
Progression unknown — 1. Bone					
Apert syndrome (acrocephalosyndactyly, type I) [71, 72]	Fixation of stapedial footplate	Craniostenosis, turribrachycephaly, hypertelorism, underdevelopment of middle one-third of face	Mental retardation, progressive synostoses of hands and feet	AD	Modeling of bone
Otopalatodigital syndrome (OPD) [73]	Thickened ossicles, short stapedial suprastructure not reaching footplate	Cleft palate, pugilistic facies, hypertelorism, small mandible	Retardation of growth, generalized dysplasia of bone, dislocation of radial head, clinodactyly	X	Modeling of bone
Progression unknown — 2. Unknown underlying developmental defect					
Ectrodactyly, ectodermal dysplasia, clefting, and mixed hearing loss (EEC syndrome) [74]	Absence of stapes and part of incus, absence of incus	Cleft lip and palate, oligodontia, absent lacrimal punctae, pinnal abnormality, sensorineural hearing loss and vestibular hypofunction	Lobster-claw deformity of hands and feet, microcephaly and mental retardation, albinoid alteration of skin and hair, renal and ureteral malformations	AD	?

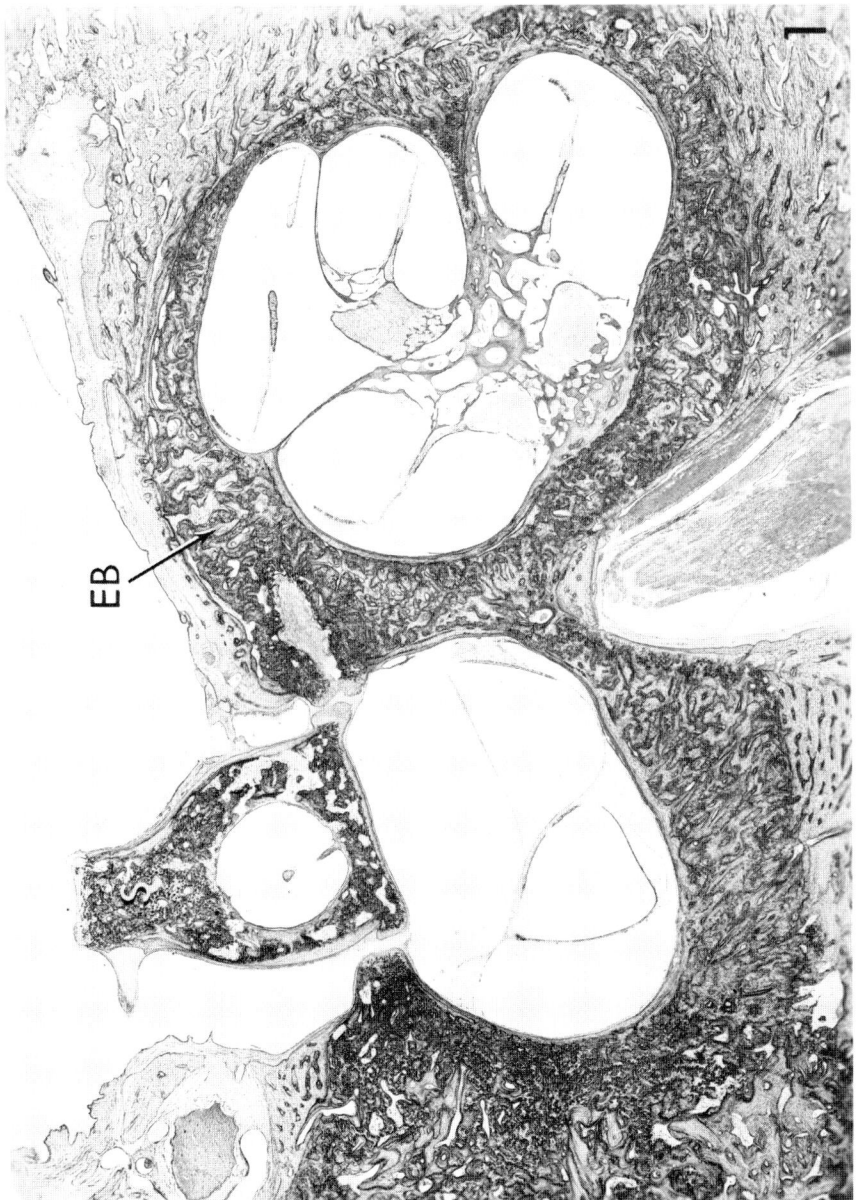

Fig. 1. *Case 1.* Albers-Schönberg disease. The stapes (S) and bone of the otic capsule modeled in cartilage (EB) demonstrated heavily calcified and persistent cartilaginous matrix.

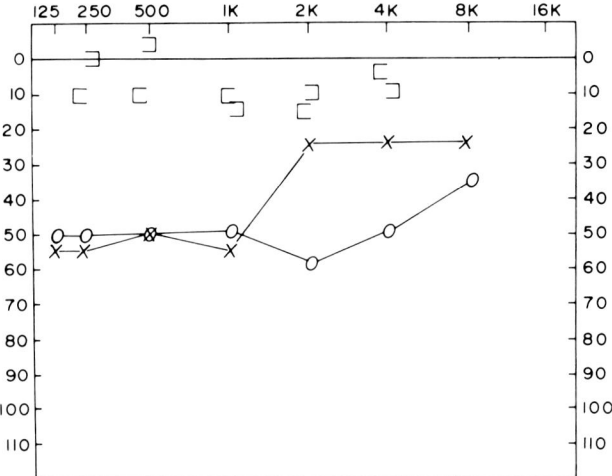

Fig. 2. *Case 2.* Sclerosteosis. Audiogram 9 years before death.

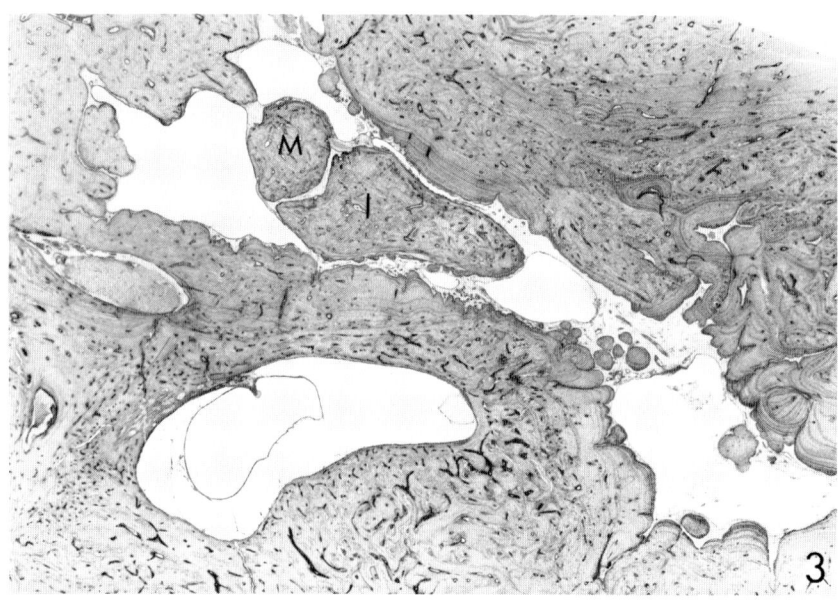

Fig. 3. *Case 2.* Sclerosteosis. In this horizontal section through the epitympanum, the malleus (M), and especially the incus (I) were crowded by bony encroachment of the epitympanic walls.

Case 2. This 30-year-old man had a progressive conductive hearing loss (Fig. 2) first detected at the age of 6 years. He and 2 of 5 sisters died of sclerosteosis. He was born with syndactyly of the 3rd and 4th fingers. He suffered recurring attacks of facial paralysis bilaterally. Other abnormalities included a large head and right-sided anosmia. He died of bacterial meningitis following craniectomy for decompression.

The temporal bone was grossly enlarged, dense, and poorly pneumatized. The external canal and epitympanum were narrowed by bony overgrowth resulting in marked narrowing of the epitympanum (Fig. 3) and bony ankylosis of the malleus to the thickened anterior epitympanic wall (Fig. 4). The stapes likewise abutted bony overgrowth in the region of the fallopian canal. The round window niche was obliterated by bone (Fig. 5). The facial and internal auditory canals were narrowed.

This group of disorders can be understood best as part of a generalized disorder of bone modeling. The dysfunction in the middle ear simply reflects the complications of dysplasia and overgrowth of bone in the limited space of the tympanic and epitympanic cavities.

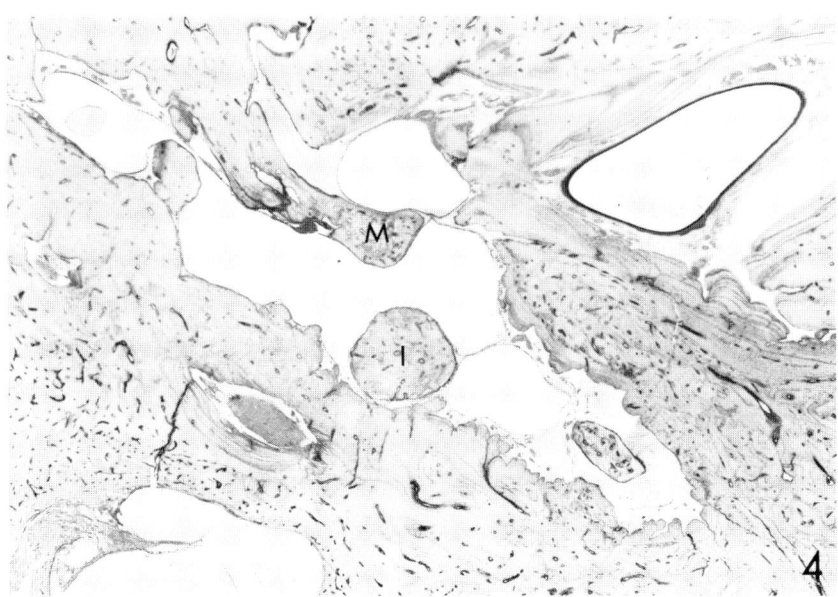

Fig. 4. *Case 2.* Sclerosteosis. The malleus (M) was fixed by bony ankylosis to the anterior epitympanic wall, and the incus (I) was close but not fused to the surrounding bone.

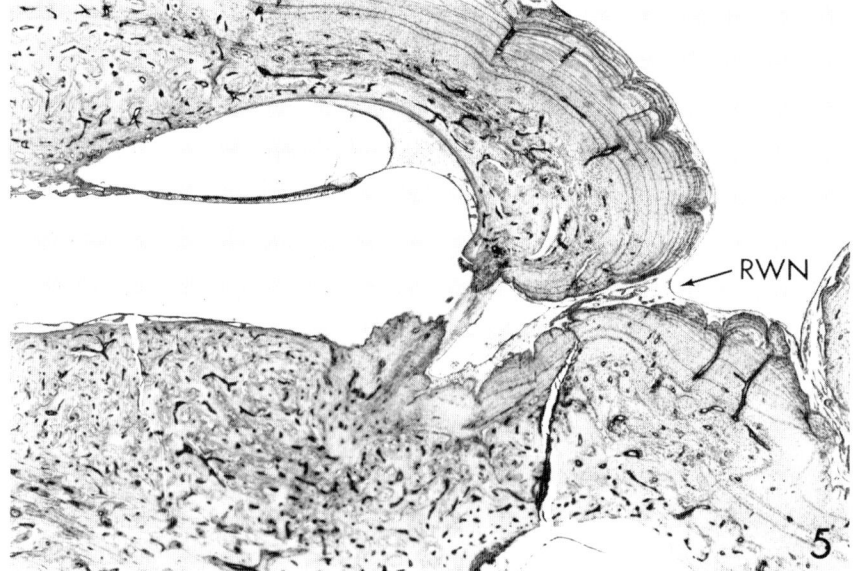

Fig. 5. *Case 2.* Sclerosteosis. The round window niche (RWN) was nearly obliterated by bony overgrowth.

Abnormalities of connective tissue. The 2nd group of genetic disorders that cause progressive conductive hearing loss demonstrates multiple defects related to connective tissues. For example, in osteogenesis imperfecta, loose joint ligaments and blue sclerae have been described in addition to a conductive hearing loss. The color of the sclerae may be due to thinness of its connective tissue matrix. Similarly, the fragility of bone characteristic of this disease is probably due to deficiencies in the mesenchymal matrix. Sensorineural hearing loss commonly seen in this disease may be due to involvement of the otic capsule and the release of toxic substances into the organ of Corti.

Findings in the middle ear have been described in only 3 of the 5 syndromes. In all 3, ankylosis of the footplate of the stapes at the stapediovestibular joint has been described as the primary cause of the conductive hearing loss. In addition, deformity of the stapedial suprastructure and of the incus have also been described in the syndrome of multiple synostoses and conductive deafness.

Mucopolysaccharidoses. The 3rd group of syndromes that cause a progressive conductive hearing loss are the mucopolysaccharidoses. The best described are the Hurler and Hunter syndromes. The underlying developmental defect is thought to be an error in metabolism of mucopolysaccharides that in turn results in an abnormal mesenchymal matrix. The abnormalities found in the middle ear include ankylosis of the incudomalleal joint, exostoses in the tympanic cavity, obliteration of the oval and round windows, and thickened mesenchyme under the epithelial lining [32–34].

Case 3. This patient with Hurler syndrome died at age 23 years of bronchopneumonia. The most striking feature in the histopathology of the temporal bones was marked thickening of the mucosa of the middle ear and mastoid that enveloped the head of the malleus and body of the incus. The thickened mucosa of the fallopian canal was reflected over the suprastructure of the stapes (Fig. 6).

Nonprogressive Conductive Hearing Loss

Abnormalities of connective tissue. The individual syndromes that form the first group of genetic disorders that produce a nonprogressive conductive hearing loss all demonstrate defects of connective tissue in the form of abnormalities of cartilage and joints and dysostoses. Although findings in the middle ear have not been described in all of the listed syndromes, fixation of the footplate of the stapes at the stapediovestibular joint is the most commonly described abnormality.

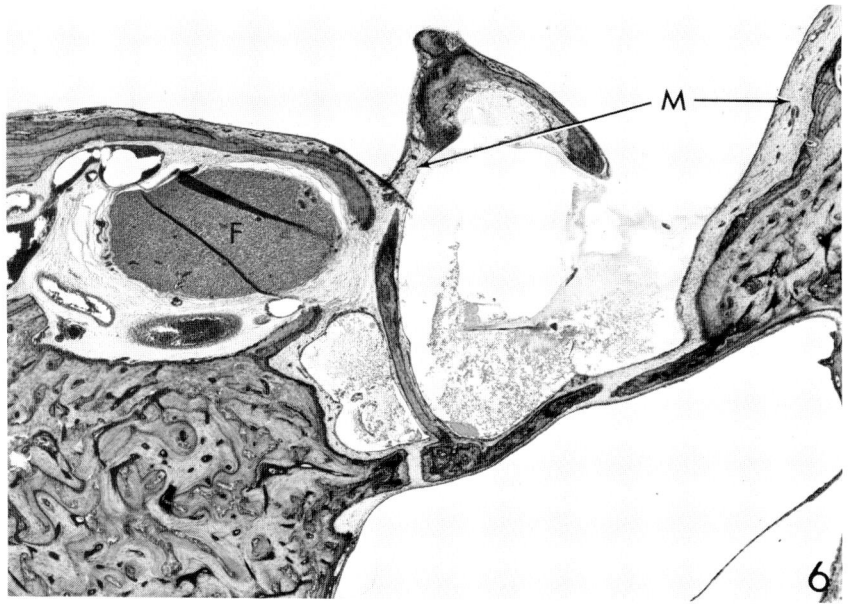

Fig. 6. *Case 3.* Hurler syndrome. The posterior crus of the stapes abutted the bony canal of the facial nerve (F), and the musoca, thickened by subepithelial mesenchyme (M), surrounded the osseous structures.

Mesodermal defects. In the 2nd group of syndromes causing a nonprogressive conductive loss, the most specific assignment of an underlying defect that can be made is "mesodermal" defects. That is, in addition to the abnormalities of the connective tissue seen in the first group, there are defects in other structures of mesodermal origin, including the genitourinary and cardiac systems. Again, the findings in the middle ear have not been described in every case. However, the architectural abnormalities generally include 2 or 3 ossicles.

Regional defects. The basis for the 3rd grouping of syndromes is the localized or regional nature of the abnormalities in each case. These may be limited to one specific area. For example, in "X-linked mixed deafness with congenital fixation of the stapes footplate and perilymphatic gusher" the abnormalities are limited to the otic capsule. In "atresia of the external auditory canal and conductive deafness" the abnormalities are limited to 1 or 2 branchial arches. Conversely, the anomalies may involve several adjacent embryologic areas or structures. For example, in Crouzon syndrome there are abnormalities of the 1st and 2nd branchial arches and tissue dorsal to them.

Although the abnormalities are limited regionally, they often involve 2 or more of the 3 primitive germ layers. To explain this group of anomalies, Poswillo [75] has expanded a hypothesis originally proposed by McKenzie [76]. The pathogenesis of these regional defects is attributed to the formation of hematomas arising from a defect in the anastomosis of the ventral pharyngeal and hyoid arteries to form the stapedial artery in the 5th week of human development. This theory was corroborated by an animal model in which pregnant rats treated with triazene produced offspring with a constellation of defects similar to the human 1st and 2nd branchial arch syndromes. Furthermore, hematomas were found in serial sections of the embryos. This hypothesis satisfactorily explains the involvement of the temporal bone, which does not arise from the branchial arches and is not supplied by the stapedial artery system, but may become involved in the spread of hematoma from contiguous areas. The relative sparing of the inner ear seen in these syndromes may be due to the formation of the cartilaginous otic capsule prior to the time of hemorrhage.

Further substantiation for this hypothesis is the finding of similar regional defects in embryos exposed to thalidomide. Similar defects were reproduced in monkey embryos treated with thalidomide, and again focal hemorrhages were found in corresponding embryologic primordia. These focal hemorrhages may cause destruction of portions of primordial tissues and delays in differentiation. The histologic findings in this group of anomalies are represented by the Treacher Collins and Crouzon syndromes.

Case 4. This patient died of pneumonia 2 months after birth. There was bilateral microtia and atresia of the external auditory canals. The facies was typical

Pathoembryology of the Middle Ear / 201

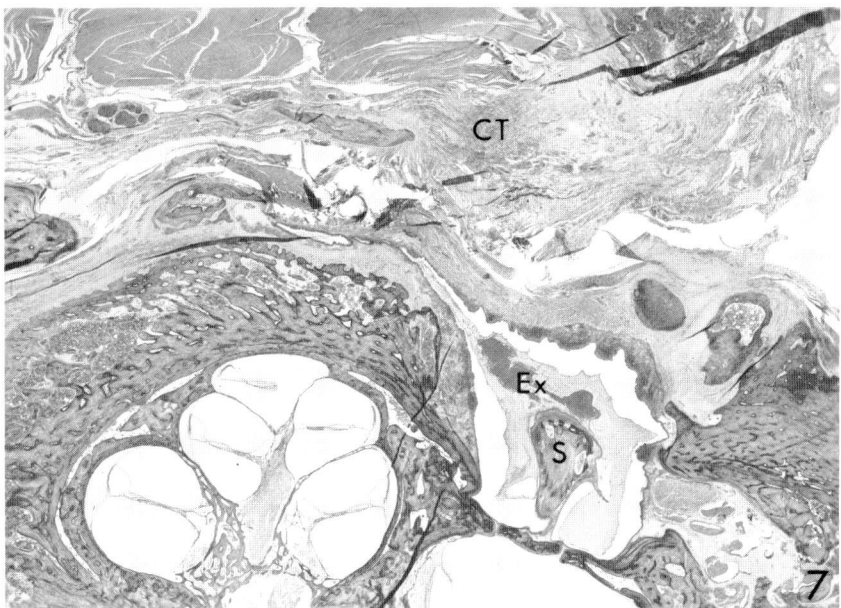

Fig. 7. *Case 4.* Treacher Collins syndrome. The external auditory canal was obliterated by connective tissue (CT). The stapedial suprastructure (S) is monopodal. There was an incidental purulent exudate (Ex) in the cleft of the middle ear.

of the Treacher Collins syndrome. The external canal was obliterated by fibrous tissue, and the stapedial suprastructure was monopodal (Fig. 7). The malleus and incus were fused.

Case 5. In this case of Crouzon syndrome there was narrowing of the external auditory canals and malformation of the suprastructure of the stapes, which was thicker than normal, deformed in shape, and possessed a narrow intercrural space (Fig. 8). In each of these cases, the bony matrix appeared normal, but there was marked abnormality in the gross architecture of the ossicles or failure in proper differentiation of a part.

Chromosomal abnormalities. Another large group of genetic syndromes resulting in a nonprogressive conductive hearing loss are the chromosomal abnormalities. As expected with multiple-gene defects, the anomalies of the middle ear are usually severe and involve all 3 ossicles.

The assignment of a specific underlying developmental defect in the chromosomal syndromes is made difficult by the multiplicity of gene defects. Similarly,

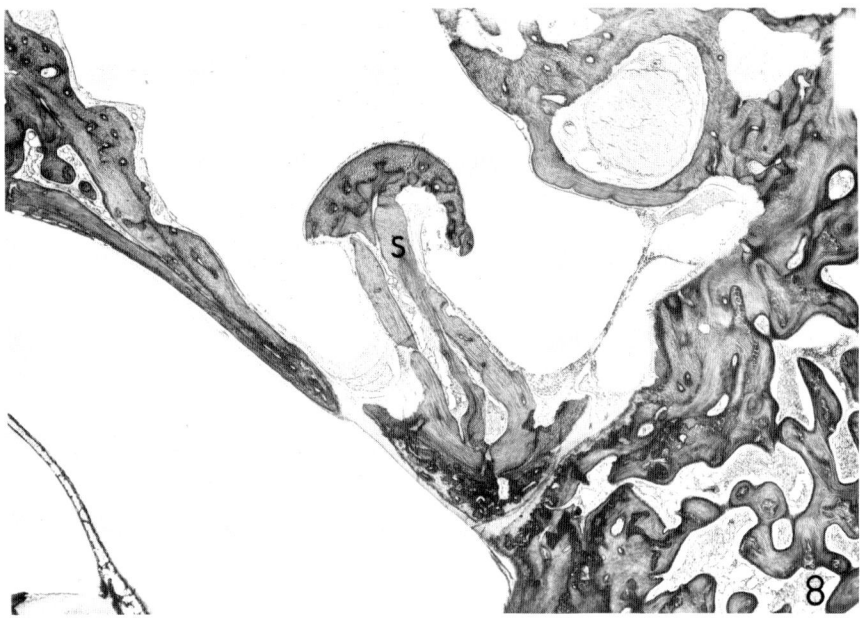

Fig. 8. *Case 5.* Crouzon syndrome. The stapedial suprastructure (S) was deformed. The crura were greatly thickened, and the intercrural space reduced.

there are a number of syndromes presumably due to a single gene defect in which even the most general of underlying developmental defects is difficult to assign (Table 2).

Case 6. This 2-week-old infant with trisomy 13 demonstrated numerous anomalies of the temporal bones. On the right, the external canal was normal, but the malleus and incus were fused. The suprastructure of the stapes was absent. On the left, there was atresia of the external auditory canal. The ossicles were malformed. There was ankylosis of the incudomalleal articulation, and the head of the stapes articulated with the lateral aspect of the incudomalleal mass (Fig. 9). The stapedial suprastructure was monopodal. The cochleae were flattened bilaterally.

FREQUENCY OF OSSICULAR MALFORMATIONS AND THE BRANCHIAL ORIGINS OF THE OSSICLES

The branchial arch derivation of the auditory ossicles is not uniformly agreed upon. Reichert [77] suggested that the malleus and incus are of 1st arch origin only and that the stapedial suprastructure is derived from the 2nd arch. However,

Pathoembryology of the Middle Ear / 203

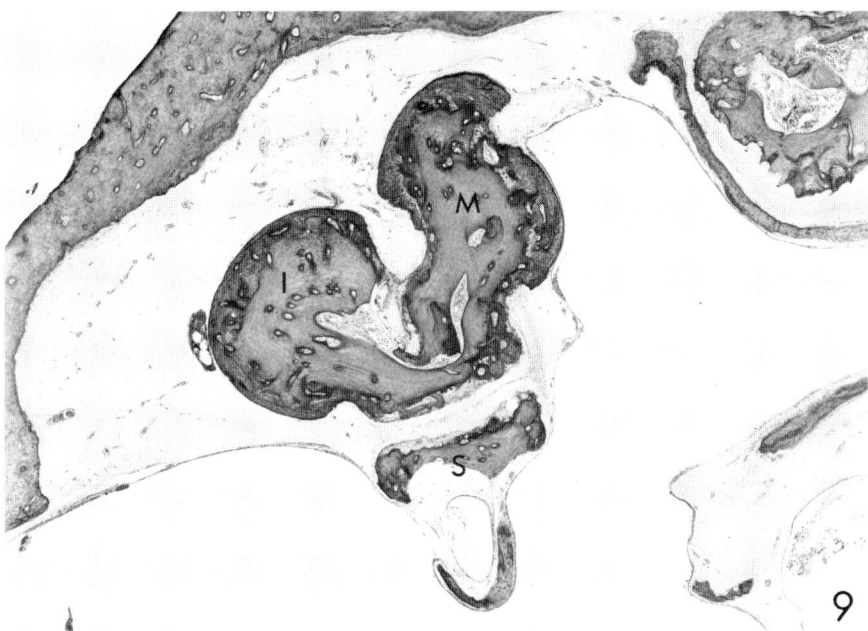

Fig. 9. *Case 6.* Trisomy 13. The ossicles were malformed. The malleus (M) and incus (I) formed a common bony mass, and the head of the stapes (S) articulated with the lateral aspect of this mass.

Anson et al [78] and Hanson et al [79] suggest that only the head of the malleus and body of the incus are of 1st arch origin, while the manubrium of the malleus, the long process of the incus, and the suprastructure of the stapes are all of 2nd arch origin, and the footplate is differentiated from the otic capsule. Hough [80], in explaining his surgical findings, has espoused the 2nd theory as being more satisfactory. Review of the genetic disorders that produce a conductive hearing loss reveals that in those syndromes in which not all ossicles are affected, ankylosis of the stapedial footplate is the most common single defect, and that anomalies of the stapes and long crus of the incus are commonly associated. However, the separation of defects is not sufficiently distinct, nor the clinical descriptions of the anomalies sufficiently specific, to warrant acceptance of one or another of the theories.

SUMMARY

Malformations of the middle ear may occur in a sporadic manner or may be genetically determined. Because the cause of sporadic anomalies is usually indeterminate, study of the genetic syndromes that lead to malformations of the middle ear, particularly those in which a single gene defect is present, offers the best opportunity to assign a probable underlying mechanism of dysmorphogenesis. Review of the literature reveals more than 50 such genetic syndromes. These have been tentatively grouped according to the characteristics of the hearing loss and the associated abnormalities, in the hope of explaining the pleiotropic effects of single gene defects by assigning a tentative underlying mechanism of dysmorphogenesis.

REFERENCES

1. Hough JVD: Malformations and anatomical variations seen in the middle ear during the operation for mobilization of the stapes. Laryngoscope 68:1337–1379, 1958.
2. Holmes LB: Inborn errors of morphogenesis. A review of localized hereditary malformations. N Engl J Med 29:763–773, 1974.
3. Caldarelli DD: Congenital middle ear anomalies associated with craniofacial and skeletal syndromes. In Jaffe BF (ed): "Hearing Loss in Children." Baltimore: University Park Press, 1977.
4. Guild SR: Histologic otosclerosis. Ann Otol Rhinol Laryngol 53:246–267, 1944.
5. Anson BJ, Wilson JG: Structural alterations in the petrous portion of the temporal bone in osteitis deformans. Arch Otolaryngol 25:560–580, 1937.
6. Clemis JD, Boyles J, Harford ER, Petasnick JP: The clinical diagnosis of Paget's disease of the temporal bone. Ann Otol Rhinol Laryngol 76:611–623, 1967.
7. Davies DG: Paget's disease of the temporal bone. A clinical and histopathological survey. Acta Otolaryngol [Suppl] (Stockh) 242:1–47, 1968.
8. Evens RG, Bartter FC: The hereditary aspects of Paget's disease: (Osteitis deformans). JAMA 205:900–902, 1968.
9. Eyring EJ, Eisenberg E: Congenital hyperphosphatasia: A clinical, pathological, and biochemical study of two cases. J Bone Joint Surg 50A:1099–1117, 1968.
10. Mitsudo SM: Chronic idiopathic hyperphosphatasia associated with pseudoxanthoma elasticum. J Bone Joint Surg 53A:303–314, 1971.
11. Thompson RC Jr, Gaull GE, Horwitz SJ, Schenk RK: Hereditary hyperphosphatasia. Studies of three siblings. Am J Med 47:209–219, 1969.
12. van Buchem FS: Hyperostosis corticalis generalisata. Eight new cases. Acta Med Scand 189:257–267, 1971.
13. van der Wouden A: Deafness caused by hyperostosis corticalis generalisata. Pract Oto Rhino Laryng 30:91–92, 1968.
14. Myers EN, Stool S: The temporal bone in osteopetrosis. Arch Otolaryngol 89:460–469, 1969.
15. Beighton P, Hamersma H, Durr L: The clinical features of sclerosteosis – A review of the manifestations in 25 affected individuals. Ann Intern Med 84:393–397, 1976.
16. Kietzer G, Paparella MM: Otolaryngological disorders in craniometaphyseal dysplasia. Laryngoscope 79:921–941, 1969.
17. Miller AL, Lehman RH, Geretti R: Unusual audiological findings in cranial-metaphyseal dysplasia. Arch Otolaryngol 89:861–864, 1969.
18. Saunders WH: Conductive deafness due to Pyle's disease. Laryngoscope 67:147–154, 1957.

19. Jackson WPU, Albright F, Drewry G, Hanelin J, Rubin MI: Metaphyseal dysplasia, epiphyseal dysplasia, diaphyseal dysplasia, and related constitutions. Arch Intern Med 94: 871–885, 1954.
20. Arenberg IK, Shambaugh GE Jr, Valvassori GE: Otolaryngologic manifestations of frontometaphyseal dysplasia. The Gorlin-Holt syndrome. Arch Otolaryngol 99:52–58, 1974.
21. Hawkins HB, Shapiro R, Petrillo CJ: The association of cleidocranial dysostosis with hearing loss. Am J Roentgenol 125:944–947, 1975.
22. Davis PL: Deafness and cleidocranial dysostosis. Arch Otolaryngol 59:602–603, 1954.
23. Fons M: Ear malformations in cleidocranial dysostosis. Acta Otolaryngol (Stockh) 67: 483–489, 1969.
24. Bretlau P, Jorgensen MB: Otosclerosis and osteogenesis imperfecta. Acta Otolaryngol (Stockh) 67:269–276, 1969.
25. Bretlau P, Jorgensen MB, Johansen H: Osteogenesis imperfecta. Light and electron-microscopic studies of the stapes. Acta Otolaryngol (Stockh) 69:172–184, 1970.
26. Robertson MS, Gregory J: Deafness, blue sclerae, and fragilitas ossium. J Laryngol 76: 655–660, 1962.
27. Greenfield G, Romano A, Stein R, Goodman RM: Blue sclerae and keratoconus: Key features of a distinct heritable disorder of connective tissue. Clin Genet 4:8–16, 1973.
28. Konigsmark BW, Gorlin RJ (eds): "Genetic and Metabolic Deafness." Philadelphia: WB Saunders, 1976, pp 128–130.
29. Maroteaux P, Bouvet JP, Briard ML: La maladie des synostosis multiples. Nouv Presse Med 1:3041–3047, 1972.
30. van Leeuwen HC: Über familiäres Vorkommen von Lipodystrophobia progressiva zusammen mit Otosklerose, Knochenzysten und geistiger Debilität. Z Klin Med 123: 534–547, 1933.
31. Roaf R, Longmore JB, Forrester RM: A childhood syndrome of bone dysplasia, retinal detachment, and deafness. Dev Med Child Neurol 9:464–472, 1967.
32. Kelemen G: Hurler's syndrome and the hearing organ. J Laryngol 80:791–803, 1966.
33. Wolff D: Microscopic study of temporal bones in dysostosis multiplex (gargoylism). Laryngoscope 52:218–222, 1942.
34. Zechner G, Altmann F: The temporal bones in Hunter's syndrome (gargoylism). Z Hals-Nas-u Ohrenheilk 192:137–144, 1968.
35. Gadoth N: Chronic progressive external ophthalmoplegia with severe cardiac dysrythmia: The value of early recognition and cardiac pacing. Isr J Med Sci 13:159–160, 1977.
36. Nassif R, Harboyan G: Madelung's deformity with conductive hearing loss. Arch Otolaryngol 91:175–178, 1970.
37. Rimoin DL, McAlister WH: Metaphyseal dysostosis, conductive hearing loss, and mental retardation: A recessively inherited syndrome. In Bergsma D (ed): Part IX. "Ear." Baltimore: Williams & Wilkins for The National Foundation-March of Dimes, BD:OAS VII(4): 116–122, 1971.
38. Vase P, Prytz S, Pedersen PS: Congenital stapes fixation, symphalangism and syndactylia. Acta Otolaryngol (Stockh) 80:394–398, 1975.
39. Forney WR, Robinson SJ, Pascoe DJ: Congenital heart disease, deafness, and skeletal malformations: A new syndrome? J Pediatr 68:14–26, 1966.
40. Gorlin RJ, Schlorf RA, Paparella MM: Cleft palate, stapes fixation, and oligodontia: A new autosomal recessively inherited syndrome. In Bergsma D (ed): Part IX. "Orofacial Structures." Baltimore: Williams & Wilkins for The National Foundation-March of Dimes, BD:OAS VII(7):87–88, 1971.

41. Spoendlin H: Congenital stapes ankylosis and fusion of tarsal and carpal bones as a dominant hereditary syndrome. Arch Otolaryngol 206:173–179, 1974.
42. Keutal J, Jorgensen G, Garbriel P: A new autosomal recessive syndrome: Peripheral pulmonary stenoses, brachytelephalangism, neural hearing loss, and abnormal cartilage calcifications/ossifications. In Bergsma D (ed): Part XV. "The Cardiovascular System." Baltimore: Williams & Wilkins for The National Foundation–March of Dimes, BD:OAS VIII(5):60–68, 1972.
43. Bart RS, Pumphrey RE: Knuckle pads, leukonychia, and deafness: A dominantly inherited syndrome. N Engl J Med 276:202–207, 1967.
44. Bixler D, Christian JC, Gorlin RJ: Hypertelorism, microtia, and facial clefting. A newly described inherited syndrome. Am J Dis Child 118:495–498, 1969.
45. Winter JSD, Kohn G, Mellman WJ, Wagner S: A familial syndrome of renal, genital, and middle ear anomalies. J Pediatr 72:88–93, 1968.
46. Stoll C, Levy JM, Francfort JJ, Roos R, Rohmer A: L'association phocomelie-ectrodactylie, malformations des oreilles avec surdité, arythmie sinusale. Arch Fr Pédiatr 31:669–680, 1974.
47. Rimoin DL, Edgerton MT: Genetic and clinical heterogeneity in the oral-facial-digital syndrome. J Pediatr 71:94–102, 1967.
48. Jorgenson RJ: Orofaciodigital syndrome II (OFD II) in brother and sister. Supra #40, p 271.
49. Nance WE, Setleff RC, McLeod A, Sweeney A, Cooper C, McConnell F: X-linked mixed deafness with congenital fixation of the stapedial footplate and perilymphatic gusher. Supra #37, p 64.
50. Escher F, Hirt H: Dominant hereditary conductive deafness through lack of incus stapes junction. Acta Otolaryngol 65:25–32, 1966.
51. Wilmot TJ: Hereditary conductive deafness due to incus-stapes abnormalities and associated with pinna deformity. J Laryngol 84:469–479, 1970.
52. Hefter E, Ganz H: Bericht über vererbte Gehörgangmissbildungen. HNO 17:76–78, 1969.
53. Supra #28, p 73.
54. McLaurin JW, Kloepfer HW, Laguaite JK, Stallcup TA: Hereditary branchial anomalies and associated hearing impairment. Laryngoscope 76:1277–1288, 1966.
55. Nevin NC: Hereditary deafness associated with branchial fistulae and external ear malformations. J Laryngol 81:709–716, 1977.
56. Sando I, Hemenway WG, Morgan WR: Histopathology of the temporal bones in mandibulofacial dysostosis. Trans Am Acad Ophthalmol Otolaryngol 72:913–924, 1968.
57. Hutchinson JC Jr, Caldarelli DD, Valvassori GE, Pruzansky S, Parris PJ: The otologic manifestations of mandibulofacial dysostosis. Trans Am Acad Ophthalmol Otolaryngol 84:520–528, 1977.
58. Boedts D: La surdité dans la dysostose craniofaciale ou maladie de Crouzon. Acta Otorhinolaryngol Belg 21:143–155, 1967.
59. Igarashi M, Filippone MV, Alford BR: Temporal bone findings in Pierre Robin syndrome. Laryngoscope 86:1679–1687, 1976.
60. Gorlin RJ, Pindborg JJ, Cohen MM Jr: "Syndromes of the Head and Neck," 2nd Ed. New York: McGraw-Hill, 1976.
61. Black FO, Sando I, Wagner JA, Hemenway WG: Middle and inner ear abnormalities 13-15 D_1 trisomy. Arch Otolaryngol 93:615–619, 1971.
62. Kos AO, Schuknecht HF, Singer AJ: Temporal bone studies in 13-15 and 18 trisomy syndrome. Arch Otolaryngol 83:439–445, 1966.
63. Fulton RT, Lloyd LL: Hearing impairment in a population of children with Down's syndrome. Am J Ment Defic 73:298–302, 1968.

64. Bergstrom L, Stewart J, Kenyon B: External auditory atresia and the deletion chromosome. Laryngoscope 84:1905–1917, 1974.
65. Fara M, Chlupackova V, Hrivnakova J: Dismorphia oto-facio-cervicalis familaris. Acta Chir Plast (Praha) 9:255–268, 1967.
66. Fraser WI, MacGillivray RC: Cervico-oculo-acoustic-dysplasia. J Ment Defic Res 12:322–329, 1968.
67. Hollister DW, Klein SH, De Jager NJ, Lachman RS, Rimoin DL: The lacrimo-auriculo-dento-digital syndrome. J Pediatr 83:438–444, 1973.
68. Mengel MC, Konigsmark BW, Berlin CI, McKusick VA: Conductive hearing loss and malformed low-set ears as a possible recessive syndrome. J Med Genet 6:14–21, 1969.
69. Ide CH, Wollschlaeger PB: Multiple congenital abnormalities associated with cryptophthalmia. Arch Ophthalmol 81:640–644, 1969.
70. Black FO, Spanier SS, Kohut RI: Aural abnormalities in partial DiGeorge syndrome. Arch Otolaryngol 101:129–134, 1975.
71. Bergstrom LV, Neblett LM, Hemenway WG: Otologic manifestations of acrocephalosyndactyly. Arch Otolaryngol 96:117–123, 1972.
72. Lindsay JR, Black FO, Donnelly WN Jr: Acrocephalosyndactyly (Apert's syndrome). Temporal bone findings. Ann Otol Rhinol Laryngol 84:174–178, 1975.
73. Buran DJ, Duvall AJ: The oto-palato-digital (OPD) syndrome. Arch Otolaryngol 85:394–399, 1967.
74. Robinson GC, Wildervanck LS, Chiang TP: Ectrodactyly, ectodermal dysplasia and cleft lip-palate. Its association with conductive hearing loss. J Pediatr 82:107–109, 1973.
75. Poswillo D: The pathogenesis of the first and second branchial arch syndrome. Oral Surg 35:302–328, 1973.
76. McKenzie J: The first arch syndrome. Dev Med Child Neurol 8:55–66, 1966.
77. Reichert C: Arch Anat Physiol Wiss Med 8:120, 1837.
78. Anson BJ, Hanson JS, Richany SF: Early embryology of the auditory ossicles and associated structures in relation to certain anomalies observed clinically. Ann Otol Rhinol Laryngol 69:427–447, 1960.
79. Hanson JR, Anson BJ, Strickland EM: Branchial sources of the auditory ossicles in man. Arch Otolaryngol 76:200–215, 1962.
80. Hough JVD: Congenital malformations of the middle ear. Arch Otolaryngol 78:335–343, 1963.

DISCUSSION

Dr. Joseph Nadol: In these 5 syndromes, middle ear findings have been described in only 3. In all 3, there is ankylosis of the stapedial footplate at the stapediovestibular joint.

Dr. David Lim: Is the sensorineural hearing loss in this group due to bony growths into the internal auditory meatus?

Dr. Joseph Nadol: The two causes that have been described are compression of the auditory nerve and hair cell loss.

Dr. Harold Schuknecht: I don't think any of these bone disorders create a retrocochlear lesion. Clinically, it doesn't look like an internal auditory canal problem. The internal auditory canal may be markedly narrowed; but there's still room for the nerve. In Paget disease, there is no clinical evidence of a retrocochlear lesion.

Dr. Heinrich Spoendlin: How about compression of the vessels?

Dr. Harold Schuknecht: It is possible, but I doubt it.

Dr. Isabelle Rapin: The internal auditory canal can be narrowed in osteopetrosis.

Dr. Robert Ruben: We have another case of osteopetrosis in which radiographs showed total obliteration of the internal auditory meatus.

Dr. Joseph Nadol: The bony overgrowth in that case might be secondary to damage of the membranous labyrinth. We often see that with vascular occlusion.

Dr. Robert Ruben: I would agree with Dr. Schuknecht on a clinical basis that typical Paget disease usually has open internal auditory meati.

Dr. Harold Schuknecht: I had the opportunity of examining some of these patients in Praetoria, South Africa.

Dr. Robert Gorlin: With Hamersma? Then they are examples of sclerosteosis.

Dr. Harold Schuknecht: Yes, he's doing facial nerve decompressions and reconstructive ear surgery on some of these cases.

Dr. Robert Gorlin: This whole area is an extremely complex one. For example, there seems to be considerable doubt that Van Buchem disease exists at all. All of Van Buchem's patients, and I believe there were 7 in his first report and 8 in the second report, stemmed from Dutch extraction. Hamersma and Beighton's sclerosteosis cases are also of Dutch extraction. The slight differences which exist between Van Buchem disease and sclerosteosis are at most dubious. Van Buchem states that he noted excrescences in the periosteum of his patients, and yet in talking to Beighton concerning older patients with sclerosteosis, these individuals also have excrescences. One cannot use elevated alkaline phosphatase levels, because there's no constancy among either group. Most patients with sclerosteosis have been abnormally tall. Many of the women among this group have been over 6 feet tall, and the majority have had some degree of syndactyly between digits 2 and 3 with a bending of the terminal phalanx of the index finger. But, again, it's not a constant feature, and I doubt that there is a true Van Buchem disease.

Dr. Joseph Nadol: The third group of syndromes that cause a progressive conductive loss is characterized by a thickness of the mucosa and its subepithelial connective tissue that envelops the middle ear and ossicular chain. This individual had Hurler syndrome.

Dr. Isabelle Rapin: How certain are you that this individual had classic Hurler syndrome? Most classic Hurler patients do not live to the age of 23.

Dr. Joseph Nadol: Well, that was the clinical diagnosis.

Dr. Harold Schuknecht: Children with Hurler syndrome frequently have serious otitis.

Dr. Joseph Nadol: In my practice I have one of these children with serious effusion and thick spongy mucosa.

Dr. LaVonne Bergstrom: I've also seen a couple of Hurler syndrome patients in state homes for the retarded who appeared to have serous otitis. Unfortunately, the circumstances did not permit us taking a biopsy. About 8 years ago, several of us from Colorado described a case of Hunter syndrome, which is an X-linked recessive disorder, who had a progressive sensorineural hearing loss without any evidence of serous or suppurative otitis.

Dr. Joseph Nadol: There is a syndrome of progressive external opthalmoplegia, retinal pigmentary degeneration, cardiac conductive defects, and mixed hearing loss. The inheritance is not known. It may not be a single gene defect, but multi-factorial, which would explain the tremendous variety of abnormalities that occur.

Dr. Isabelle Rapin: The most recent evidence is that this syndrome is not genetic.

Dr. Jon Aase: Is there an eponym for this?

Dr. Robert Gorlin: Yes, Kearns-Sayre syndrome.

Dr. David Smith: One of the most remarkable things to me is the short distance from the middle ear to the meatus. Is that true in other instances of atresia?

Dr. Joseph Nadol: Well, the soft tissue of external ear has been removed. Sometimes the atretic plate may be several millimeters in thickness.

Dr. Robert Gorlin: It has been shown that azothiaprine and thalidomide produce conditions similar to hemifacial microsomia or oculoauriculoverterbral (Goldenhar) syndrome, but that Treacher Collins syndrome was caused by selective death of cells within the neural crest.

Dr. David Lim: Dr. Schuknecht, do you know the status of the otoconia or the gravity receptors in the mucopolysaccharidoses?

Dr. Harold Schuknecht: No, I haven't looked at it.

Discussion of Middle Ear Anomalies —
Reply to Dr. Nadol

Isamu Sando, MD, DMS

As an addition to Dr. Nadol's presentation, I would like to report on our recent study and review of the literature on anomalies of the middle ear, and present representative illustrations of anomalous structures. We found 48 diseases which involve anomalies of the middle ear (Table 1). Anomalies of the ossicles were observed most commonly, occurring in 42 of 48 diseases that were reviewed. Anomalies of the tympanic cavity were less frequent, being observed in 18 of the diseases, and anomalies of the nerves of the middle ear were seen to be associated with 14 of the diseases studied. Of the ossicular anomalies, the stapedial anomalies were the most commonly observed, occurring in 34 of the 42 diseases studied. Anomalies of the facial nerves were the most commonly encountered of all anomalies of the nerves, occurring in 11 of the 14 diseases. Of anomalies of the intratympanic muscles, those involving the stapedial muscle occurred more frequently than those of the tensor tympani muscle and were found in 7 out of 8 diseases. Persistence of the stapedial artery was the most frequently observed anomaly of the vessels of the middle ear and was associated with 6 out of 10 diseases.

Figure 1 is a photomicrograph of a section of temporal bone from a 10-day-old boy with Treacher Collins syndrome. A bony tympanic plate has replaced the area usually occupied by the tympanic membrane, the malleus, and the incus; and a columelliform stapes is present. Figure 2 shows a photomicrograph of a slide from the temporal bone from the same boy with Treacher Collins syndrome. The facial nerve may be seen exiting the temporal bone laterally, instead of transversing it.

Figure 3 is a photomicrograph of a section of temporal bone from a 10-day-old girl with trisomy 18 syndrome. Absence of the stapedial tendon and its bony pyramidal eminence has resulted in exposure of the stapedial muscle to the middle ear space. Figure 4 is a photomicrograph of a section of temporal bone from a 6½-week-old girl with trisomy 13 syndrome, showing a persistent stapedial artery in the area of the stapedial obturator foramen. In Figure 5, an extremely small epitympanic cavity may be seen in the temporal bone of a 10-day-old boy with Treacher Collins syndrome. Figure 6 is a photomicrograph of a section of temporal bone from a 4-day-old girl with trisomy 13 syndrome and demonstrates the absence of the bony portion of the eustachian tube and the bony carotid canal.

Table 2 is a summary of the relationships of the anomalies of the middle ear, with or without associated anomalies in other parts of the body, to the etiologies of the diseases studied. E, M, I, and O represent anomalies observed in the external ear, the middle ear, the inner ear, and the other parts of the body, respectively. Through this study we noted the following trends:

1) Hereditary characteristics of disease are very commonly associated with anomalies of the middle ear. Of the 48 diseases studied, 32 were hereditary. The second most common association of anomalies of the middle ear is with diseases of unknown etiology; this was the case in 12 of the 48 diseases studied.

2) Most of the diseases associated with anomalies of the middle ear are diseases also associated with anomalies in parts of the body other than the ear. Among these diseases, those involving anomalies of the external ear, of the middle ear, of the inner ear, and of other parts of the body are the most common (33 of 48 diseases studied).

TABLE 1. Anomalies of the Middle Ear (48 Diseases)

Tympanic membrane		7
Ossicles		42
Malleus	20	
Incus	25	
Stapes	34	
Nerves		14
Facial nerve	11	
Chorda tympani nerve	5	
Superficial petrosal nerve	2	
Muscles		8
Tensor tympani muscle	4	
Stapedial muscle	7	
Vessels		10
Internal carotid artery	2	
Stapedial artery	6	
Jugular bulb	3	
Tympanic cavity		18
Mastoid		6
Eustachian tube		1
Carotid canal		1

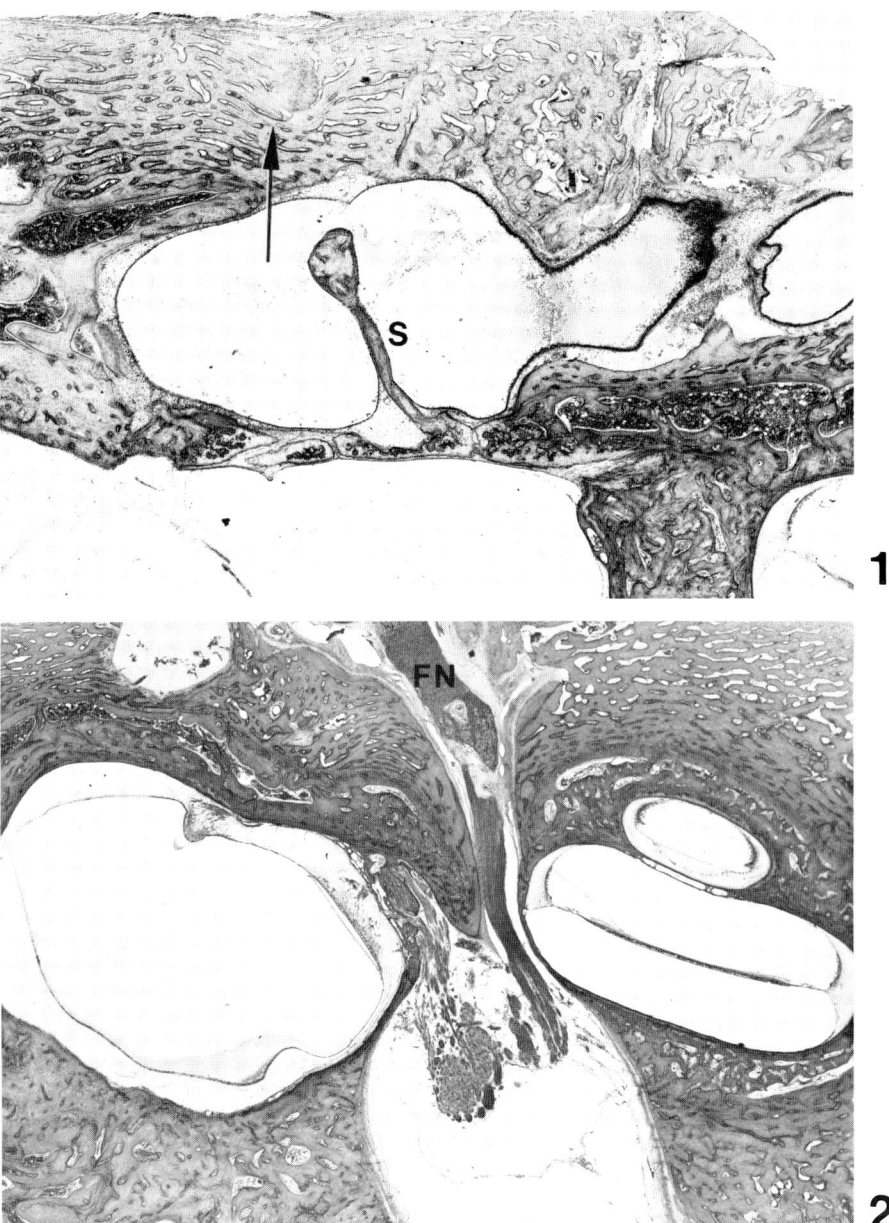

Fig. 1. Human temporal bone: horizontal histologic section showing bony tympanic plate (arrow) and the columella type of stapes (S). (H & E ×13)

Fig. 2. Section of human temporal bone: horizontal histologic slide. FN indicates abnormal course of facial nerve. (H & E ×8)

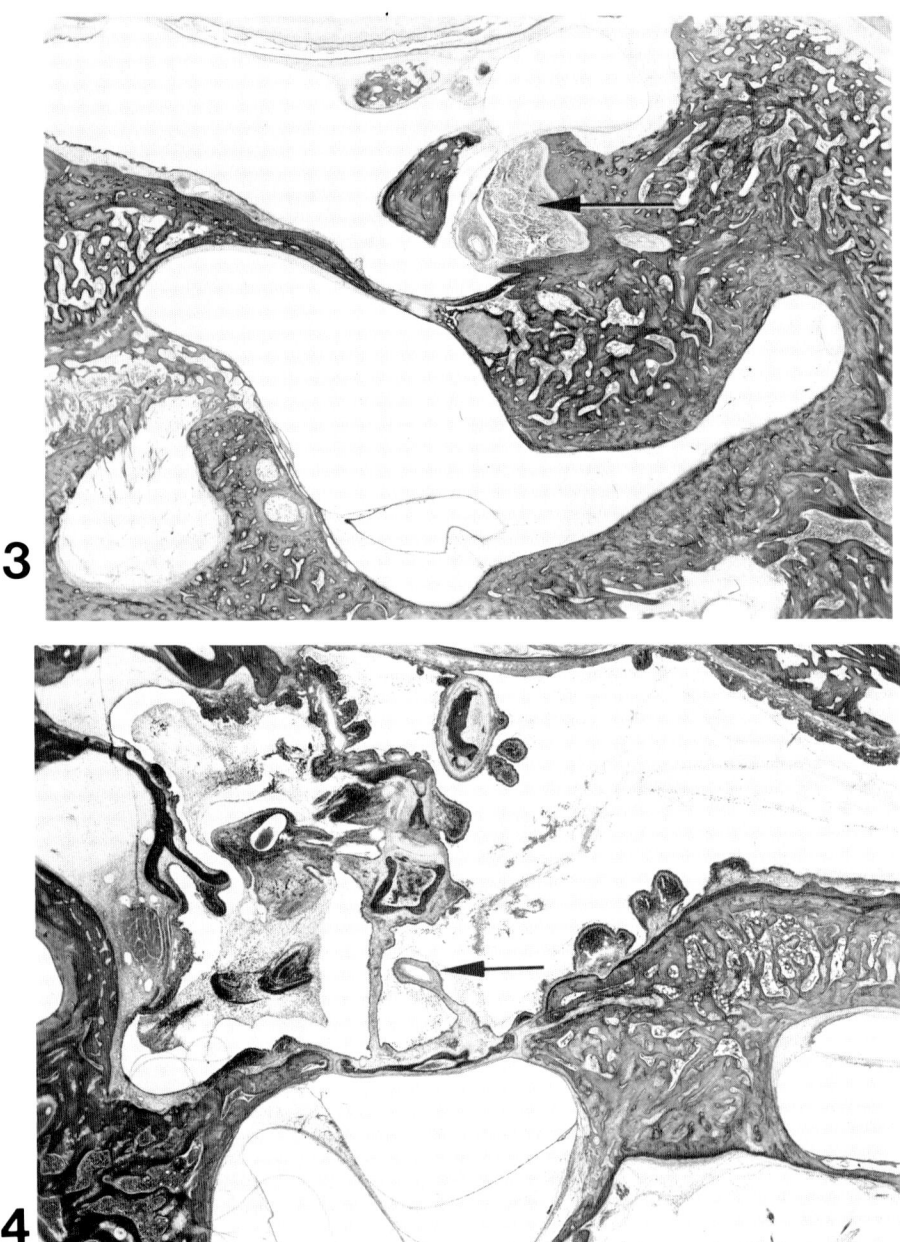

Fig. 3. Human temporal bone: histologic section showing exposure of the stapedial muscle to the space of the middle ear (arrow). (H & E ×14)

Fig. 4. Human temporal bone: horizontal histologic section showing persistent stapedial artery (arrow). (H & E ×8)

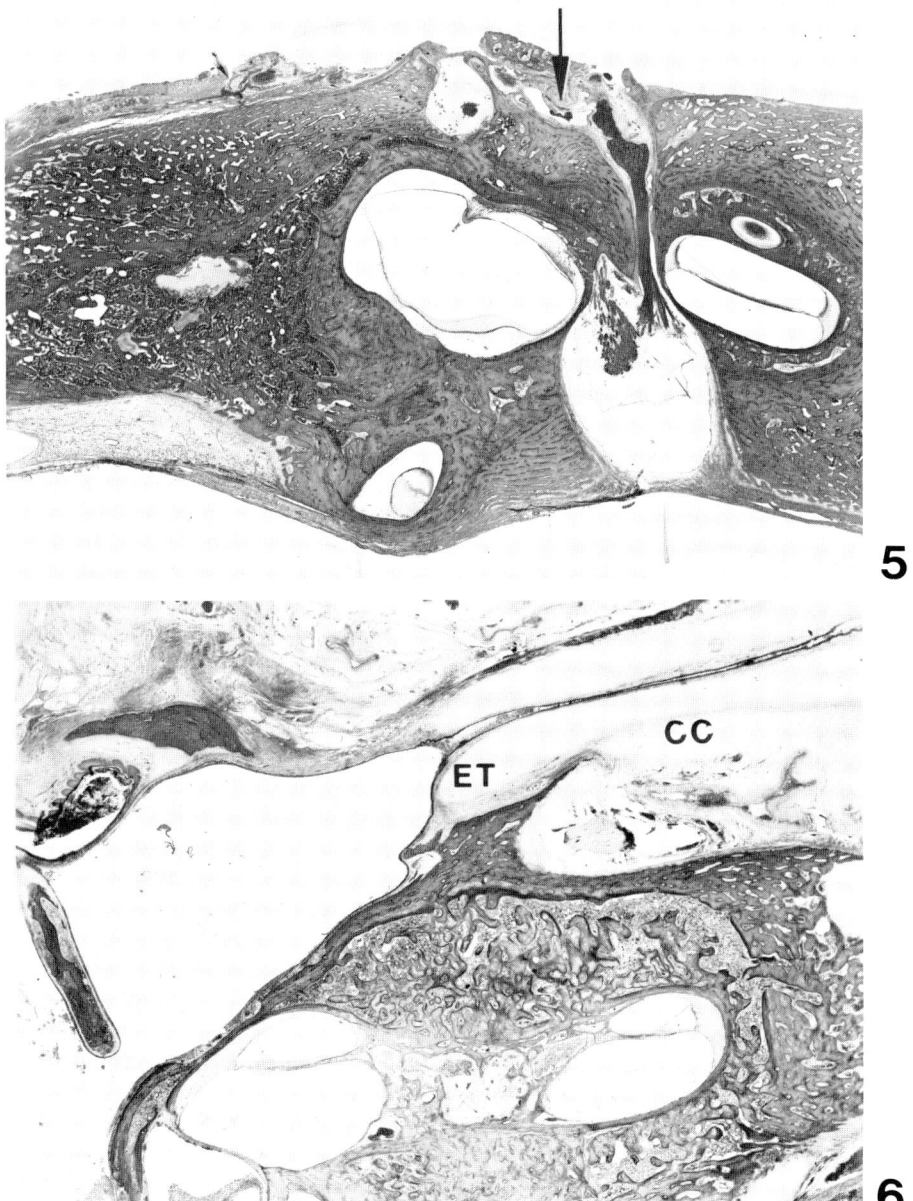

Fig. 5. Human temporal bone: horizontal section showing extremely small epitympanic cavity (arrow). (H & E ×4.5)

Fig. 6. Human temporal bone: histologic section showing eustachian tube (ET) and carotid canal (CC) in very close proximity, both lacking their bony canals. (H & E ×12)

TABLE 2. Relation of Anomalies of the Middle Ear to Etiologies of Diseases

Etiologies Anomalies	Unknown etiologies	Hereditary characteristics	Prenatal infections	Iatrogenic ototoxicities	Environmental factors	Total
M	6	1				7
E, M		1				1
M, I						0
E, M, I						0
M, O		7	1			8
E, M, O	2	9				11
M, I, O	1	5	1		1	8
E, M, I, O	3	9		1		13
Total	12	32	2	1	1	48

ACKNOWLEDGMENT

I would like to express my appreciation to the University of Colorado Medical Center for making available to me the materials used for this discussion.

Assessment and Consequence of Malformation of the Middle Ear

LaVonne Bergstrom, MD, FACS

Conductive hearing loss from an early age has long been felt to be important, but recently more and more studies have shown significant delays in language from even mild or fluctuating conductive hearing losses dating from early life [1]. New urgency has been added to the problem by recent work in experimental animals, suggesting that such impairments may result in changes in second order neurons in the cochlear nuclei [2, 3]. The early detection of isolated congenital conductive hearing loss is not easy, and significant delays may occur. Even when a child has obvious concomitant anomalies or findings of otitis media, the first formal diagnosis of hearing loss may be delayed for up to 18 years (Table 1). It would appear that priorities in assessment include: 1) upgrading our teaching of medical students, family physicians, pediatricians, and otolaryngologists in recognizing children who may be at risk for malformations of the middle ear, and 2) indoctrinating primary care physicians with the no-longer-new idea that it is possible to perform audiometry in infants and young children.

Assessment begins at birth. Of a series of children ultimately found to have congenital hearing loss, 17% were found to have defects of the conducting mechanism (Table 2). Of these, 50% have other congenital anomalies, a statistic probably somewhat unrepresentative of the population as a whole, since two-thirds of all those cases of congenital hearing loss are derived either from multidisciplinary clinics devoted to the diagnosis and care of children with birth defects or from a residential school for the retarded. Those children, who have isolated middle ear defects and appear otherwise normal, generally go to regular schools and are hard to find in published surveys of hearing or otologic problems in public schools. Available statistics suggest an incidence of approximately 0.4% in children in public schools [4].

The first step in assessment is suspecting the problem. Very frequently family history is not believed to be positive where isolated defects of the middle ear are

TABLE 1. Treatment Delay in Congenital Conductive Hearing Loss

	Mean	Median
With associated defects[a] Range 0.7 to 18 yrs	4.2 yrs	4.5 yrs
No associated defects[a] Range 0.1[b] to 44 yrs	13.4 yrs	

[a]One patient had positive family history.
[b]Patient's mother thought to have had prenatal rubella, disproven.

TABLE 2. Incidence of Middle Ear Defects in 687 Children Having Congenital Hearing Loss

	No. of Cases
Isolated	8
With external ear defects	33
With systemic defects	15
With external ear and systemic defects	24
With inner ear defects	14
With external and inner ear defects	7
With inner ear and systemic defects	4
With external and inner ear and systemic defects	12
Total	117

present. In this series, 2.7% of the patients had isolated ossicular defects and had a family history of congenital conductive hearing loss without associated anomalies. A number of familial entities in which congenital anomalies of the middle ear occur have been described in the literature, but most have at least a mild pinnal or branchial abnormality. Inheritance may be autosomal dominant, autosomal recessive, or X-linked [5]. Where family history is positive, its nature should be ascertained if possible, and the infant or child examined and tested to rule out congenital conductive hearing loss.

Another risk factor for congenital middle ear anomalies is the presence of pinna or craniofacial defects. Certain syndromes such as Treacher Collins, Goldenhar, and otopalatodigital are fairly well known and recognizable in the neonatal period, but many are seldom recognized or little known. A large number of syndromes are known (Table 3), and undoubtedly there are many more. The proliferation of syndromes is confusing and difficult for all but the relatively few clinicians who do genetic counseling or consulting in cases of birth defects, in spite of the availability of several excellent, well-illustrated compendiums for reference. It is probably useful to remember the branchial origin of the middle ear, its bony and cartilaginous

TABLE 3. Syndromes Which May Be Associated With Middle Ear Defects or Progressive Conductive Hearing Loss*

Pierre Robin [6, 7]	Otopalatodigital [42]
Treacher Collins [8, 9]	Hemifacial microsomia [43]
Apert [10, 11]	First and second branchial syndrome [43]
Orofaciodigital II [12]	Frontonasal dysplasia
Pfeiffer [13]	Oculodentodigital [44]
Hallermann-Streiff	Ocular hypertelorism
Otofaciocervical [14]	Chondrodystrophia calcificans
Malformed, low-set ears [15]	Congenital facial palsy
Saethre-Chotzen [16]	Lop ears, micrognathia
Osteogenesis imperfecta [17]	Kniest syndrome [45]
Trisomy 21 [18]	Cryptophthalmia [46]
Chromosome 18 deletion syndrome [19]	Proximal symphalangism [47]
Familial branchial fistula [20–23]	VATER [48, 49]
Cleidocranial dysostosis [24]	Recurrent meningitis/stapes
Hypertrophied, thickened ear lobules [25, 26]	footplate fistula [50, 53]
Microtia and atresia [27–34]	Crouzon [54]
Osteopetrosis [35, 36]	Moebius [55]
Craniometaphyseal dysplasia [37]	Klippel-Feil [56]
Fanconi anemia syndrome [38]	Knuckle pads with leukonychia [57]
Diastrophic dwarfism [39]	Madelung deformity [58]
Thalidomide embryopathy [40, 41]	DiGeorge [59, 60]
Goldenhar [61, 62]	
Forney [63]	
Congenital cholesteatoma [64]	
Renal, genital and middle ear anomalies [65, 66]	

*Entities not having a reference number are the author's cases.

nature, and its close geographic relation to the base of the skull. Hearing loss is an important potential functional byproduct of these external anomalies, but it is surprising that visual and dental problems are often points of concentration, together with cosmetic considerations. Congenital hearing loss as a concomitant of multisystem syndromes becomes a more likely diagnosis as the number of major defects seen in an individual increases (Fig. 1). Anomalies of the middle ear make up a substantial number of the findings in these patients [67].

Prenatal injuries account for an unknown number of anomalies of the middle ear. Agents found in the histories of our patients and others include thalidomide, diphenylhydantoin, thyroid hormone, contraceptive pills, lututrin, other progestational agents, diuretic, steroid, sulfisoxazole, nitrofurantoin, cephalexin monohydrate, demethylchlortetracycline, dicyclomine HCl-doxylamine succinate, meprobamate, maternal diabetes, maternal rubella, maternal syphilis, influenza, hepatitis, hyperemesis gravidarum, toxemia of pregnancy, bleeding in the 1st trimester, pyelonephritis, irradiation in the 1st trimester, and abdominal injury in the 1st trimester [6, 10, 19, 40, 48, 60, 68–72]. Since some of these entities also have

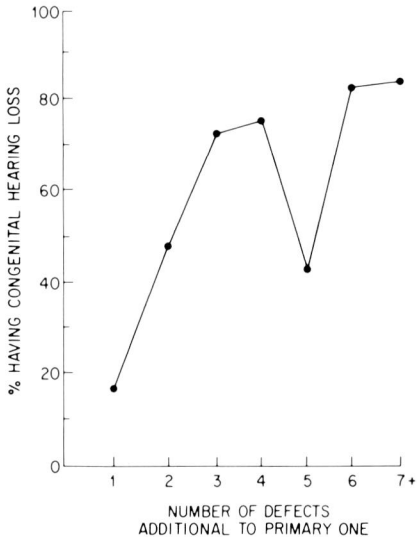

Fig. 1. Correlation of number of congenital defects and the likelihood of having congenital hearing loss. (From Bergstrom L: Congenital and acquired deafness in clefting and craniofacial syndromes. Cleft Palate J 15:254–261, 1978, with permission.)

occurred during pregnancies that result in normal children, their impact is difficult to assess. Large prospective studies would be required to detect any significant incidence of these factors in malformational syndromes. The theoretic possibility of interaction between genetic makeup and altered intrauterine environment makes evaluation of the effect of these factors even more difficult. Further, in pregnant animals, experimental exposure to trypan blue, vitamin A deficiency, irradiation [57], and corticosteroids has resulted in offspring with otic or craniofacial anomalies. Human chromosomal defects, most notably deletion of the long arm or ring formation of chromosome 18 [19], trisomy 21 [18], deletion of the long arm of chromosome 13 [6], trisomy 13 [71], trisomy 18 [69], and Turner XO syndrome [73] may cause defects of the middle ear. Some of these infants are not viable, and their anomalies remain of theoretic interest.

ASSESSMENT OF THE PATIENT

Once a defect of the middle ear has been suspected, assessment follows 2 more-or-less simultaneous courses: 1) to assess the patient, and 2) to assess the ear. Assessment of all patients includes a thorough family, prenatal, perinatal, and routine medical history. This may well include obtaining physicians' and hospitals' records of the prenatal, perinatal, and subsequent medical course, including a record of prescription and "street" drugs taken by both parents at the time of conception and subsequently, by the mother. A general physical examination is important for preanesthesia preoperative assessment, but it is more important in ruling out associated congenital defects of areas other than the head and neck (Table 4).

The young infant is ideal for specific determination of etiology. Within the 1st weeks after birth, cultures and serologic determinations for congenital viral infections and syphillis are most likely to be fruitful. They should be done if any of the following are present: microcephaly, hydrocephaly, cataract, cloudy cornea, pigmented retina, rash, petechiae, low birthweight, jaundice, hepato- or splenomegaly, depressed nasal septum, rhagades, "snuffles," bony defects, hypotonia, delayed development, poor growth, spasticity, other neurologic deficits, or heart murmurs. Appropriate consultations with other specialists should be obtained. Such an evaluation may occasionally be helpful in the workup of anomalies of the middle ear, but more frequently will be useful in the assessment of congenital sensorineural hearing loss. However, in 5 of our patients having congenital conductive or mixed hearing loss, there was a history of maternal rubella or exposure to rubella early in the 1st trimester, and in 2, congenital rubella was proven. If the child's general physical examination is unremarkable, routine blood count and urinalysis will probably suffice, and attention may be turned to assessing the ear.

The physical examination of the head and neck should be as complete as is consistent with the child's age and physical status. Oral examination will reveal defects of the stoma, teeth, and palate; pharyngeal and nasopharyngeal examination will reveal infection or hypertrophy that may adversely affect function of the eustachian tube or predispose to otitis media. Examination of the nose may reveal defects of external contour or posterior choanal atresia. Palpation of facial bones and parotid glands, and testing for mobility in the temporomandibular joint are important in looking for hemifacial microsomia and are also important in such syndromes as Pierre Robin, Treacher Collins and Goldenhar. The frontal and orbital areas and the area of the nasal bridge should be inspected to look for hypertelorism, frontal bossing, proptosis, strabismus, and other abnormalities often seen in craniofacial defects associated with anomalies of the middle ear. The neck should be inspected for branchial fistulae, webbing, shortness, immobility or torticollis, defects associated with such syndromes as hereditary branchial defects, Turner, Klippel-Feil, Wildervanck, Goldenhar, and VATER. Stridor and hoarseness may occur in the G syndrome [74, 75] (which one of our affected patients has: a laryngeal web was present). Direct or indirect laryngoscopy may be important in the examination of some children.

However, if gross otic or craniofacial anomalies are present, a number of considerations are urgent. If there is microtia with atresia or other gross defects of the external ear, especially if combined with hemifacial microsomia, the status of the kidneys should be assessed early. Urinalysis may be normal, but this fact should not deter one from pressing on with evaluation of the renal status. Ultrasonography

TABLE 4. Incidence of Inapparent Internal Defects in Patients Having Middle Ear Anomalies

Syndrome or Otic defect	No.	Internal defect	No.
Microtia/atresia	37	None	24
		Renal	7
		Cardiac	1
		Renal and skeletal	1
		Vertebral	2
		Sacral lipoma	1
		Esophageal	1
Microtia only	2	Cardiac	1
		Cardiac, ribs	1
Atresia only	9	Chromosomal	4
		Ureteral	1
Other pinna anomalies	3	Cardiac	1
		Renal	1
Pinna and craniofacial, non-syndromal	4	Esophageal	1
Ossicular defects	10	None	10
Goldenhar	3	Renal and vertebral	1
		Renal and cardiac	1
		Cardiac, skeletal	1
Klippel-Feil	2	None	2
Apert	6	None	
Pfeiffer	1	None	
Crouzon	4	Cardiac	1
		Choanal atresia	1
Treacher Collins	8	None	8
Pierre Robin	2	Cardiac, GI, skeletal	1
		Cardiac	1
Fanconi pancytopenia	4	Renal	2
Diastrophic dwarfism	1	None	
Oculodentodigital	2	Endocrine	1
Misc. multidefect, non-syndromal	10	Vertebral	2
		Multiple GI, GU CNS	1
		Paretic vocal cord	1

will demonstrate the presence and gross anatomy of the kidneys, but an IVP is the most reliable way to assess renal function and patency of the drainage system. In our series, 22.5% had significant renal defects. In isolated atresia of the external otic canal, renal defects may also occur. In the presence of atresia of the osseous canal, abnormal facies, hematologic or immunologic deficiencies, or other defects, genetic consultation and chromosomal testing may be indicated [19].

Children with gross craniofacial defects will benefit from multispecialty consultations. If there is evidence of hydrocephalus, stridor, craniostenosis or proptosis, prompt neurosurgical and ophthalmologic intervention may prevent or arrest cerebral or ocular damage or may even save the child's life. In these, as well as in less dramatic cases, x rays will be an important part of the assessment. Films of the skull may add considerably to the otologist's evaluation if a base view is included. In the infant or young child whose cranial and facial bones are not yet heavily ossified, the normal or anomalous internal auditory canal, labyrinth, malleus, incus, and mastoid often will be demonstrated beautifully. In any event, those assessing the child should try to coordinate radiographic examinations so that duplication, overlap, and inconvenience are minimized. We have often gained considerable information from careful perusal and review of existing films with the head and neck radiologist. Every effort should be made to borrow films taken previously, which may be quite helpful in evaluating the child.

Malformations of digits and limbs are seen in thalidomide embryopathy, Apert acrocephalosyndactyly, oculodentodigital syndrome, Fanconi pancytopenia, proximal symphalangism, and Madelung deformity, just to mention a few of the less subtle ones. Dwarfism is seen in Hurler and Fanconi syndromes; and gross skeletal deformities in diastrophic dwarfism, Kniest syndrome, and osteogenesis imperfecta (congenital type). X rays will be important in their overall assessment; screening for mucopolysaccharides in diagnosing Hurler and similar storage disorders; hematologic and renal workups are indicated in Fanconi syndrome. The presence of a heart murmur, cyanosis, or known or previously operated cardiac defects will suggest the congenital rubella syndrome, trisomic syndromes, and Forney syndrome. The apparent presence of retardation or dull facies should be carefully considered from the standpoint of a facial anomaly which may give such a false appearance and also point to the possibility of hearing loss [76]. Of course, assessment of developmental and intellectual level and potential are important in the overall picture, if there is any question regarding retardation.

ASSESSMENT OF THE EAR

The pinna and its symmetry of form, size, and position with its mate should be evaluated. Examination of the otic canal and tympanic membrane is not complete until it is examined under the operating microscope, although in most cases most of the information can be obtained on routine otoscopy. Occasionally an ossicular anomaly may be seen through a translucent ear drum, or a retraction pocket or small attic cholesteatoma visualized.

In the patient with microtia/atresia where the pinna is quite defective, the height of the hairline on the involved and normal sides should be compared. Palpate and inspect the space between mastoid and mandibular condyle; in general, if the mastoid is noticeably small or the space very narrow or nonexistent, the middle ear defect is severe and the likelihood of successful reconstruction of the middle ear is small. Assess the mobility of the facial muscles; if there is facial paresis or paralysis, surgery may be inadvisable. If the mandible, maxilla, and parotid are hypoplastic, middle ear hypoplasia and severe ossicular defects can be anticipated.

Testing with a tuning fork to augment or check on the audiometric result is important. Earphones may be inadvertently reversed; machines may be malfunctioning or out of calibration; or the audiologist may have recorded results for the wrong ear or wrong patient. Patients who have a profound unilateral sensorineural hearing loss may give both tuning fork and audiometric findings that falsely indicate a conductive hearing loss in the involved ear. Masking may pose a dilemma in some patients. If the patient is an older child or adult, his ability to read lips, the quality of voice, modulation, and articulation may help resolve the issue of whether the patient's loss is sensorineural, conductive, mixed, of infantile or adult onset.

Bone and air conduction, speech audiometry, and acoustic bridge testing are essential in patients who have middle ear malformations. Repeated testing may be necessary if the patient's responses are inconsistent or confusing. Testing of the infant and young child is not for the occasional pediatric audiologist. The acoustic bridge test is now routine in most otologic practices, but must be correlated with the otologic examination. Middle ear effusions make it impossible to get accurate results, and medical and surgical efforts to clear the fluid may be frustrated for so long that this portion of the evaluation may have to be done after amplification has been provided. However, where the middle ear is clear, diminished static compliance in the presence of normal tympanometry may be seen, and the acoustic reflex may be absent. The development of ipsilateral testing has made it possible to assess these parameters in the opposite "normal" ear of patients with microtia/atresia, an ear that may have a significant congenital conductive or sensorineural hearing loss in up to 20% of patients [29, 67]. Brainstem audiometry and cortical evoked response audiometry may not differentiate conductive from sensorineural hearing loss, but may at least indicate whether the child has a hearing loss. Transtympanic electrocochleography cannot be done in an atretic or severely stenotic ear, although techniques utilizing the ear lobe or mastoid process may be feasible.

Polytomography of the ears need not be part of the initial assessment of an infant or young child, since heavy sedation might be required, but routine mastoid

Assessment of Middle Ear Malformations / 225

views, especially the Stenvers, transorbital and base views, can be helpful in determining whether the essential components of the ear are present. However, if the child proves difficult to test audiometrically and is not responding to sound nor producing speech or language, or if the child appears to be retarded, blind, or neurologically handicapped, all diagnostic modalities should be utilized promptly. Hypocycloidial polytomography has reached a high level of precision when done meticulously, and surprisingly good resolution of middle and inner ear structures is possible. Part of the assessment of the middle ear is, of course, to assess inner ear structure and function as well. Views are taken in the lateral and Guillen projections, but supplemental cuts from the basal aspect or other angles may be required at times. Both ears should be studied, even if only one appears to be abnormal.

X ray of the ear has 2 purposes — diagnosis, and as a guideline for surgery. With the latter in view it may be preferable to obtain polytomography closer to the proposed time of surgery. The child is better able to cooperate; roentgenograms have less time to become misplaced prior to surgery, and the family is more likely to be in the city where the surgery will be performed. There is some difference of opinion among otologic surgeons, but if the child is otherwise normal and his middle ear deficit is bilateral, the surgery may be done just prior to his entering school. There is, however, good rationale for waiting until the age of 8 or 10 when frequency of otitis media decreases, thus lessening the likelihood of one cause of postoperative complication.

The child must be assessed for his readiness for surgery. If he has had multiple hospitalizations for other congenital or medical problems, he may need a summer for fun rather than another operation. Or if he has missed a lot of school, surgery might better be postponed. The child himself should want the surgery and have some elementary understanding of postoperative care and temporary restrictions. Whether or not the possibilities of complications or poor results should be, to some degree, shared with the child is hard to say. If he has had previous operations or hospitalizations he may, in fact, be sophisticated beyond his years in that regard. The surgeon should talk alone with the child to explore his or her hopes, fears, and understanding of the realities and goals of the operation. The surgeon also needs to be sure that the parents have been thoroughly oriented.

In general, the ear with the poorer hearing is selected for surgery, but the bone conduction should be normal or near-normal so as to give the greatest potential for gain. There are certain anatomic situations that may dampen enthusiasm for surgery. They include marked hypoplasia of the middle ear space, absence of the oval or round window, severe abnormalities in or absence of the ossicles, severe malposition of the fallopian canal in an unfavorable position (although this may not be determinable preoperatively if the fallopian canal cannot be visualized well), poor-to-near absence of mastoid air-cell pneumatization, displacement of the middle cranial fossa into the epitympanum, and an abnormal inner ear. The findings in our series of cases are presented in Table 5.

TABLE 5. Type of Middle Ear Anomalies Found in Determinate Cases

Ossicular malformation	6
Ossicular fixation	6
Fusion of malleus and incus	1
No ossicles	1
Absent malleus	1
Anomalous incus	1
Stapes malformation	7 (1 also fixed)
Stapes fracture	1
Stapes fixation	8*Δ
Rudimentary stapes and oval window	1
Absent or occluded oval window	4
Anomalous stapes and incus	1

* 4 associated with wide cochlear aqueduct.
Δ 1 Pendred syndrome with mixed HL.

There is a difference of opinion on when to operate the 2nd ear, assuming it is suitable for surgery. One group of distinguished, experienced otologists prefers to defer surgery on the 2nd ear until the patient is old enough to give a truly informed consent, whether or not he or she is legally of age. Another group, given an equal anatomic situation, would prefer to operate both ears in childhood. The first group, in general, would not operate unilateral cases until the patient is mature; the second group probably would operate unilateral cases early.

Until surgery can be performed, or if surgery is going to be postponed indefinitely, the child should have early amplification, binaural if possible. There may be indication in some children to aid the impaired ear even if one ear is normal, especially if the child has limited vision, neurologic deficits, is retarded, or is otherwise handicapped. In some instances where the results of repeated hearing tests have been equivocal and where acoustic bridge testing and polytomography have been unsuccessful because of the child's hyperactivity or because poor health makes sedation or anesthesia inadvisable, a hearing aid may be fitted temporarily as a test to see if the child's responsiveness or performance improves. For the school child who has no hearing aids, preferential seating in school, training in lip reading, or special classes may be needed.

Polytomography has some risks — those of sedation or even general anesthesia in young children, and of irradiation, especially to the cornea, which may receive as much as 60 times the permissible dose [77]. With shielding, this can be cut to one-tenth that dose, but not all radiologists are happy with the resulting quality of the radiograph. The necessary information could perhaps be obtained with fewer cuts. At any rate it is apparent that the radiologic team must be skilled, meticulous, and able to get cooperation from the patient, and if not, to try another day rather than to produce a series of blurred radiographs and irradiate the patient needlessly.

The otologist must assess the films and share clinical information with the head and neck radiologist. Both must recognize the limitations of tomography; for example, it does not show the stapes well, and unless a footplate is thickened, fixation cannot be determined. Minor discontinuity in the ossicular chain can cause major hearing loss, but little or nothing will be seen on the tomogram. The specific situations in which various middle ear defects have been reported are tabulated in Table 6. Ultrasonography does not as yet have capabilities equal to tomography, but computerized tomography may soon surpass it as far as the temporal and petrous bones are concerned.

A surprising number of patients having middle ear anomalies, whose ears have been studied radiographically or at autopsy, have been found to have structural abnormalities of the vestibular system, often with a normal cochlea. This has been reported in auditory atresia, Treacher Collins, preauricular pit and cervical fistula syndrome, in some of the cases in which spontaneous fistulae have been found in the stapes footplate, in trisomy 13, and in a number of unclassified cases [8, 9, 23, 29, 34, 50, 71]. The horizontal semicircular canal seems to be the most frequently affected. Routine preoperative functional assessment of the vestibular system has not been done. Vestibular testing is, of course, limited in its technology and its scope, and may be difficult in children. Nevertheless, since injury to the vestibular labyrinth is a potential postoperative complication, it seems that preoperative documentation of function, within the state of the art, might be prudent and possibly interesting. Where one or both external auditory canals are atretic, caloric examination cannot be done; but techniques are being developed to quantify the ocular responses to rotation so that it may be possible to detect significant asymmetries in response. Two young patients in our series have had dysequilibrium during bouts of otitis media and are being worked up for fistulae.

CONSEQUENCES

The consequences of middle ear malformations might be divided into 2 groups – those subsequent to the defect itself, and those subsequent to the treatment. We have discussed delay in development of language and the possibility of impaired development of the brain, both probably secondary to delayed intervention and early auditory deprivation in bilateral losses. Even where hearing loss is detected early, its seriousness may not be appreciated because of coincidental serous or suppurative otitis media to which the hearing impairment may be attributed. Although most children adapt very well to conditions present from birth, some children with unilateral conductive hearing losses have problems with sound localization and with conversations, particularly in noise or in group situations. The child who has an undetected conductive loss may be thought to be a slow learner, or to be inattentive or lazy. The stigmas thus applied early may haunt him for years to come.

TABLE 6. Specific Middle Ear Anomalies and Their Known Associations

Structure	The Anomaly	Its Associations
Tympanic membrane	Absence or hypoplasia	Microtia/atresia or atresia alone [31]
Malleus	Absence	Microtia/atresia [27, 31]
		Madelung deformity [58]
		Treacher Collins [8, 9, 78, 79]
		Knuckle pads, leukonychia, deafness [57]
		DiGeorge [60]
	Deformed	Microtia/atresia [31]
		Goldenhar [80]
		Otopalatodigital [42]
		Trisomy 18 [68]
		Trisomy 13, [70]
	Fixation	Isolated finding
	Fused to incus	Microtia/atresia [31, 38, 81]
		Fanconi pancytopenia [38]
	Fused to incus and atretic plate	Treacher Collins [8]
		Crouzon [54]
		Moebius [55]
Incus	Hypoplastic long or lenticular process	Thalidomide ears [82]
		Isolated [83]
		Otopalatodigital [42]
		First branchial cleft syndromes [84]
		Hypertrophied, thickened ear lobules [25, 26]
		Treacher Collins
	Fixation to stapes	Isolated
	Fixation to aditus	Klippel-Feil [56]
	Fixation to aberrant styloid process	Microtia/atresia [27]
	Absence	Microtia/atresia [32, 81]
		Treacher Collins [8]
	Long process coursing anteriorly	Thalidomide [40]
		Trisomy 18 [68]
	Amorphous	Microtia/atresia [31]
		Madelung deformity [58]
		Treacher Collins [8]
Stapes	Bulkiness	Pierre Robin [6]
		Rubella [86, 87]
		Osteopetrosis [35, 36]
	Monopod	Treacher Collins [8, 9]
		Isolated [83]
	Absent or hypoplastic footplate	Isolated [83]
		Treacher Collins [8]
		Goldenhar [71]
	Two footplates	Curled pinna [88]

(continued next page)

TABLE 6. (Continued)

Structure	The Anomaly	Its Associations
Stapes	Crura fail to meet footplate or fuse to otic capsule or fallopian canal	Otopalatodigital [42] Thickened, hypertrophied ear lobule [25, 26]
	Absence or hypoplasia	Isolated [83] Michel aplasia [89] Isolated [83]
Incus	Displaced	Treacher Collins [78]
Stapes	Tilting resulting in contact with fallopian canal	Isolated [24]
	Bony bridges projecting from adjacent tympanic walls, fusing with stapedial crus	Thalidomide [40] Klippel-Feil [56] Microtia [27] Madelung deformity [58] Mixed deafness [85] Proximal symphalangism [47]
	Absence of obturator foramen with resultant bulkiness or small size of stapes	Trisomy 18 [68] Isolated [83]
	Head and crura separated	Treacher Collins [78]
	Fixation of footplate	Microtia/atresia [31] Fanconi pancytopenia [38] Apert acrocephalosyndactyly [10, 11] Crouzon [54] Isolated [83]
	Fixation of footplate with perilymph gusher	Isolated [83] Familial [90, 91] Apert acrocephalosyndactyly [10, 11] Otopalatodigital [42] Goldenhar [92]
	Fistula of stapes footplate	Isolated With labyrinthine defects
	Fracture	Osteogenesis imperfecta [17]
Multi-ossicular defects	Absence of malleus, incus and stapes	Microtia/atresia [31, 32] Treacher Collins [8] Knuckle pads – leukonychia [42] DiGeorge [60]
	Fusion of ossicles	Diastrophic dwarfism [39] Treacher Collins [8] Cryptophthalmia [46] DiGeorge [93]
Facial nerve	Interrupting continuity of ossicular chain	Subarachnoid-tympanic fistulae [94] Treacher Collins [95]

(continued next page)

TABLE 6. (Continued)

Structure	The Anomaly	Its Associations
	Crossing or obstructing stapes footplate	Isolated [83]
Oval window	Narrow, hypoplastic or absent	Pierre Robin [6]
		Thalidomide [40]
		Waardenburg [96]
		Goldenhar [92]
		Moebius [55]
		With round window closure and Mondini malformation [97]
		DiGeorge [60]
		Crouzon [54]
		With middle ear choristoma [24]
Round window	Absence	See above
Muscles and tendons	Ossification of stapedius tendon	Isolated [83]
Middle ear space	Aplastic or hypoplastic	Atresia [31]
		Thalidomide [41]
		Pierre Robin [6, 18]
		Goldenhar [20]
		Microtia/atresia [31]
		Treacher Collins [8, 9, 78, 79]
		Crouzon [54]
	Compartmentalized	Knuckle pads – leukonychia [57]
		Treacher Collins [9, 78]

Case 1. A 16-year-old male had a bilateral 60 dB air bone gap which had been discovered several years previously. He had been truant from school, and after a previous operation on the right ear had not improved his hearing, he became delinquent. At the time of admission for a 2nd ear operation, he was in the custody of the juvenile court authorities. The record of the previous surgery was not available, and polytomography was unremarkable. General physical examination was negative.

The right ear was explored under general anesthesia. The stapedial superstructure was absent; incus and malleus were normal and mobile. A control hole was picked in the center of the footplate, which was somewhat thick and fixed. Perilymph gushed from the control hole and quickly filled the middle ear and ear speculum. Gelfoam and fat from the earlobe placed over the control hole did not stem the flow until the incus was transposed with its short process over the fat in the hole in the stapes. The long process was positioned under the manubrium of the malleus. A postoperative audiogram showed a stable bone line, and there was no vertigo or unsteadiness. A partial improvement in air conduction was seen during short-term follow-up, but unfortunately the patient did not return for further follow-up.

Case 2. Failure to recognize hearing loss contralateral to an atretic ear because an audiogram was not done can have serious educational sequelae, as illustrated in the following case. A 7-year-old boy had unilateral grade III microtia/atresia. The opposite pinna was somewhat protuberant, but canal and tympanic membrane were normal. He was referred for evaluation because he had failed first grade. His poor progress in school had been partly attributed to the fact that English was not the language spoken in the home. Audiometry revealed bilateral conductive hearing loss with excellent cochlear reserve. Polytomography showed an adequate middle ear space on the right, an atretic plate, and what appeared to be a fused monobloc malleus and incus. The left ear showed a narrow oval window and thickened footplate area.

Case 3. Associated defects may be underestimated or overlooked in the desire to rehabilitate hearing, as in the following presentation. A rather diminutive 10-year-old boy had normal speech and language development, and had done well in school without amplification, even though it had been known for several years that he had a bilateral conductive hearing loss. Otoscopic examination was normal. He was found to be somewhat anemic, was treated with iron, and then underwent right stapedectomy for fixation of the footplate. It was felt that he had a good hearing result, but an audiogram 2 years later was virtually identical to the preoperative one. A younger sister was also tiny and anemic, but also had hypoplastic thumbs. Her audiogram was similar to his, and she underwent right stapedial mobilization about a year later. Two years later she went into severe renal failure; nonfunctioning fused presacral kidneys were found, and she received chronic hemodialysis. A diagnosis of Fanconi pancytopenia was made; subsequently her brother was found to have a hypoplastic right kidney.

This pair of sibs illustrates another problem, that of surgical failure. The surgery on these 2 patients was done by a skilled, experienced otologist and there were no intraoperative problems. The causes of failure in middle ear surgery are not always clear, but results may be less than optimum. However, children often do surprisingly well with improved hearing even if it is at borderline levels.

Case 4. Sometimes a congenital physical finding in the ear can be overlooked or misinterpreted, and diagnosis of hearing loss delayed. The following case is illustrative. A female child had not walked until 25 months and was suspected of being retarded. Physical examination at 27 months showed a small child who had epicanthal folds, a flat nasal bridge, slightly low pinnae, hyperextensible joints, and a small umbilical hernia. She walked clumsily.

Otologic examination under the microscope revealed that the cartilaginous canals narrowed to a pinpoint. Audiogram showed a 25 dB bilateral conductive hearing loss. Petrous pyramid polytomography revealed an atretic plate at the level of the tympanic membrane, but ossicles appeared normal. A karyotype was done and revealed a partial deletion of the long arm of chromosome 18. After being fitted with a hearing aid, she progressed well and ultimately was able to keep up in regular classes in school [19].

Case 5. A female child, born in a small village in Mexico, had a cleft lip which was subsequently repaired. The right pinna was cupped, and the parents were told that there was a hearing loss in the right ear. Speech developed adequately. A younger sib had a defect of the lip and alveolar ridge, but the family history was otherwise negative for clefts and craniofacial defects. No other family member was thought to have a hearing problem.

Weber tuning fork tests referred to the right ear, and Rinne tests were negative bilaterally. Tympanic membranes were normal, but the right malleus could not be well visualized. The palate was high-arched but intact. The remainder of the head and neck examination was normal. Audiogram showed a pure conductive hearing loss in the right ear with a speech awareness threshold of 36 dB. There was a mixed hearing loss in the left ear and speech reception threshold of 81 dB (Fig. 2). Oto-admittance testing showed high resistance, absent acoustic reflexes, and normal tympanometry. Polytomograms of the ear showed an absent left malleus, large vestibule bilaterally, and no semicircular canals. The left cochlea showed disproportion between the basal and the apical and middle turns.

This case illustrates the wisdom of otologic workup even in cases of apparently unrelated malformation and mild pinna malformation. The patient could have undergone corrective otologic surgery on her better-hearing ear. It is possible that the poorer ear once had much better hearing and that the loss has increased in that ear and may continue to do so.

Complications of middle ear surgery include high-tone sensorineural loss from mechanical stimulation of the ossicular chain with a drill; sensorineural or even total loss across the frequencies as a result of inner ear damage; vertigo or permanent vestibular paralysis of the operated ear; poststapedectomy otitis media which may lead to suppurative labyrinthitis if the labyrinth has been inadvertently opened; facial paresis or paralysis; injury to the dura; leakage of cerebrospinal fluid; perilymphatic fistula; stenosis of the external auditory canal; perforation of the tympanic membrane or failure of a graft to take; lateralization of a grafted tympanic membrane; refixation of mobilized or repositioned ossicles, and slipping of stapes or other prostheses for ossicular replacement.

Fitting of hearing aids presents problems in some children with middle ear anomalies, particularly those with bilateral microtia/atresia who need hearing aids when they are very young. Bone conduction hearing aids need to be snugly applied, but devices to accomplish this are not always reliable. If the child has a significant cranial abnormality or has recently undergone surgery for craniostenosis, wearing the aids may not be possible for awhile. Children who have relatively normal pinnae, but microcanals, may have trouble wearing an aid at

Assessment of Middle Ear Malformations / 233

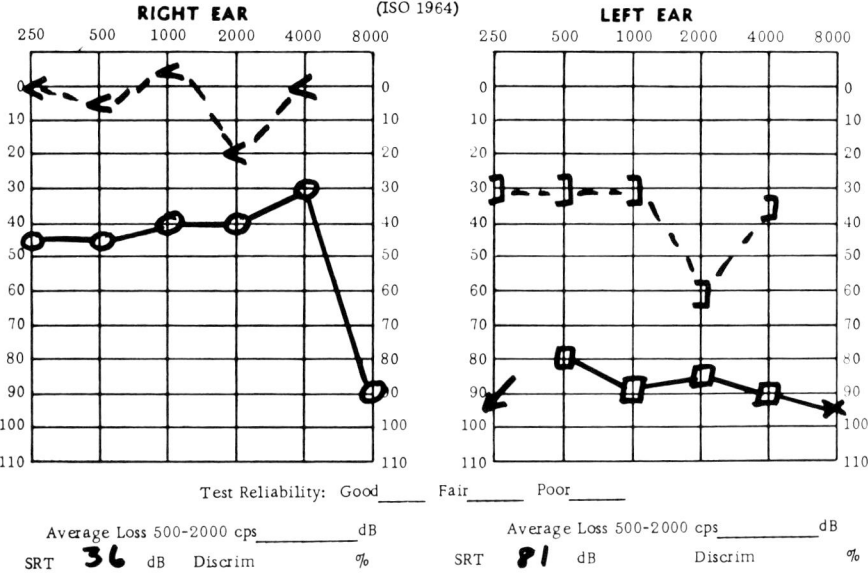

Fig. 2. *Case 5*. Audiogram.

ear level because of difficulties in keeping the earmold in place. Malfunctioning hearing aids, dead batteries, cracked tubing, poorly fitting earmolds, ear canal irritation from the mold, loss of or violence to the aids by the child or his companions, rejection of hearing aids by children and by many teenagers, and parents who are not firm in their approach to the wearing of the aid by the child, are familiar problems to audiologists, dispensers of hearing aids, speech therapists, teachers, and otolaryngologists. The need to resume use of a hearing aid after unsuccessful ear surgery is particularly frustrating to youngsters and teenagers.

Cholesteatoma behind an atretic plate is one consequence that is serious, and for that reason surgery is mandatory. The tympanic membrane is present and there is desquamation of keratinizing squamous epithelium. Such a cholesteatoma is not easy to diagnose, and overt signs of pressure and infection may be present before detection. X-rays may show erosion of bone or a soft tissue mass, and are more valuable if there are previous ones for comparison. Gill found a high incidence of mastoid infection in 46 of 83 atretic ears he explored [31]. This finding has not been mentioned often in other series, and, therefore, it cannot be interpreted regarding probable frequency nor as an indication for surgery, especially since it apparently had been an unexpected finding preoperatively.

Middle ear malformations may exist by themselves, and the consequences for the patient may be only hearing loss, although the loss may be mixed in nature or conductive in one ear, while a sensorineural hearing loss is present in the other ear. The main objectives of treatment in such a patient are to restore functional hearing, first by amplification and training, and later, if possible, by surgical correction. The child who has other defects, as well as congenital conductive hearing loss, lives on a merry-go-round of visits to doctors, tests, hospitalizations, hearing aids and other appliances, surgery, and possible death or additional disability. Occasionally we, as clinicians, may be so busy "fixing things" that we forget the child and his basic needs. A final case may suffice to illustrate.

Case 6. Bilateral microtia/atresia prompted comprehensive workup of a young boy at the age of 5 years. He also had left facial paresis, slight antimongoloid obliquity of the orbits, increased interocular distance, and bifid uvula. Mastoid tomograms showed bilateral Mondini cochlear malformation and minor anomalies of the vestibule. There was a thick crista in each internal auditory canal. There were marked anomalies of the right middle ear. There was no response to audiometry in the right ear and responses at 90 dB in the left ear which could be brought up to 50–55 dB with a hearing aid.

Special training was begun. At the age of 6, pinna reconstruction was started, since it was recognized that he was not a candidate for middle ear surgery. Over the ensuing years, he underwent 14 procedures in attempts to create acceptable looking pinnae. His mother's life was spent taking him to doctors' offices and to clinics and being with him during hospitalizations. During this time the boy's father left, never to return, and the mother was forced to go to work. During much of the time he was undergoing or recovering from otoplasty procedures he was unable to wear one or both of his bone conduction hearing aids. At age 12 his only language was gestural. When he was 14 years old, further attempts to create new external ears for him were abandoned.

CONCLUSION

Anomalies of the middle ear comprise a small, but significant, proportion of congenital hearing losses, but figures are difficult to obtain. Large school surveys seldom include enough diagnostic information for the category to be recognized. There are as yet insufficient statistics from neonatal screening or high-risk registry studies. Congenital conductive losses present technical and threshold problems in detection.

The presence of other anomalies, especially of the head and neck region, is an indicator of their probability. Asymmetry of anomalies of the air conduction mechanism is frequent. An obvious unilateral defect may be associated with an occult contralateral defect of equal severity.

Association with inner ear defects is surprisingly common, considering the differences in embryologic origin of middle ear and inner ear. Heredity, a teratogen, or chromosomal defect are demonstrated or thought to be a likely cause in a relatively small number of patients. Etiology in most patients remains unknown.

The diagnostic work-up is similar to that for congenital sensorineural hearing loss, including family, prenatal, perinatal history, a careful physical examination, especially of the head and neck area, laboratory tests and x rays and may include several specialty consultations.

Surgery may be undertaken in the first 5–10 years of life if the loss is bilateral, with correction of the second ear after the individual has reached the age when he is capable of giving an informed consent. Severe inner ear anomalies, middle ear window defects, gross malposition of the facial nerve or a severe combined loss are among contraindications to middle ear surgery. Prior to the time of surgery, if the loss is bilateral, and at any time, if the defect is deemed inoperable, or if surgical results are poor, amplification and other habilitative measures may be indicated. The long-term results of surgery seem to be poorer than the initial results, for unknown reasons, but many patients derive both subjective and objective benefit.

There is a small but significant association of middle ear defects with anomalies of the vestibular portion of the labyrinth, although these vestibular anomalies may be asymptomatic.

Middle ear anomalies show great diversity, and any structure of the middle ear may be involved. Those involving nonauditory structures may be only curiosities or may present major obstacles to successful middle ear surgery.

REFERENCES

1. Downs MP: The expanding imperatives of early identification. In Bess FH (ed): "Childhood Deafness: Causation, Assessment and Management." New York: Grune & Stratton, 1977, pp 95–106.
2. Webster DG, Webster M: Brainstem auditory nuclei after sound deprivation. J Accoust Soc Am 59 (Suppl. 1):91, 1976.
3. Webster DB, Webster M: Neonatal conductive hearing loss: Central consequences and critical period in mice. Presented at the Forum of the Association for Research in Otolaryngology, November, 1978, Las Vegas, Nevada.
4. Hildyard VH, Stool SF, Valentine MA: Tuning fork tests as aid to screening audiometry. Arch Otolaryngol 78:151–154, 1963.
5. Konigsmark BW: Hereditary deafness with external ear abnormalities: A review. Johns Hopkins Med J 127:228–244, 1970.
6. Bergstrom L, Hemenway WG, Sando I: Pathological changes in congenital deafness. Laryngoscope 82:1777–1792, 1972.
7. Igarashi M, Filippone MV, Alford BR: Temporal bone findings in Pierre Robin syndrome. Laryngoscope 86:1679–1687, 1976.
8. Maran AGD: The Treacher Collins syndrome. J Laryngol Otol 78:135–151, 1964.
9. Sando I, Hemenway WG, Morgan WR: Histopathology of the temporal bones in mandibulofacial dysostosis (Treacher Collins syndrome). Trans Am Acad Ophthalmol Otolaryngol 72:913–924, 1968.
10. Bergstrom L, Neblett LM, Hemenway WG: Otologic manifestations of acrocephalosyndactyly. Arch Otolaryngol 96:117–123, 1972.

11. Lindsay JR, Black FO, Donnelly WH Jr: Acrocephalosyndactyly (Apert's syndrome): Temporal bone findings. Ann Otol Rhinol Laryngol 84:174–178, 1975.
12. Rimoin DL, Edgerton MT: Genetic and clinical heterogeneity in the oral-facial-digital syndromes. J Pediatr 71:94–102, 1967.
13. Martsolf JT, Cracco JB, Carpenter GG, O'Hara AE: Pfeiffer syndrome. An unusual type of acrocephalosyndactyly with broad thumbs and great toes. Am J Dis Child 121:257–262, 1971.
14. Fara M, Chlupackova V, Hrivnakova J: Dismorphia otofacio-cervicalis familiaris. Acta Chir Plast 9:255–268, 1967.
15. Mengel MC, Konigsmark BW, Berlin CI, McKusick VA: Familial conductive hearing loss and malformed, low-set ears, prabably a new entity. J Med Genet 6:14–21, 1969.
16. Aase JM, Smith DW: Facial asymmetry and abnormalities of palms and ears: A dominantly inherited developmental syndrome. J Pediatr 76:928–930, 1970.
17. Bergstrom L: Osteogenesis imperfecta: Otologic and maxillofacial aspects. Laryngoscope 87 (Suppl):6, 1977.
18. Igarashi M, Takahashi M, Alford BR, Johnson PE: Inner ear morphology in Down's syndrome. Acta Otolaryngol (Stockh) 83:175–181, 1977.
19. Bergstrom L, Stewart JM, Kenyon B: External auditory atresia and the deleted chromosome. Laryngoscope 84:1905–1917, 1974.
20. Fourman P, Fourman J: Hereditary deafness in family with ear-pits (fistula auris congenital). Br Med J 2:1354–1356, 1955.
21. McLaurin JW, Kloepfer HW, Laguaite JK, Stallcup TA: Hereditary branchial anomalies and associated hearing impairment. Laryngoscope 76:1277–1288, 1966.
22. Rowley PT: Familial hearing loss associated with branchial fistulas. Pediatrics 44:978–985, 1969.
23. Fitch N, Lindsay JR, Srolovitz H: The temporal bone in the preauricular pit, cervical fistula, hearing loss syndrome. Ann Otol Rhinol Laryngol 85:268–275, 1976.
24. Pou JW: Congenital anomalies of the middle ear: Presentation of two cases. Laryngoscope 81:831–839, 1971.
25. Escher F, Hirt H: Dominant hereditary conductive deafness through lack of incus-stapes junction. Acta Otolarynol (Stockh) 65:25–32, 1968.
26. Wilmot TJ: Hereditary conductive deafness due to incus-stapes abnormalities and associated with pinna deformity. J Laryngol Otol 84:469–479, 1970.
27. Altmann F: Problem of so-called congenital atresia of the ear. Arch Otolaryngol 50:759–788, 1949.
28. Sullivan JA, McAskile K, Smith B: Surgical management of congenital atresia of the ear. J Laryngol Otol 73:201–222, 1959.
29. Naunton R, Valvassori GE: Inner ear anomalies: Their association with atresia. Laryngoscope 78:1041–1049, 1968.
30. Potter GD: Inner ear abnormalities in association with congeital atresia of the external auditory canal, including a case of Michel deformity. Ann Otol Rhinol Laryngol 78:598–604, 1969.
31. Gill NW: Congenital atresia of the ear. J Laryngol Otol 83:551–587, 1969.
32. Harada O, Ishii H: The condition of the auditory ossicles in microtia. Plast Reconstr Surg 50:48–53, 1972.
33. Schuknecht HF: Reconstructive procedures for congenital aural atresia. Arch Otolaryngol 101:170–172, 1975.
34. Jafek BW, Nager GT, Strife J, Gayler RW: Congenital aural atresia: An analysis of 311 cases. Trans Am Acad Ophthalmol Otolaryngol 80:588–595, 1975.
35. Myers EN, Stool S: The temporal bone in osteopetrosis. Arch Otolaryngol 89:460–469, 1969.

36. Suga F, Lindsay JR: Temporal bone histopathology of osteopetrosis. Ann Otol Rhinol Laryngol 85:15–24, 1976.
37. Kietzer G, Paparella MM: Otolaryngological disorders in craniometaphyseal dysplasia. Laryngoscope 79:921–941, 1969.
38. McDonough EG: Fanconi anemia syndrome. Arch Otolaryngol 92:284–285, 1970.
39. Walker BA, Scott CI, Hall JG, Murdoch JL, McKusick VA: Diastrophic dwarfism. Medicine 51:41–59, 1972.
40. Jørgensen MB, Kristensen HK, Buch NH: Thalidomide-induced aplasia of the inner ear. J Laryngol Otol 78:1095–1101, 1964.
41. Takemori S, Tanaka Y, Suzuki JI: Thalidomide anomalies of the ear. Arch Otolaryngol 102:425–427, 1976.
42. Buran DJ, Duvall AJ: The oto-palato-digital syndrome. Arch Otolaryngol 85:394–399, 1967.
43. Converse JM, Coccaro PJ, Becker M, Wood-Smith D: On hemifacial microsomia: The first and second branchial arch syndrome. Plast Reconstr Surg 51:268–279, 1973.
44. Gorlin RJ, Meskin LH, St. Geme JW: Oculodentodigital dysplasia. J Pediatr 63:69–75, 1963.
45. Roaf R, Longmore JB, Forrester RM: A childhood syndrome of bone dysplasia, retinal detachment and deafness. Dev Med Child Neurol 9:464–472, 1967.
46. Ide CH, Wollschlaeger PB: Multiple congenital abnormalities associated with cryptophthalmia. Arch Ophthalmol 81:640–644, 1969.
47. Strasburger AK, Hawkins MR, Eldridge R, Hargrave RL, McKusick VA: Symphalangism: Genetic and clinical aspects. Bull Johns Hopk Hosp 117:108–127, 1965.
48. Rapin I, Ruben RJ: Patterns of anomalies in children with malformed ears. Laryngoscope 86:1469–1502, 1976.
49. Quan L, Smith DW: The VATER association, Vertebral defects, Anal atresia, TE-fistula with esophageal atresia, Radial and Renal dysplasia: A spectrum of associated defects. J Pediatr 82:104–107, 1973.
50. Stool S, Leeds NE, Shulman K: The syndrome of congenital deafness and otic meningitis: Diagnosis and management. J Pediatr 71:547–552, 1967.
51. Rice WJ, Waggoner LG: Congenital cerebrospinal fluid otorrhea via a defect in the stapes footplate. Laryngoscope 77:341–349, 1967.
52. Stroud MH, Calcaterra TC: Spontaneous perilymph fistulas. Laryngoscope 80:479–487, 1970.
53. Bennett RJ: Subarachnoid fistula due to a congenital defect in the stapedial footplate. J Laryngol Otol 85:169–175, 1971.
54. Baldwin JL: Dysostosis craniofacialis of Crouzon. A summary of recent literature and case reports with emphasis on involvement of the ear. Laryngoscope 78:1660–1676, 1968.
55. Livingstone G, Delahunty JE: Malformation of the ear associated with congenital ophthalmic and other conditions. J Laryngol Otol 82:495–304, 1968.
56. McLay K, Maran AGD: Deafness and the Klippel-Feil syndrome: 3 cases. J Laryngol Otol 83:175–184, 1969.
57. Bart RS, Pumphrey RE: Knuckle pads, leukonychia and deafness. N Engl J Med 276:202–207, 1967.
58. Nassif R, Harboyan G: Madelung's deformity with conductive hearing loss. Arch Otolaryngol 91:175–178, 1970.
59. Adkins WY, Gussen R: Temporal bone findings in the third and fourth pharyngeal pouch (DiGeorge) syndrome. Arch Otolaryngol 100:206–208, 1974.

60. Black FO, Spanier SS, Kohut RI: Aural abnormalities in partial DiGeorge's syndrome. Arch Otolaryngol 101:129–134, 1975.
61. Singh SP, Rock EH, Shulman A: Klippel-Feil syndrome with unexplained apparent conductive hearing loss. A case report. Laryngoscope 79:113–117, 1969.
62. Bergstrom L, Thompson P, Wood RP II: New patterns in congenital otonephropathies. Laryngoscope 89:177–194, 1979.
63. Forney WR, Robinson SJ, Pascoe DJ: Congenital heart disease, deafness and skeletal malformations: A new syndrome? J Pediatr 68:14–19, 1966.
64. Peron DL, Schuknecht HF: Congenital cholesteatomata with other anomalies. Arch Otolaryngol 101:498–505, 1975.
65. Turner G: A second family with renal, vaginal and middle ear anomalies. J Pediatr 76:641, 1960.
66. Winter JSD, Kohn G, Mellman WJ, Wagner S: A familial syndrome of renal, genital and middle ear anomalies. J Pediatr 72:88–93, 1968.
67. Bergstrom L: Congenital and acquired deafness in clefting and craniofacial syndromes. Cleft Palate J 15:254–261, 1978.
68. Karmody CS, Schuknecht HF: Deafness in congenital syphilis. Arch Otolaryngol 83:18–27, 1966.
69. Sando I, Bergstrom L, Wood RP II, Hemenway WG: Temporal bone findings in trisomy 18 syndrome. Arch Otolaryngol 91:552–559, 1970.
70. Lindsay JR: Inner ear pathology in congenital deafness. Otol Clin North Am 4:249–290, 1971.
71. Sando I, Leiberman A, Bergstrom L, Izumi S, Wood RP II: The temporal bone histopathological findings in trisomy 13 syndrome. Ann Otol Rhinol Laryngol 84 (Suppl):21, 1975.
72. Milkovich L, van den Berg BJ: Effects of prenatal meprobamate and chlordiazemoxide hydrochloride on human embryonic and fetal development. N Engl J Med 291:1268–1271, 1974.
73. Partsch C, Schmidt-Wittkamp E: Pterygium – Syndrom und Schwerhörigkeit. Arch Ohr Nas Kehlkopfheilk 183:336–338, 1964.
74. Gilbert EG, Visekud C, Mossman HW, Opitz JM: The pathologic anatomy of the G syndrome. Z Kinderheilkd 3:290–298, 1972.
75. Kasner J, Gilbert EG, Visekul C, Deacon J, Herrmann JPR, Opitz JM: Studies of malformation syndromes VID: The G syndrome. Further observations. Z Kinderheilkd 118:81–85, 1974.
76. Crysdale WS: Abnormal facial appearance and delayed diagnosis of congenital hearing loss. J Otolaryngol 7:349–352, 1978.
77. Chin FK, Anderson WB, Gilbertson JD: Radiation dose to critical organs during petrous tomography. Radiology 94:623–627, 1970.
78. Ruben RJ, Toriyama M, Dische MR, Bransilver B, Daly JF: External and middle ear malformations associated with mandibulo-facial dysostosis and renal abnormalities: A case report. Ann Otol Rhinol Laryngol 78:605–624, 1969.
79. Hutchinson JC, Caldarelli DD, Valvassori GE, Pruzansky S, Parris PJ: The otologic manifestations of mandibulo-facial dysostosis. Trans Am Acad Ophthalmol Otolaryngol 84:520–528, 1977.
80. Budden SS, Robinson GC: Oculoauricular vertebral dysplasia. Am J Dis Child 125:431–433, 1973.
81. Burcher JA, Rumbaugh CL, Stroud MH: Some radiographic and clinical observations in bony atresia of the external auditory canal. Laryngoscope 78:216–226, 1968.
82. Takemore S, Tanaka Y, Suzuki J-I: Thalidomide anomalies of the ear. Arch Otolaryngol 102:425–427, 1976.

83. Hough JVD: Malformations and anatomical variations seen in the middle ear during the operation for mobilization of the stapes. Laryngoscope 68:1337–1379, 1958.
84. Cavo JW Jr, Pratt IL, Alonso WA: First branchial cleft syndromes and associated congenital hearing loss. Laryngoscope 86:739–745, 1976.
85. Schlosser WD, Goldman BR, Winchester RA: Further experience with diagnosis and management of congenital mixed deafness. Laryngoscope 74:773–788, 1964.
86. Richards CS: Middle ear changes in rubella deafness. Arch Otolaryngol 80:48–59, 1964.
87. Hemenway WG, Sando I, McChesney D: Temporal bone pathology following maternal rubella. Arch Klinische Exp Ohr Nas Kehlkopfheilk 193:287–300, 1969.
88. Murphy KWR: A unique stapedial abnormality. J Laryngol Otol 85:501–503, 1971.
89. Ormerod FC: The pathology of congenital deafness. J Laryngol Otol 74:919–950, 1960.
90. Olson NR, Lehman RH: Cerebrospinal fluid otorrhea and the congenitally fixed stapes. Laryngoscope 78:352–360, 1968.
91. Glasscock ME: The stapes gusher. Arch Otolaryngol 98:82–91, 1973.
92. Nenzelius C: On spontaneous cerebrospinal otorrhea due to congenital malformations. Acta Otolaryngol 39:314–327, 1951.
93. Kretschmer R, Say B, Brown D, Rosen FS: Congenital aplasia of the thymus gland (DiGeorge's syndrome). N Engl J Med 279:1295–1301, 1968.
94. Bennett RJ: On subarachnoid-tympanic fistulae. A report of two cases of the rare indirect type. J Laryngol Otol 80:1242–1252, 1966.
95. Edwards WG: Congenital middle ear deafness with anomalies of the face. J Laryngol Otol 78:152–170, 1964.
96. Jensen J: Tomography of the inner ear in a case of Waardenburg's syndrome. Am J Roentgenol 101:828–833, 1967.
97. Adkins WY, Gussen R: Oval window absence, bony closure of round window and inner ear anomaly. Laryngoscope 84:1210–1224, 1974.

DISCUSSION

Dr. David Smith: Two things I'd appreciate any comments about: the role of the muscles in the middle ear, and the effect of lack of mobility in ossicular articulations. Do the ossicles become fixed in time, due to deficit of function?

Dr. Charles Berlin: One of the textbook explanations of middle ear muscles is that they are noise protectors. They are, in fact, voice protected, ie protected from one's own voice. Every time you talk, just before you talk, those muscles pull in and protect you from the very high intensity of your own vocal tract, which has about 115 dB sound pressure right inside the mouth. It's much too intense to tolerate.

Dr. David Lim: Are you talking about the stapedial muscle, or the tensor tympani?

Dr. Charles Berlin: In humans, mostly it's stapedial, but in a lot of other animals, it's both.

Dr. Ralph Wedgwood: Would there be any defined defect with the muscles of the middle ear? If you're correct, you can't stabilize them, you should probably not give up the speech patterns because you can't stand the sound of your own voice.

Dr. Harold Schuknecht: Congenital absence of the stapedius muscle is not uncommon, and these patients exhibit no evidence of acoustic trauma as a result of not having this muscle. Additionally, you can cut it in a stapedectomy operation and the patients are not more susceptible to acoustic trauma. In congenital aural atresias, where the ear is partly deprived of environmental sound stimulation, the stapes is always mobile.

Dr. Walter Nance: I can think of many useful purposes in trying to define hereditary deafness syndromes that appear to be transmitted as a monogenic trait. This is not to say that genes are acting in isolation, and it is not to say that that the problems of trying to decide if you have two genetic syndromes, or one genetic syndrome, or whether there are variations between one family and another is due to different alleles, different modifier genes, and so on. But I do think that there are a growing number of monogenic syndromes that contribute to deafness.

Dr. Thomas Van De Water: The earlier the effect, the more environmental interaction one single gene is going to have on the whole developmental scheme. Take for example neural crest, using a teratogen. If you hit it very early, you're probably going to affect otoplacode formation, then the contribution to visceral arches, and then you're going to hit the contribution to the otocapsule; the otocyst is going to be malformed because the otic placode was malinduced and, therefore, you have the effect of the otocyst upon the mesenchyme producing its cartilaginous capsule. So you really get all these components, perhaps because of a single gene action.

Dr. Ralph Wedgwood: It seems to me that the influence of teratogens on the production of malformations of the middle ear or the inner ear is greatly influenced by timing.

Dr. Thomas Van De Water: I think timing is essential, especially in the case of teratogens.

Dr. Ralph Wedgwood: Do we know enough about timing to use timing landmarks in the formation of the middle ear in man?

Dr. LaVonne Bergstrom: There's a lot of information on this subject.

Dr. David Lim: Do the sacculus and cochlea develop at the same time, while the utricle and the semicircular canal have different timing?

Dr. Thomas Van De Water: No, the sacculus and utricle develop at about the same time. The cochlea develops later.

Dr. Heinrich Spoendlin: I just want to make a short comment on timing. We found a malformation in a family in 5 generations having the fusion of the carpal bones and stapedial ankylosis.

Dr. LaVonne Bergstrom: This symphalangism syndrome is very famous, of course — it has been traced back to English nobility. The carpal bones have the same period of development as the stapedial footplate.

Dr. Robert Gorlin: You couldn't possibly interpret it on the basis of time because the carpal and tarsal bones appear at varying times, up to the age of almost 16 years. This is not initial coalition, it is progressive fusion.

Dr. Richard Bobbin: I'd like to make a comment about aspirin. Both Dr. Thalmann and I have shown that aspirin acts on the cochlea. It may be acting on the transmitter agent between the hair cells and the VIIIth nerve, and if it is taken during development, it may affect the hair cells or the VIIIth nerve.

Genetic Malformations of the Inner Ear in the Mouse and in Man

Malkiat S. Deol, PhD, DSc

About 50 mutant genes are known to affect the inner ear in the mouse, and the number would be much larger but for the laborious task of ascertaining whether a newly arisen mutation is indeed new or merely a recurrence of an old one. These genes can be roughly divided into 2 groups. In one group, the morphogenesis of the inner ear is defective, and gross or cytoarchitectural abnormalities appear at various stages of development. In the other group, the morphogenesis proceeds along normal lines until the organ is fully developed or very nearly so, but then degeneration of various structures, especially the neural epithelium, sets in at various times. There are some mutants in which both types of abnormalities may occur together, but in general it is possible to decide into which group a particular mutant falls. This brief survey is concerned only with genes falling into the morphogenetic group and with comparable situations in man.

GENETIC MALFORMATIONS IN THE MOUSE

The mutant genes causing malformations in the inner ear in the mouse are listed below roughly in the order of the severity of their effects, beginning with the severest. Although no gene causing congenital hypothyroidism has been described in the mouse, this disorder has been included here because at least one such gene is known in man, and experimental induction of congenital hypothyroidism in the mouse has shed light on the human condition. The name of each gene is followed by its standard symbol in parentheses. The abnormalities described are illustrated by schematic drawings, and the pattern of these is shown in Figure 1, which represents the normal inner ear.

Kreisler (kr)

The effects of this recessive gene are highly variable and generally asymmetric [1–3]. In severe cases, no part of the inner ear bears any resemblance to the normal (Fig. 2). In others, many of the normal features may be recognizable. In gen-

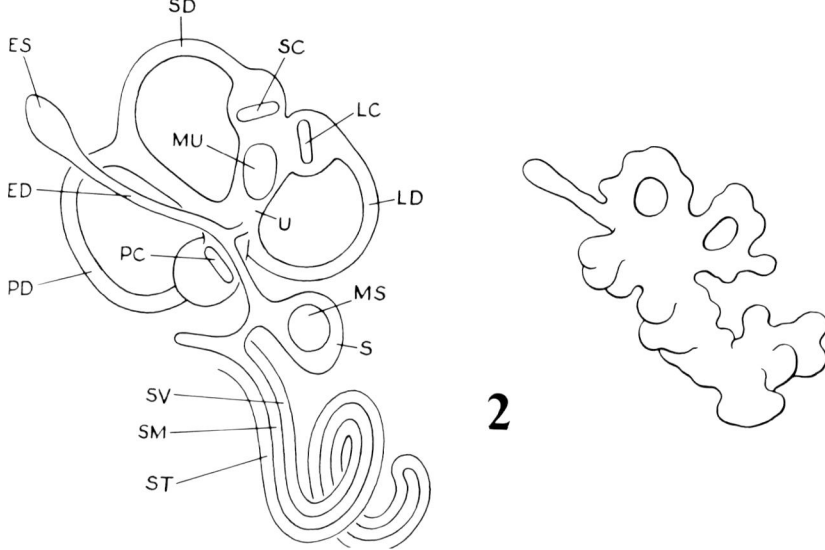

Fig. 1. Schematic drawing of the membranous inner ear of a normal mouse. In the following drawings modeled on this one, abnormalities of form are shown by simple modification of the outline and abnormalities of cytoarchitecture by stippling. ED = endolymphatic duct; ES = endolymphatic sac; LC = lateral crista; LD = lateral semicircular duct; MS = macula of saccule; MU = macula of utricle; PC = posterior crista; PD = posterior semicircular duct; S = saccule; SC = superior crista; SD = superior semicircular duct; SM = scala media; ST = scala tympani; SV = scala vestibuli; U = utricle.

Fig. 2. Kreisler homozygote.

eral, almost every part of the organ is affected to some extent. The bony capsule may be incomplete, and the inner ear may extend out of the gap in the form of a cyst into the cranial cavity or into the muscles of the neck. Ganglion cells and stretches of neural epithelium may lie scattered in the walls of the cysts.

These abnormalities can be traced back to the otic vesicle stage, and are preceded by abnormalities of the neural tube in that region [2]. The last 3 neuromeres of the rhombencephalon in kreisler embryos do not form, and their place is taken by a single abnormally large thickening of the neural tube (Fig. 3). The ganglion cells in this region do not become organized into the facial-acoustic and glossopharyngeal-vagal complexes, which in the normal embryo are found adjacent to the 4th and 6th neuromeres, respectively, but lie irregularly distributed along the sides of the neural tube. The otic vesicle, which normally adjoins the 5th neuromere, is separated from the neural tube by this uninterrupted ganglionic mass. It is known from experiments with amphibian and avian embryos that the inductive

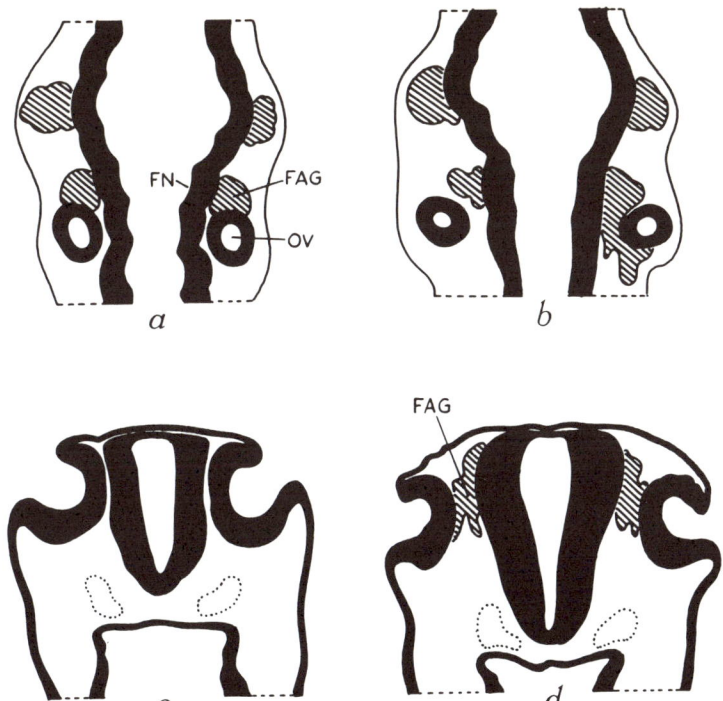

Fig. 3. a, b) Longitudinal and c, d) transverse sections of 9-day-old normal (a, c) and kreisler (b, d) embryos. FAG = facial-acoustic ganglionic complex; FN = 4th neuromere; OV = otic vesicle.

influence of the neural tube is essential for the normal differentiation of the otic vesicle [4–6], and as the neural tube in kreisler embryos is not only abnormal in this region but is not even in contact with the otic vesicle, it is not surprising that the subsequent development of the otic vesicle follows an erratic course without any clear pattern. It would seem that the kreisler gene has resulted in the loss of some morphogenetic directions rather than in their modification, as appears to be the case in some other mutants.

Sightless (*Sig*)

This semidominant gene affects all parts of the inner ear in the homozygote (Fig. 4). The cochlea is very poorly coiled, and its fine differentiation is grossly abnormal. The utricle and the saccule are confluent, and only the utricle has a macula. There is only one semicircular duct with an abnormally wide lumen. It has no crista and its position does not correspond to that of any of the normal semicircular ducts. The endolymphatic duct and sac are missing. The abnormalities are usually, but not always, symmetric [7].

It seems probable that the abnormalities of the inner ear in this mutant are also consequent to the anomalous relationship between the neural tube and the otic vesicle when it first forms. In normal embryos at the 9-day stage, the otic vesicle lies opposite the 5th neuromere, but in sightless homozygotes its position is shifted posteriorly and it lies opposite the cleft between the 5th and the 6th neuromeres (Fig. 5). As the facial-acoustic ganglionic complex retains its normal position adjacent to the 4th neuromere, it is separated dorsally from the otic vesicle and only its ventral part is in contact with it [7]. It is possible that the position of the otic vesicle in relation to the neural tube is abnormal because the otic placode is induced in a slightly anomalous position.

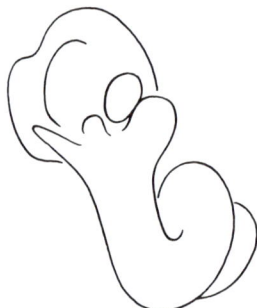

Fig. 4. Sightless homozygote.

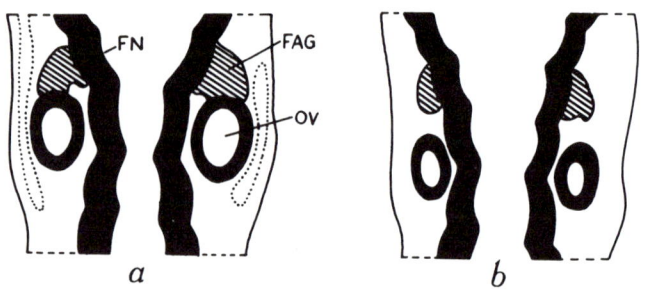

Fig. 5. Longitudinal sections of 9-day-old a) normal and b) sightless embryos. FAG = facial-acoustic ganglionic complex; FN = 4th neuromere; OV = otic vesicle.

Dreher (dr)

This recessive gene causes widespread malformations in the inner ear. No part is actually missing, but none is normal either (Fig. 6). The cochlea is poorly coiled, and the organ of Corti has severe cytoarchitectural abnormalities. The utricle and saccule are imperfectly separated. The lumen of the semicircular ducts is severely reduced or missing altogether. The differentiation of the maculae and the cristae is also affected. The endolymphatic duct is short and the sac is confined to the otic capsule [8].

Developmental studies have shown that the abnormalities of the inner ear are preceded by those of the neural tube [9]. In 9-day-old normal embryos the thin roof of the rhombencephalon extends caudally beyond the 6th neuromere, whereas in dreher embryos it comes to an end in the region of the 4th neuromere, and the thick walls meet dorsally in the region of the otic vesicle (Fig. 7). The abnormal morphogenesis of the otic vesicle could be ascribed to interference with the normal inductive function of the neural tube consequent to its own malformation.

Dancer (Dc)

The effects of this semidominant gene are variable and are confined to the vestibular part of the inner ear in the heterozygote, the cochlear part being normal. The lateral and superior semicircular ducts may be severely constricted, discontinuous, or altogether absent, but the superior duct is less frequently affected than the lateral one. When a duct is altogether absent, its crista is also missing. The posterior duct is unaffected. The utricle is invariably abnormal: it is severely reduced and lacks a macula (Fig. 8). The saccule is somewhat smaller than normal, but is otherwise unaffected. The utricle and the saccule are sometimes confluent. The superior vestib-

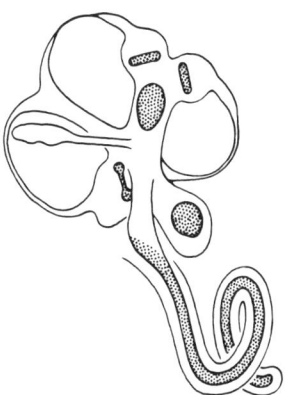

Fig. 6. Dreher homozygote.

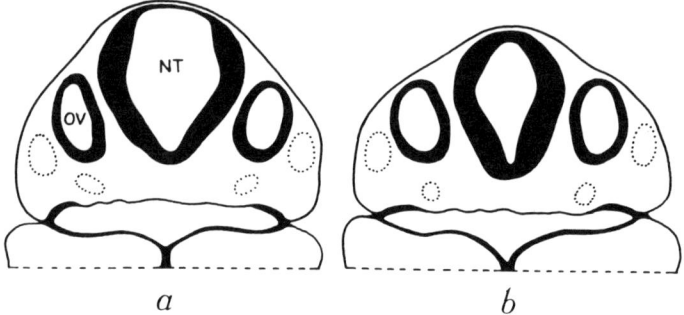

Fig. 7. Transverse sections of 10-day-old a) normal and b) dreher embryos. NT = neural tube; OV = otic vesicle.

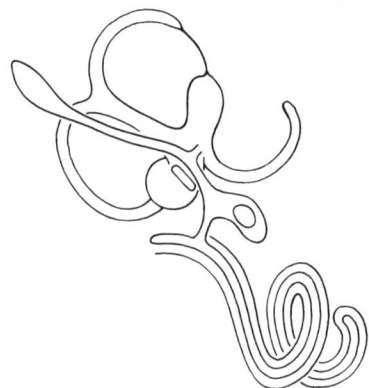

Fig. 8. Dancer heterozygote.

ular ganglion is severely reduced or missing. The abnormalities of the utricle are symmetric but those of the semicircular ducts may not be. The homozygotes die before birth [10].

The abnormalities of the inner ear can be traced back to 10-day-old embryos. The acoustic ganglion in dancer embryos at this stage is smaller than normal (Fig. 9). Investigation at later stages shows that the ganglion is smaller because the cells that are to give rise to the superior vestibular division are missing. As the abnormalities of the adult inner ear are confined to the parts that are normally innervated by this division, it is reasonable to assume that they are in some way consequent to the absence of the ganglion. This relationship may indicate some inductive function on the part of the ganglion, but may also mean that the superior vestibular ganglion is of placodal origin, and the region of the placode that gives rise to it is the

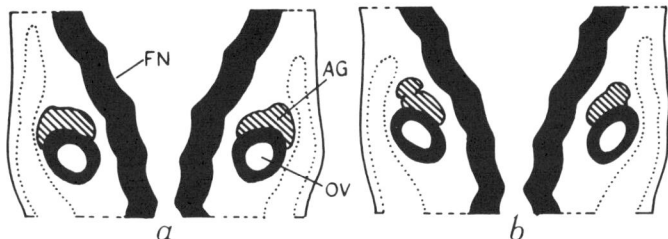

Fig. 9. Longitudinal sections of 10-day-old a) normal and b) dancer embryos. AG = acoustic ganglion; FN = 4th neuromere; OV = otic vesicle.

region from which the parts that this ganglion innervates develop. If this latter possibility is correct then it is easy to see how a placode that cannot give rise to the ganglion would also fail to develop the parts that the ganglion innervates.

Fidget (fi)

This recessive gene inhibits the formation of all 3 semicircular ducts. The utricle is much larger than normal, as if the fusions necessary for the formation of the ducts had not occurred, and that part of the vesicle had remained a single large chamber (Fig. 10). The crista of the lateral duct is always missing. The other 2 cristae are present, but since they are not situated in different ampullae (but in the same chamber), they are unlikely to function normally. The macula of the utricle is normal, but that of the saccule is somewhat reduced. The 2 sides are symmetric, and the abnormalities are always the same, as if the gene had led to a specific modification of the directions for the morphogenesis of the inner ear [11].

Developmental studies have failed to suggest a cause for the abnormal morphogenesis. However, as the behavior of fidget mice is also affected, and as there are strong arguments for regarding the behavior of this and other similar mutants as having a central cause [12], it is possible that the neural tube is not entirely normal in fidget embryos. The fact that fidget mice also have reduced eyes appears to support this assumption, because the primary optic vesicles are essentially an extension of the forebrain.

Waltzer-type (Wt)

This semidominant gene affects the morphogenesis of the lateral and posterior semicircular ducts in the heterozygote (Fig. 11). These ducts may be severely constricted in the middle or be discontinuous. While the terminal parts of the lateral duct, including the crista, are always present, the posterior duct may be missing altogether; when this happens, its crista is also absent. The superior duct is normal, as are other parts of the inner ear. The 2 sides may be asymmetrically affected. The homozygotes die before birth [13].

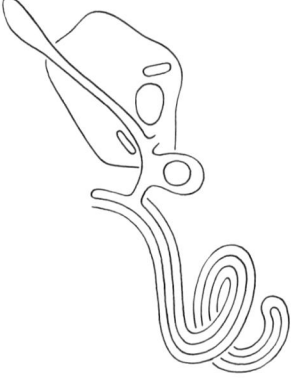 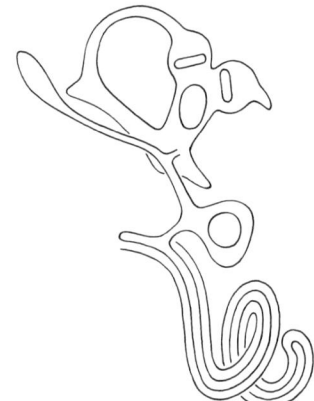

Fig. 10. Fidget homozygote.   Fig. 11. Waltzer-type heterozygote.

The development of these abnormalities in the heterozygote has not been studied, but it is known that the homozygotes, which die too early in embryonic life to show any malformations of the inner ear, have abnormal neural tubes [14]. The ganglia are also likely to be affected. It is reasonable to assume that the abnormalities in the heterozygous embryos are similar in nature, but not quite so severe. The developmental basis of the malformation of the inner ear in the waltzer-type heterozygote may then be essentially similar to that of the mutants described above.

Histidinemia (*his*)

This recessive gene leads to a deficiency of the enzyme histidase in the homozygote, which results in an excessively high concentration of histidine and its imidazole derivatives. The offspring of such histidinemic mothers may have widespread abnormalities of the inner ear, depending on their genetic background. In severely affected organs, no part may be normal (Fig. 12). The semicircular ducts may be extremely narrow, the endolymphatic duct very wide, and the endolymphatic sac grossly distended. The saccule and the utricle may be malformed. The scala tympani may be severely reduced, and the scala vestibuli correspondingly enlarged. The cytoarchitecture of the organ of Corti, the maculae, and the cristae may be grossly abnormal. The 2 sides are frequently dissimilar, and the inner ear is sometimes quite normal [15–17, and unpublished observations].

As these abnormalities can be produced experimentally by feeding the mother a diet rich in histidine [17], they are obviously teratogenic effects of maternal histidinemia. In the absence of developmental studies it is not possible to say how they originate. However, in view of the fact that the behavior of the offspring of histidinemic mothers is also affected and the correlation between behavior and abnormalities of the inner ear is not very good, it may be assumed that the neural tube is in some way involved in this case as well.

Shaker-with-syndactylism (sy)

This recessive gene has severe effects on all parts of the inner ear in the homozygote (Fig. 13). Most of the abnormalities appear after birth. The semicircular ducts lose their lumen and are represented by simple strands of cells. The ampullae as well as the utricle and saccule become highly irregular in shape. The endolymphatic duct is virtually closed in the middle, and the endolymphatic sac remains very small. The cytoarchitecture of the organ of Corti, of the maculae, and of the cristae becomes grossly disorganized. In advanced stages virtually all the chambers of the inner ear are found to be filled with dedifferentiated cells. These abnormalities are all symmetric [18].

Developmental studies show that the earliest detectable abnormalities occur in the mesenchymal condensations around the primitive otic labyrinth, and for a considerable period they remain confined to the periotic structures which are derived from these condensations [18]. This would seem to suggest that in this mutant the primary defect lies in the mesenchyme; but as the induction of the mesenchymal condensation is in turn dependent on the otic labyrinth, it is not possible to say how the two might be related.

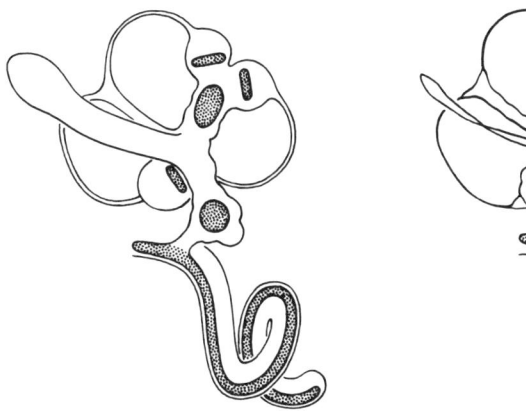

Fig. 12. Effects of maternal histidinemia.

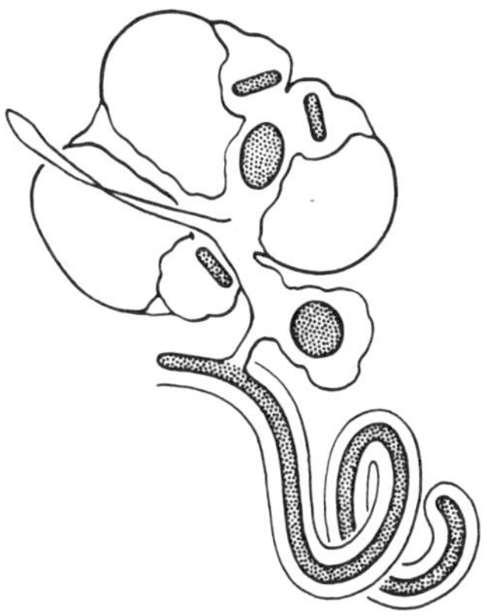

Fig. 13. Shaker-with-syndactylism homozygote.

Kinky (Fu^{ki})

The effects of this semidominant gene in the heterozygote are extremely variable. In severe cases no part of the inner ear remains normal (Fig. 14). The lumen of the semicircular ducts is greatly reduced or altogether eliminated. The utricle and the saccule are distorted. The endolymphatic duct and sac are much wider, and may be confined to the otic capsule. The cochlea is poorly coiled. The cytoarchitecture of the organ of Corti, the maculae, and the cristae is strikingly abnormal. The 2 sides are frequently different [12]. The development of this mutant has not been studied, but it is known that the homozygotes die in early embryonic stages.

Twirler (*Tw*)

The effects of this semidominant gene are variable, and are confined to the vestibular part of the inner ear (Fig. 15). The most common abnormalities are a reduction or absence of the lateral semicircular duct and absence of otoliths in the maculae. The other 2 ducts are present, but have an irregular outline. The cristae are all present. The cochlea is not affected [19]. The homozygotes die soon after birth. The development has not been studied.

Nijmegen waltzer (*nv*)

This recessive gene affects only the morphogenesis of the lateral semicircular duct, which may be severely constricted in the middle, discontinuous, or altogether absent (Fig. 16). Its 'crista' is always present, although it may not bear any resemblance to the normal structure; for instance, it may take the form of a deep cup in-

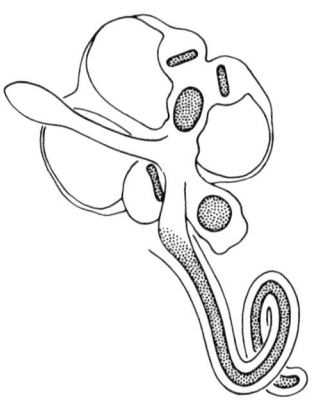

Fig. 14. Kinky heterozygote.

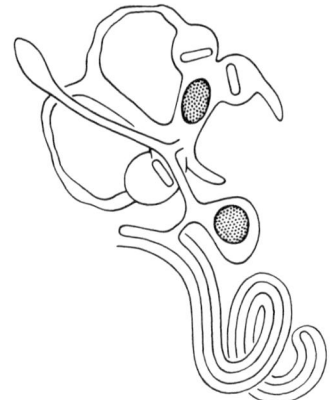

Fig. 15. Twirler heterozygote.

stead of a ridge. Its neural epithelium, however, is always greatly reduced and the associated nerve is much thinner than normal. The 2 sides are frequently different [20].

The development of this mutant has not been studied, but the reduction of the lateral crista and its nerve would suggest a reduction in the number of ganglion cells associated with it. This could mean, by analogy with the mutant dancer, that the part of the placode that is to give rise to this ganglion and the lateral semicircular duct is affected.

Zigzag

It is not certain whether we are concerned here with a single gene with incomplete penetrance or more genes acting together; for this reason no symbol has been given. Moreover, the mutant is believed to be extinct. In affected animals the lateral semicircular duct was found to be constricted or discontinuous on either one side or both (Fig. 17). Its ampulla was always present, as was the crista, which appeared to be normal [21]. Nothing is known about the development of this mutant.

Rotating (rg)

This recessive gene causes malformation of all 3 semicircular ducts. Their lumen is abruptly reduced in the middle of the arc (Fig. 18). In severe cases, the duct may be entirely blocked. The lateral duct is always affected but one or both of the others may be normal. The 2 sides are often different [22]. The development has not been studied.

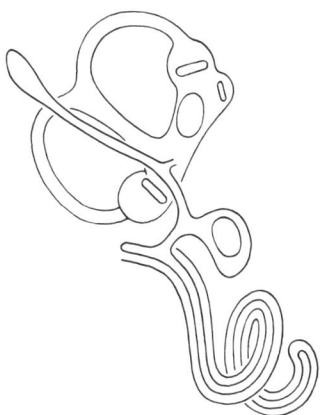
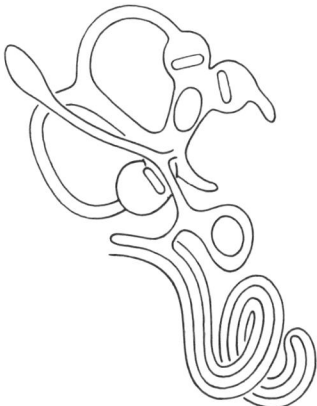

Fig. 16. Nijmegen waltzer homozygote.   Fig. 17. Zigzag homozygote.

Pallid (pa)

The effects of this recessive gene are highly variable, and are confined to the 2 maculae (Fig. 19). The otoliths may be missing in one or in both, but in any particular ear if they are missing in the saccule they are also missing in the utricle, while the converse does not hold [23]. The cytoarchitecture of the maculae appears to be normal. The 2 ears often are affected differently. Several other genes have similar effects: among these are mocha [24], muted [25], and tilted head [26].

Developmental studies have shown that the abnormality of the otoliths can be detected as early as the 16th day of gestation [27], although its cause is not clear. However, it has been found that not only can a similar abnormality be produced in the offspring by feeding the mother a manganese-free diet, but also that administration of manganese to the mother during pregnancy can lead to the formation of normal otoliths in mutant offspring [26]. Evidently, manganese is essential for the development of the otoliths, and the pallid gene raises the manganese requirements of the embryo because normal and pallid embryos can occur in the same litter; but the precise role of manganese is not understood.

Hypopigmentation

There are many genes in the mouse that cause various types of hypopigmentation, that is, loss of pigment in a manner distinct from albinism, such as spotting or dilution [28]. The loss of pigment may be localized or total. Most of the genes that lead to at least a moderate degree of hypopigmentation also affect the inner ear [29]. The abnormalities are essentially similar in all cases, although they may vary in extent. They are largely cytoarchitectural, generally appear after birth, and are confined to the cochlea and the saccule (Fig. 20).

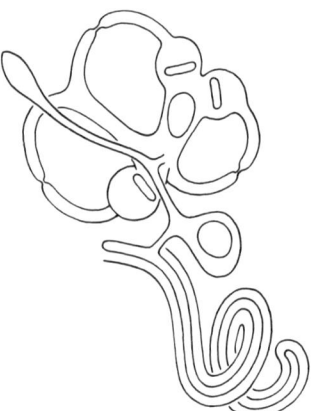

Fig. 18. Rotating homozygote.

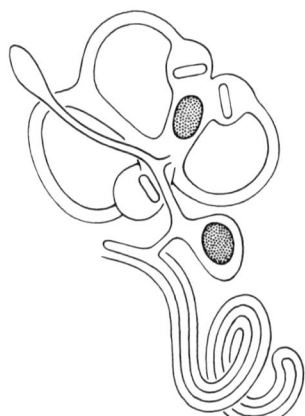

Fig. 19. Pallid homozygote.

In the cochlea there is a dedifferentiation of the organ of Corti, which may result not only in the loss of many types of cells, but also in fusions of the Reissner membrane with the organ of Corti, with the tectorial membrane and with the stria vascularis, to the virtual elimination of the cochlear duct (scala media). The stria vascularis is greatly reduced even if it is free of the Reissner membrane. In some cases the basal part of the cochlea is unaffected. The abnormalities of the saccule are similar in principle: a process of dedifferentiation leads to the elimination of its chamber, with the roof resting on the otoliths. In general, the cochlea may be affected without the involvement of the saccule, but if the saccule is affected, then so is the cochlea. These abnormalities may be asymmetric.

In some cases there is experimental evidence [30, 31] that the genes affect the neural crest, and hypopigmentation occurs because melanocytes originate in the neural crest. Since these same genes affect the inner ear, the abnormalities of the latter can be explained best on the assumption that the spiral ganglion and a part of the vestibular ganglion supplying the saccule are of neural crest origin. The abnormalities of the inner ear could then be seen as consequences of those of the ganglia [29, 32].

Hypothyroidism

As mentioned earlier, induced hypothyroidism in the mother during pregnancy leads to abnormalities of the inner ear in the offspring. These appear to be confined to the cochlea, and are generally constant (Fig. 21). There is a slight dis-

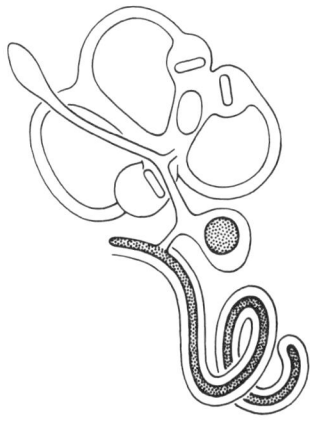
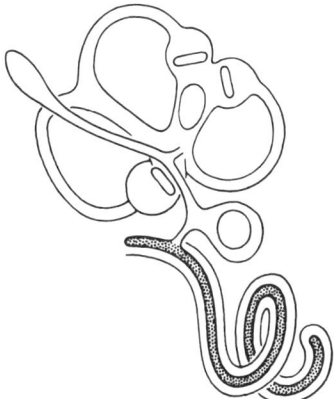

Fig. 20. Effects of hypopigmentation.   Fig. 21. Effects of hypothyroidism.

organization of the cytoarchitecture of the organ of Corti, even loss of some hair cells on occasion, but the most striking abnormality is a severe distortion of the tectorial membrane [33]. There is no contact between the membrane and the hair cells, and consequently hearing is affected.

Developmental studies suggest that the abnormality of the tectorial membrane is due to a malfunction of the columnar epithelium of the inner spiral sulcus [34]. These cells are believed to be responsible not only for the secretion of the membrane, but also for its maturation. As the secretion of the membrane does not appear to be interfered with and only the maturation is faulty, it would seem that thyroxine is necessary for the normal function of the epithelium only in the later stages of the development of the tectorial membrane.

GENETIC MALFORMATIONS IN MAN

Genetic disorders of the inner ear are common in man [35–39]. Their pathology is very poorly understood because it is extremely difficult to find suitable material for study, but it is clear that both types of abnormalities, degenerative as well as morphogenetic, occur [38, 40–45]. Everberg's extensive investigations in Denmark [42–45] have shown that morphogenetic abnormalities gross enough to be detectable by radiography are much more widespread than is realized: the vast majority of cases with asymmetric defects pass unnoticed because the less affected or normal side has retained enough function to hide the disorder.

Malformations of the inner ear observed in man have been reviewed by Ormerod [46]. He classifies them into 5 types, all of which are believed to occur in genetic conditions, although some are much more frequent than others. It is of great interest to note that all 5 types of malformations are represented among the mouse mutants described above. The same is true of the unilateral abnormalities observed by Everberg [42–45]. Indeed, the similarities between the human and murine disorders are so striking that it is difficult not to regard them as homologous conditions originating in much the same manner. However, pathologic similarities by themselves are not enough to form a basis for presumptive homology. Some other line of evidence, such as constant association with some feature independent of the inner ear, is necessary for this purpose. Such evidence is available for 3 types of disorders, those associated with hypopigmentation, hypothyroidism, and histidinemia.

There are at least 4 genes in man that cause deafness associated with abnormalities of pigmentation [29, 37, 39]. Two of these are autosomal dominant, one autosomal recessive, and one X-linked recessive. Very little is known about the pathology of the inner ear, but the 2 sides are often affected to different extents, and some residual hearing is frequently present in one or both ears. A strong case can be made for regarding these disorders as homologous to those observed in the mouse and several other species of mammals [29, 47]. It is therefore probable that their manner of origin is also similar.

There is an autosomal recessive gene that causes deafness associated with hypothyroidism in man [33, 38]. It is almost certain that there are more genes of the same type, for congenitally deaf persons have a higher frequency of hypothyroidism than the general population, and in a high proportion of cases their relatives are also affected [48]. Although very little is known about the abnormalities of the inner ear in this syndrome, it is a reasonable assumption that they are similar to those produced in the mouse by means of induced hypothyroidism, and that the basis of the association between deafness and hypothyroidism is also the same. The situation in man, however, is different in one respect: the mother may be euthyroid and it is the fetus that is hypothyroid because of its genetic constitution.

The evidence for hereditary histidinemia in man is less clear, but it is believed that an autosomal recessive gene is involved [39]. Again, nothing is known about the inner ear, but the fact that speech defects are frequent in affected persons suggests that the inner ear may not be normal. As described above, studies on mutant mice have shown that the inner ear abnormalities in an animal are not the result of its own histidinemia but that of the mother. The human condition is rather rare and its discovery is too recent to permit anything but speculation; but it may be discovered one day that speech defects (and presumptive disorders of the inner ear) are in fact teratologic consequences of maternal histidinemia.

REFERENCES

1. Hertwig P: Erbliche Missbildungen des Gehörorgans bei der Maus. Verh Anat Ges 53: 256–269, 1956.
2. Deol MS: The abnormalities of the inner ear in kreisler mice. J Embryol Exp Morphol 12: 475–490, 1964.
3. Ruben RJ: Development and cell kinetics of the kreisler (kr/kr) mouse. Laryngoscope 83: 1440–1468, 1973.
4. Zwilling E: The determination of the otic vesicle in *Rana pipiens*. J Exp Zool 86:333–342, 1941.
5. Detwiler SR, van Dyke RH: The role of the medulla in the differentiation of the otic vesicle. J Exp Zool 113:179–200, 1950.
6. Yntema CL: An analysis of the induction of the ear from foreign ectoderm in the salamander embryo. J Exp Zool 113:211–244, 1950.
7. Khaze'i N: Developmental genetics of a new neurological mutant in the mouse. PhD Thesis, University of London, 1974.
8. Fischer H: Untersuchungen am Innenohr einer bewegungsgestörten, tauben Hausmausmutante im Vergleich mit der vererbbaren, labyrinthären Hörstörung des Menschen. Arch Ohr Nas Kehlk Heilk 170:411–433, 1957.
9. Deol MS: The origin of the abnormalities of the inner ear in dreher mice. J Embryol Exp Morphol 12:727–733, 1964.
10. Deol MS, Lane PW: A new gene affecting the morphogenesis of the vestibular part of the inner ear in the mouse. J Embryol Exp Morphol 16:543–558, 1966.
11. Truslove GM: The anatomy and development of the fidget mouse. J Genet 54:64–86, 1956.
12. Deol MS: The probable mode of gene action in the circling mutants of the mouse. Genet Res 7:363–371, 1966.

13. Stein KF, Huber SA: Morphology and behaviour of waltzer-type mice. J Morphol 106: 197–204, 1960.
14. Stein KF, Filosa SH: The lethal effect of homozygosity of the gene for waltzer-type, a neurological mutant in *Mus musculus*. Dev Biol 19:358–367, 1969.
15. Kacser H, Bulfield G, Wallace ME: Histidinaemic mutant in the mouse. Nature 244:77–79, 1973.
16. Bulfield G, Kacser H: Histidinaemia in mouse and man. Arch Dis Child 49:545–552, 1974.
17. Kacser H, Mya KM, Duncker M, Wright AF, Bulfield G, McLaren A, Lyon MF: Maternal histidine metabolism and its effect on foetal development in the mouse. Nature 265: 262–266, 1977.
18. Deol MS: The development of the inner ear in mice homozygous for shaker-with-syndactylism. J Embryol Exp Morphol 11:493–512, 1963.
19. Lyon MF: Twirler: A mutant affecting the inner ear of the house mouse. J Embryol Exp Morphol 6:105–116, 1958.
20. Deol MS: Genes affecting behaviour and the inner ear in the mouse. In van Abeelen JHF (ed): "The Genetics of Behaviour." Amsterdam: North-Holland, 1974, pp 259–271.
21. Lyon MF: Zigzag: A genetic defect of the horizontal canals in the mouse. Genet Res 1: 189–195, 1960.
22. Deol MS, Dickie MM: Rotating, a new gene affecting behaviour and the inner ear in the mouse. J Hered 58:69–72, 1967.
23. Lyon MF: Hereditary absence of otoliths in the house mouse. J Physiol 114:410–418, 1951.
24. Lane PW, Deol MS: Mocha, a new coat color and behavior mutation on chromosome 10 of the mouse. J Hered 65:362–364, 1974.
25. Lyon MF, Meredith R: *Muted*, a new mutant affecting coat colour and otoliths of the mouse, and its position in linkage group XIV. Genet Res 14:163–166, 1969.
26. Erway LC, Fraser AS, Hurley LS: Prevention of congenital otolith defect in pallid mutant mice by manganese supplementation. Genetics 67:97–108, 1971.
27. Lyon MF: The developmental origin of hereditary absence of otoliths in mice. J Embryol Exp Morphol 3:230–241, 1955.
28. Searle AG: "Comparative Genetics of Coat Colour in Mammals." London: Logos Press Ltd, 1968.
29. Deol MS: The relationship between abnormalities of pigmentation and of the inner ear. Proc R Soc Lond Biol 175:201–217, 1970.
30. Mayer TC: The development of piebald spotting in mice. Dev Biol 11:319–334, 1965.
31. Mayer TC, Green MC: An experimental analysis of the pigment defect caused by mutations at the *W* and *Sl* loci in mice. Dev Biol 18:62–75, 1968.
32. Deol MS: The neural crest and the acoustic ganglion. J Embryol Exp Morphol 17:533–541, 1967.
33. Deol MS: An experimental approach to the understanding and treatment of hereditary syndromes with congenital deafness and hypothyroidism. J Med Genet 10:235–242, 1973.
34. Deol MS: The role of thyroxine in the differentiation of the organ of Corti. Acta Otolaryngol 81:429–435, 1976.
35. Brown KS: The genetics of childhood deafness. In McConnell FC, Ward PH (eds): "Deafness in Childhood." Nashville: Vanderbilt University Press, 1967.
36. Deol MS: Inherited diseases of the inner ear in man in the light of studies on the mouse. J Med Genet 5:137–158, 1968.
37. Deol MS: The ear. In Sorsby A (ed): "Clinical Genetics," 2nd Ed. London: Butterworths, 1973.

38. Fraser GR: "The Causes of Profound Deafness in Childhood." London: Baillière Tindall, 1976.
39. McKusick VA: "Mendelian Inheritance in Man," 4th Ed. Baltimore: The Johns Hopkins University Press, 1975.
40. Friedmann I: "Pathology of the Ear." Oxford: Blackwell Scientific Publications, 1974.
41. Altmann F: The inner ear in genetically determined deafness. Acta Otolaryngol (Suppl) (Stockh) 187, 1964.
42. Everberg G: Hereditary unilateral deafness. Acta Otolaryngol (Stockh) 47:303–311, 1957.
43. Everberg G: Unilateral anacusis. Clinical, radiological and genetic investigations. Acta Otolaryngol (Suppl) (Stockh) 158:366–374, 1960.
44. Everberg G: Further studies on hereditary unilateral deafness. Acta Otolaryngol (Stockh) 51:615–635, 1960.
45. Everberg G: Investigations into unilateral total deafness and absence of vestibular function with a particular view to the X-ray appearances in the inner ear. Acta Otolaryngol (Stockh) 52:47–62, 1960.
46. Ormerod FC: The pathology of congenital deafness. J Laryngol 74:919–950, 1960.
47. Brown KS, Bergsma DR, Barrow MV: Animal models of pigment and hearing abnormalities in man. In Bergsma D (ed): Part IX. "The Ear." Baltimore: Williams & Wilkins for The National Foundation–March of Dimes, BD:OAS VII(4):102, 1971.
48. Baschieri L, Benedetti G, de Luca F, Negri M: Evaluation and limitations of perchlorate tests in the study of thyroid function. J Clin Endocrinol 23:786, 1963.

DISCUSSION

Dr. Malkiat Deol: Any gene that can have different effects on the two sides is bound to be subject to changes in genetic background.

Dr. Thomas Van De Water: From doing organ culture studies on the Kreisler mouse, I've noticed two things—one is that heterogeneity that you've spoken of, where one side does not look at all like the other side; but sometimes there is some homogeneity of development on both sides. I have to select certain breeds in order to get it. There are two distinct types: one in which you can see asymmetry on the sides, while the other appears relatively symmetric, where you have almost the same sides, otic cups to otic vesicles.

Dr. David Lim: What kind of mouse is this?

Dr. Malkiat Deol: This is sightless, a blind mouse. The symbol is Sig and the homozygote is affected. The heterozygote has some abnormalities, but they're very slight. A colleague has a strain of mouse, Dreher, with abnormal eyes and ears. In general, almost every structure could be recognized. There is sort of an endolymphatic duct and sac, and an abnormal organ of Corti. The coiling is rather poor. No part of the epithelium is normal enough to be regarded as having normal function. The abnormality of the inner ear is tied to those structures that are innervated by the ganglion that is missing. Originally, I thought that the ganglion itself plays an inductive role in differentiation so that the superior vestibular part induces the structures that are abnormal. But now Drs. Van de Water and Ruben tell me that you can grow a perfectly normal, or nearly normal, labyrinth without the ganglion. So perhaps the ganglion does not play a role. If so, we have to find another explanation – why the absence of the particular ganglion should lead to gross malformations later on of only those structures that are innervated by it. The only other explanation that I can think of is that when the ganglion is just a single structure, it appears to be homogenous, but it is not--there is somewhat biochemical differentiation in it. But why does the elimination of the particular type of cell give rise to abnormalities only of certain structures and not others? Possibly each specific part of the vesicle gives rise to a specific part of the ganglion.

The homozygote, which dies, usually about 8 or 9 days after gestation or at birth, frequently has a cleft palate. We were dealing here with the heterozygote. Now this next is a mutant called Fidget. In this case, the homozygotes die long before the palate is formed. You see in the other mutant, the homozygotes lived long enough to show cleft palate. In this case, they die too early.

Many of the ears that I have seen remind me of the Mondini type of change. In the Pallid mouse, we find abnormalities of the inner ear that are associated with hypopigmentation. Mutations at a locus that has at least one allele that can cause spotting can cause this type of abnormality. This is a normal organ of Corti.

Dr. David Lim: You say the tectorial membranes were abnormal: what about the cupola?

Dr. Malkiat Deol: Normal. But the abnormalities of the tectorial membrane I could not miss. I try to cut sections at a thickness of 7 microns, that gives me only a single layer of hair cells. In this case, as you can see, the pillars of Corti are missing. Everything else is there. The hair cell is occasionally distorted, occasionally missing, but very often there.

Dr. Heinrich Spoendlin: You have considerable degeneration of the neurons.

Dr. Malkiat Deol: There's degeneration of many other things. But at the moment, I'm talking about morphogenetic abnormalities. The abnormality in the organ of Corti that is morphogenetic is confined to the malformation or malfunction of the cells that are going to give rise to the pillars of Corti. I will now show you three consecutive sections from the Bronx Waltzer mouse. In this case, there is no inner cell and there is no rod, either the inner or the outer. In this next case, you find the outer rod is very nearly perfect, while the inner one is slightly distorted.

Dr. Charles Berlin: Can I ask if anybody has recorded action potentials or single units on this animal?

Dr. David Lim: I think it is an extremely exciting animal model. There is a considerable controversy as to the function of the inner and outer hair cells. This is genetic surgery.

Dr. Robert Ruben: As you go through this very impressive list of mutants, is it possible to give an estimate of the number of different genes that control the development of the membranous and bony labyrinth? You've described 14 mutants having different errors of development.

Dr. Malkiat Deol: I think that if you want to estimate the number of loci that may be involved in the morphogenesis of the inner ear, it might have been possible to do it. For years at the Jackson Laboratory they kept strict records of the occurrence of such mutants. If they had carried that work for many years longer, some clever statistician may have been able to work out the possible number of new mutations that are yet to arise in times to come. But that hasn't happened, and I see no way of finding out how many there might have been.

The Genetic Analysis of Profound Prelingual Deafness

Walter E. Nance, MD, PhD

I would like to describe some of the methods of genetic analysis that can be applied in situations where we cannot recognize a specific hereditary deafness syndrome by either clinical or audiologic criteria, and must rely solely on the available pedigree information, that is to say, the detailed history of the number of affected and normal family members, including parents, sibs, and other more remote relatives. The problem of a deaf child who is brought for evaluation by hearing parents with no known family history of deafness is commonly confronted in clinics. The results of many careful genetic studies suggest that at least 50% of children in schools for the deaf have hearing losses that are genetic in etiology, although it may not be possible to identify every hereditary case individually. In 1968, through the collaboration of the Office of Demographic Studies of Gallaudet College, we were able to collect family history data on approximately 16,000 deaf children in 12,000 families. Some of the results of our analyses of these data which constitute, in all likelihood, the largest study of a single genetic condition that has ever been attempted, are presented here. The results of these analyses are contained in much greater detail in the Ph.D. dissertation of my former student, Dr. Susan Rose.

The method of analysis that one applies to data of this type is known as segregation analysis. In this procedure, the sibships with deaf children are first subdivided according to the mating type of the parents, the number of children, the number of affected family members, and the number of probands. The proband is the index case through whom the family was identified. Anyone who collects family history data with the intention of using the pedigrees for a sophisticated genetic analysis must indicate how each family was identified, ie who was the proband in the family. For example, if a study of 4th grade students in schools for the deaf were conducted, every deaf child in the 4th grade would be a proband. Deaf sibs in the 7th grade, 3rd grade, or 12th grade would be secondary rather

than index cases. However, a family that had 2 deaf children in the 4th grade would have 2 probands. In some situations one cannot be certain whether a particular family was referred because there were 2 affected children, or whether the 2nd affected child should be regarded as a secondary case.
a secondary case.

After we subdivide the families by the total number of children, the number of affected members, and the number of probands, we try to obtain estimates of 3 different parameters. These are π, the ascertainment probability; p, the segregation ratio; and x, the proportion of sporadic cases. π is the probability that an affected child is a proband; its value can vary from one to nearly zero, and its importance can best be understood as follows. First, assume that all affected individuals in a population are represented by pingpong balls in a large container, and that affected sibs are joined together by strings. If we randomly sample "deaf children" from this total population of "pingpong balls," there would be, for example, 3 balls that we could pick to draw out a family with 3 affected individuals in it but only one way to select families with a single affected child. If our ascertainment probability π is very low, that is if we select only a small proportion of the total population of affected individuals – there will be a bias toward collecting families with multiple affected individuals; thus, it is important to identify how the families are ascertained and what proportion of the affected individuals are probands. While the value of π is of little intrinsic interest, it is important to estimate it and to include the estimate in further analyses to obtain unbiased results.

The two parameters in which we are most interested are the segregation ratio, p – the proportion of affected individuals – and x, the proportion of sporadic cases. A major goal of segregation analysis is to search for evidence of familial aggregation of the trait in question. We may suppose that many cases of deafness are sporadic; that is to say, they arise largely from environmental causes which are associated with a negligible recurrence risk. However, there may also be a subpopulation in which there is a high recurrence risk. Thus, we are interested in estimating what proportion, x, of all cases is sporadic and what proportion, $1-x$, is nonsporadic or high-risk cases; among the latter, we would also like to know the value of p, the recurrence risk.

I think it is important to emphasize that this method of analysis does not impose any genetic model on the data but rather searches only for evidence of familial aggregation. The process by which we obtain the estimates of π, p, and x is known as maximum likelihood estimation. In other words, if we try hundreds of values of these 3 parameters, which combination best fits the data we have actually collected? Fortunately, efficient computer programs have been developed to find the best-fitting values of the 3 variables by iterative techniques.

Alternately, we may say, "I don't want to estimate p; I want to test the hypothesis that p is 0.25, because if the deafness in these families results from a recessive trait, that is the recurrence risk I would expect." We could then assume a trial value for one of the parameters and see whether it fits the data, ie see whether the data allow you to reject any particular trial value of p.

An example of the results of such an analysis is summarized in Table 1. Among the normal by normal matings, there was a subpopulation of 86 families where there was evidence of consanguinity. We would ordinarily consider the presence of parental consanguinity as strong evidence that we are dealing with an autosomal recessive trait. When we ask the questions, "Are all the cases with consanguineous parents genetic (ie $x = 0$)?" and is the segregation ratio in these families 0.25 (ie $p = 0.25$)?" we see on the first line of Table 1 that these two assumptions fit the data reasonably well as indicated by the small values of X^2 on the right of the Table. Turning next to the normal by normal matings without consanguinity, we can break these down into 2 groups: Cases in which there is a positive family history and those in which there is a negative family history.

Smith: How many generations were you using?

Nance: Basically we were dealing with 2-generation data. In all of the families under discussion, both parents had normal hearing but there was at least one affected child. When I use the term "positive family history," however, I am referring to an anamnestic history of deafness or profound hearing loss in some relative outside the nuclear family unit, possibly in a previous generation. The negative family history cases were those in which there was no known family history of deafness outside the nuclear family.

TABLE 1. Segregation Analysis of Normal by Normal Matings With at Least One Deaf Child ($\pi = 0.325$)*

Mating type and hypothesis tested	No. of Families	No. of Children Deaf	Hearing	$x^2 p$	$x^2 x$
Consanguineous $H_0: p = 0.25, x = 0.0$	86	150	148	2.17	3.44
Nonconsanguineous Positive family Hx $H_0: p = 0.25, x = 0.0$ $H_1: p = 0.25, x = 0.20$	1,391 1,391	2,142 2,142	3,496 3,496	96.97 0.95	103.85 —
Negative family Hx $H_0: p = 0.25, x = 0.0$ $H_1: p = 0.25, x = 0.65$	10,509 10,509	12,712 12,712	28,739 28,739	5,290 1.93	5,833 —

*(Adapted from Nance We, et al: In Lubs HA, de La Cruz F (eds): "Genetic Counseling." New York: Raven Press, 1977.)

On line 2 of Table 1 we see that a test of the hypothesis that all of the deaf children born to these hearing, nonconsanguineous parents are the result of fully penetrant recessive genes, with no sporadic cases, can be resoundingly rejected, as shown by the very large value of χ^2 which indicates that this hypothesis does not fit the data well. Therefore, the hypothesis that $x = 0$ is probably not valid, and we then ask the computer to determine the best-fitting value of x under the assumption that p is still 0.25. In cases with a positive family history, the value of x that fits the data best is 0.2. In the negative family history cases, the value of x that fits best is 0.65.

What does this mean? It means that among deaf children produced by nonconsanguineous normal by normal matings, with a remote history of deafness, only about 20% are nongenetic. In similar matings without such a history, 65% are estimated to be nongenetic and about 35% genetic. By simply inquiring about remote family history of deafness we can considerably improve our ability to predict correctly whether the case is genetic or not. In both subgroups of the normal by normal nonconsanguineous matings, when x is fixed at its maximum likelihood value, the assumption that p is 0.25 gives a very good fit as indicated by the small values of the "goodness of fit" X^2s. It looks, then, as if these families include recessive cases, with a variable proportion of nongenetic cases as well, and one of the important uses for these kinds of data is to obtain accurate empiric risk estimates for genetic counseling.

DISCUSSION

Dr. Robert Ruben: In your negative family history, you're assuming approximately 65% are nongenetic. Now when you define sporadic, you've got one of 2 choices: a) you're wrong, b) you're right, b_1) some of these are new mutations, b_2) you have known exogenous cause, eg rubella. How do you handle something like that?

Dr. Walter Nance: It's interesting, useful, and important to define precisely what is mean by a sporadic case. We can divide all the sibships into multiplex families in which there are 2 or more affected children and simplex families in which there is only 1 affected child. The basic assumption we make in all these analyses is that all the multiplex cases are genetic until proven otherwise. This is probably a reasonable assumption in almost all cases. For example, if the incidence of nongenetic deafness in the population is assumed to be 1:1000, very roughly, we might expect that only 1: 1,000,000 2-child families would have 2 deaf children "by chance" or as independent events. Thus, the assumption that all such cases are genetic in etiology will not be in error very frequently.

The simplex cases, on the other hand, consist of 2 types. They may be genetic cases. Dr. Ruben is correct when he points out that, in addition to deafness from sporadic. By sporadic, we mean a case in which there is a very low recurrence risk, on the order, perhaps of, 1:1000. We know that even if we are dealing with a recessive trait, for every 2-child sibship in which both children are affected; there will be 6 families in which only 1 of the 2 children is affected. Therefore, if we wait until there are 2 affected children in the family before we even consider the possibility that we might be dealing with a recessive trait, we will be missing the part of the iceberg that is below the water. Segregation analysis looks at the number of cases in which there are multiple affected sibs and estimates what proportion of the simplex families must be chance-isolated genetic cases. The cases that are "leftover," so to speak, provide an estimate of x, the proportion of sporadic cases, Dr. Ruben is correct when he points out that, in addition to deafness from such environmental causes as rubella, the sporadic cases also include any new mutations that may have occurred since these cases would also be associated with a negligible recurrence risk within the nuclear sibship, although not, perhaps, among the offspring of the affected child.

We can use estimates of p and x to obtain useful comparative risk figures. The data shown in Table 2 reflect the composite results of an analysis of several large bodies of data, including deaf by normal and deaf by deaf, as well as the normal by normal mating types I have discussed. Normal parents, of course, will ordinarily not come to see an otolaryngologist or genetic counselor unless they already have had an affected child. The appropriate recurrence risk if there is a negative family history is about 10%, while the recurrence risk if there is a positive family history is approximately 20%. If a couple comes for counseling with their first child affected, but a specific cause or syndrome cannot be identified, I think these would be the appropriate risk figures to use. Confronted with this uncertainty, intuition would tell you that the more normal children the couple have had beyond the

TABLE 2. Empiric Risk of Deafness in Offspring of Various Mating Types*

Mating type	No. of deaf offspring	No. of tested offspring					
		0	1	2	3	4	5
Normal by normal							
Positive family history	1	–	0.20	0.19	0.17	0.16	0.14
Negative family history	1	–	0.10	0.08	0.07	0.05	0.04
Deaf by normal							
All normal children	0	0.07	0.04	0.03	0.02	0.01	0.01
At least 1 deaf child	>1	–	0.41	0.41	0.41	0.41	0.41
Deaf by deaf							
All normal children	0	0.10	0.04	0.03	0.02	0.01	0.01
All deaf children	S	0.10	0.61	0.80	0.92	0.97	0.99
Deaf and normal child	>0>S	–	–	0.37	0.37	0.37	0.37

*(Adapted from Bieber J, Nance WE: In Jackson LG, Schimke RH (eds): "Clinical Genetics." New York: John Wiley, 1979.)

affected child, the less likely it is that the case was genetic in the first place. In Table 2, we have adjusted the empiric risk figures to take into account the number of normal children in the sibship. For example, in cases with a positive family history, the recurrence risk falls to about 14% for couples with 5 normal children in addition to their affected child. If there is a negative family history, the risk would tail off to about 4%.

Dr. Robert Ruben: Does birth order make a difference? Let's say that the 5th child happens to be affected, and the other 4 were not; is their risk of recurrence 14% and not 20% even with a positive family history?

Dr. Walter Nance: We have not taken birth order into account. If a 4th child is affected after 3 previous normal children, we would give the parents a risk appropriate for one affected child with 3 normal sibs. Other than Rh incompatibility, I think no cause of deafness would be expected to show a parity effect.

A deaf parent by normal parent mating is rather interesting. In this situation, the couple might well come for premarital counseling and the best guess of the risk that their first child would be affected is about 7%, rapidly falling to about 0.6% after they have had 5 normal children. This statistic assumes, of course, that no other diagnostic information allows the recognition of a specific cause for the parent's deafness.

Dr. Charles Berlin: In a deaf by normal mating in which the first child is deaf, the likelihood should seem very high . . .

Dr. Walter Nance: It is 41%. If it is a deaf by normal mating that has already produced a deaf child, we would ordinarily consider the family's disorder to represent an example of dominantly inherited deafness. The reason the recurrence risk is only about 41% instead of 50% is that many dominant forms of deafness have low penetrance. Waardenburg syndrome is a classic example, where only a fraction of people who inherit the gene actually manifest profound bilateral deafness.

The deaf by deaf matings are more complex, and there are several possibilities to consider. Both parents obviously could have nongenetic deafness, in which case the risk would be very low. Or one parent could have dominant deafness, in which case the risk would be close to 50% regardless of the marriage partner. Finally, if both parents have recessive deafness, their children would either be all deaf or all hearing, depending on whether the parents have the same type or different type of recessive deafness.

In a deaf by deaf mating, the phenotype of the first child profoundly alters the genetic counseling for subsequent children. Before the first child is born, the empiric risk in our data is very close to 10%, although I imagine most laymen and many professionals would consider the risk of having a deaf child in a deaf by deaf mating to be substantially higher than that. Once the couple has had a single normal child, their risk for deafness in subsequent children is cut to about 4% and rapidly decreases as more normal children are born. After 5 normal children, the risk is less than 1%. If the first child is deaf, however, the risk for the next child jumps to 66% and rapidly approaches 100% as more deaf children are born into the family. Finally, if the deaf couple has had both deaf and normal children, we are dealing with a segregating sibship and, at least for our data, the empiric risk was 32%.

Although these Tables are applicable for cases in which no definite cause for the the deafness can be established, they cannot and should not replace a careful clinical and genetic evaluation. In practice, we use the Tables as a starting point for counseling. If, on the basis of our evaluation we are suspicious of a genetic etiology even though we cannot prove it, we would be inclined to cite the appropriate figure in the Table as a lower limit to the risk. On the other hand, if we have reason to suspect an environmental cause, we would cite the data in the Table as an upper limit to the recurrence risk. In this way, we attempt to combine the subtle clinical impressions derived from a careful medical evaluation with factual risk estimates which are based on the analysis of large bodies of pedigree data. When accompanied by a discussion of the ubiquity of recessive genes for deafness and other hereditary diseases in the general population, most parents of deaf children respond favorably to this type of genetic counseling.

Neurophysiology of Auditory Deprivation*

Ben M. Clopton, PhD

Conductive or sensorineural hearing impairments early in life threaten the normal development of neural processing capabilities in the auditory system. It is important that we understand the nature of this threat if we are to ameliorate these aural defects fully. A point of reference for all peripheral management of hearing impairments is the maintenance of the possibility of central function. The lack of this possibility restricts any treatment to the cosmetic, regardless of the importance of the results to the patient. The clinical problem posed by auditory deprivation due to early deafness is only beginning to be assessed, and it is clear that the opportunity is great for contributions to our understanding from basic science.

A number of observations indicate that early auditory deprivation in humans has a deleterious effect on development of language and other mental capacities. Even a few years of auditory input before the onset of hearing loss has a noticeably positive effect on a variety of estimations of intelligence, capacities for language, and correlated indices, such as that of earning power [1]. Congenital deafness has a severe impact on socialization because of its vital role in acquisition of language. The concept of a critical period for some aspects of development of language is being increasingly invoked, and the sensitivity of the developing nervous system to even slight hearing loss during this period is gaining growing recognition.

This recognition is illustrated by the concern about the insidious effects of fluctuating hearing loss due to recurring bouts of otitis media in childhood. This kind of hearing loss presents a significant problem in about 15% of children [2], and it often goes unnoticed due to its episodic nature and correlation with minimal behavioral changes. The hearing loss incurred is usually less than the level of 25 dB previously accepted as the criterion beyond which there should be serious

---

*Supported by NIH grant NS-13052.

concern [3]. Sounds may be reduced by only 10–15 dB in the frequencies used for speech. While this loss is minimal and in most situations might be tolerated easily by adults, it can severely compromise the input to a developing auditory system, and has prompted use of a 15 dB critical level for ascertaining impairment in children [4].

Language is a complex matrix of components varying in duration and intensity that must be classified by the receiver if it is to be successfully decoded. This recognition of components must occur at a number of levels, each having rules of probability for sequencing and combination that differ across languages. Recognition of some components may be partially innate, perhaps even common to many species [5], but experiential factors are also at work [6]. This recognition is often made difficult due to noise, individual variations in speakers, and other limitations. Some features of speech having low energy, such as unvoiced consonants, are detected largely by the use of acquired rules for such cases. The acquisition of these rules is possible only if high quality speech is available during early learning, and even minimal losses can prevent this. Adequate hearing for an adult is not necessarily adequate hearing for a child.

The concept of a critical period for the development of basic hearing capabilities has some disturbing implications for all classes of hearing impairments in childhood, especially the more severe ones associated with congenital defects, and those with postnatal onset. The lesser attenuations in hearing can be alleviated in many cases by amplification of the signal, but malformations of the outer and middle ear require surgical treatments that are more conveniently accomplished later in life, if they are at all feasible. Sensorineural losses due to genetic abnormalities or metabolic insult are especially challenging and must await new treatments (for example, a cochlear prosthesis), if indeed any plausible means of restoring auditory input is possible. The question in all these instances is, what urgency must be attached to supplying at least minimal input to the system so as to maintain a semblance of future function. The very existence of fibers of the 8th nerve is threatened in cases of complete loss of hair cells [7], but equally debilitating changes may arise from deprivation of sound due to early conductive attenuation of sounds. A critical period implies that early loss is not reversible by later experience with sound. It is not presently known how valid this concept is in development of hearing. Of course, it can apply to some central auditory functions and not to others.

It is imperative that we gain more precise definitions of auditory plasticity. Observations on humans may be highly suggestive, but many will discount such evidence as being indicative of "deficits in learning" that can be corrected by later remedial therapy. Anatomic and neurophysiologic observations are now beginning to reveal extensive sequelae of early deprivation of sound in the auditory centers of the brainstem. Such effects of deprivation can influence all aspects of auditory function and must be viewed as detrimental to hearing as any cochlear lesion.

ANIMAL MODEL

The neurophysical and anatomic observations that will be described often involve myomorphic rodents, such as the laboratory rat. These animals have relatively restricted and predictable postnatal sequences for peripheral auditory development under normal conditions [8, 9]. Figure 1 illustrates the major limitations on hearing, the disappearance of these near the end of the 2nd week after birth, and the onset of normal indices of hearing in the rat. This schedule allows experimentation with variables in stimulation that would be more difficult with the more precocious development characterizing other common experimental animals, especially primates.

It must be emphasized that cochlear changes continue up to a month after birth. For example, changes in the cells of the inner spiral sulcus and pillar cells have been reported until 20 days after birth (DAB), and Hensen cells show some morphologic changes until 25 DAB [10, 11]. The onset of overall function, however, is rapid from about 10–15 DAB, and it is nearing completion according to most criteria by 21 DAB when the animals are normally weaned. The possibility of auditory deprivation affecting developing cochlear function cannot be discounted. Efferent innervation of the cochlea, for example, is a relatively late event in the sequence, appearing after 10 DAB [12], and early stimulation could conceivably influence its function.

Ultimately a correlation will be possible among the histogenetic and migratory processes, and those establishing interconnectivity of auditory neurons and neurophysiologic observations. Only minimal correspondences can be designated at present, most observations having been made on anatomic development.

The sites of the auditory centers of the brainstem are marked with neural elements quite early in development [13, 14]. The large and medium-sized neurons destined for the ventral and dorsal cochlear nuclei form on the 10th–13th days of gestation in the mouse [13]. The granular neurons of both nuclear divisions form later. In the ventral nucleus the granular cells form as late as the 14th day, and in the dorsal division these cells are forming as late as birth on the 18th or 19th day. Their schedules of migration and connection are somewhat uncertain, but dynamic changes in neuronal populations of the cochlear nuclei continue for weeks after birth [15]. Morest [16] has observed the formation of calyces of Held in the medial nucleus of the trapezoid body and found persistent growth cones at presynaptic sites a week after birth in the cat, and a month after birth in the rat. While some neuronal projections [17] may be established at the onset of auditory function and be relatively resistant to reorganization, other synapses are likely to take longer to stabilize and thereby be more subject to stimulation influences. This should be especially true for the intranuclear pathways mediated by those neurons with short axons that are late in developing.

An anatomic study of changes in the brainstem after postnatal deprivation of sound from 3–45 DAB found significant changes in neuronal morphology [18]. Neurons in the region of the globular cells of the ventral cochlear nucleus and

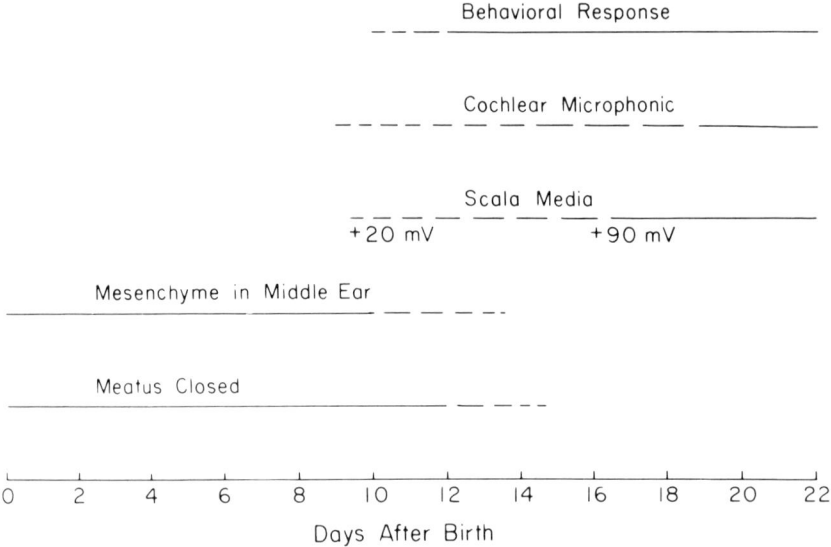

Fig. 1. Typical schedule for onset of hearing in the laboratory rat.

medial nucleus of the trapezoid body were smaller in deprived animals than in controls that experienced normal stimulation by sound during development. In addition, deprivation produced a decrease in the number of neurons in the dorsal cochlear nucleus. Similar, but more severe changes were seen in a human brain from a congenitally deaf person. Such findings suggest that important distortions of auditory processing will be present, if normal hearing is restored after early hearing impairment.

EXPERIMENTAL OBSERVATIONS

The following experiments concern the effects of developmental deprivation of sound in rats. This deprivation was produced by ligation of the external auditory meatus when the pups were 10 days old. This procedure produced a conductive hearing loss comparable to that in congenital malformation of the external or middle ear. In most cases, the procedure is reversible so as to allow stimulation of the ear some time later. At the time of electrophysiologic recording, the closed meatus was opened, cerumen and epithelial debris cleared from the tympanic membrane, and the middle ear inspected for obvious pathology. The experiments will be described in reverse of the order in which they were conducted, so as to provide a more cohesive sequence; thus the reader must anticipate some demonstrations of hindsight.

Some recent observations on the tuning curves for single neurons in the coch-

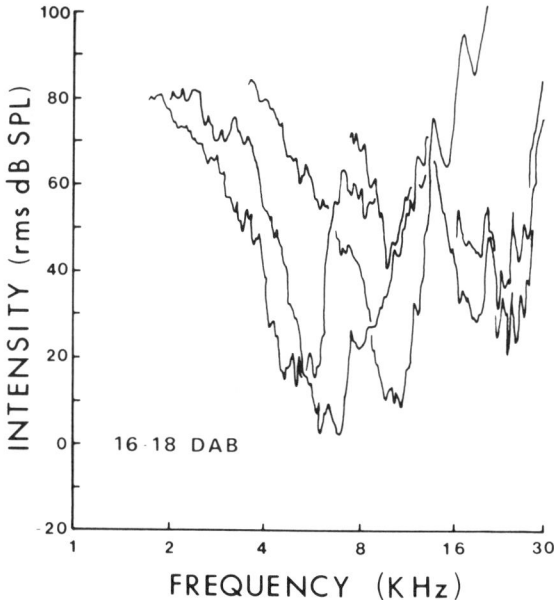

Fig. 2. Tuning curves for single units in rat pups at 16–18 DAB. Each curve represents approximately 128 determinations of threshold by a computer-directed process. Tuning curves shown in this and the following 3 figures are from the cochlear nucleus.

lear nuclei are illustrated in Figures 2 through 5. Figure 2 shows tuning curves for pups 16–18 DAB. While the threshold curves for these units demonstrate selectivity of frequencies even at this early stage of development, they have characteristics that clearly distinguish them from unit threshold curves in the adult. Units with high characteristic frequencies (CFs) have especially unusual responses. Their minimum thresholds are elevated, and they often have multiple peaks such that no one frequency dominates their response. Units with lower CFs have less elevated minimum thresholds, but they are less sensitive than would be expected in the mature animal.

These tuning curves are more symmetric and broader than adult curves, primarily due to a lack of a sharp cutoff on the side for high frequencies. Only slight indications of tails in the low frequencies are present. These observations are in agreement with others indicating an initial sensitivity to low frequencies with a progressive spread to high frequencies [9, 19]. A purely conductive loss due to remnants of peripheral attenuation cannot account for the shapes of the curves. Immaturity in cochlear or neural structures must be responsible.

Selected tuning curves from various stages of development are illustrated in Figure 3. The unit with the highest CF was recorded 22 DAB and demonstrates

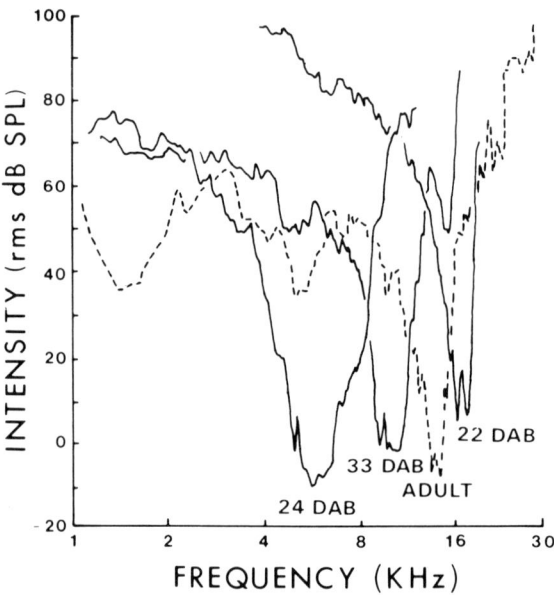

Fig. 3. Tuning curves from rats at various stages of development under normal conditions for sound. A typical adult curve is shown with dashed lines for comparison.

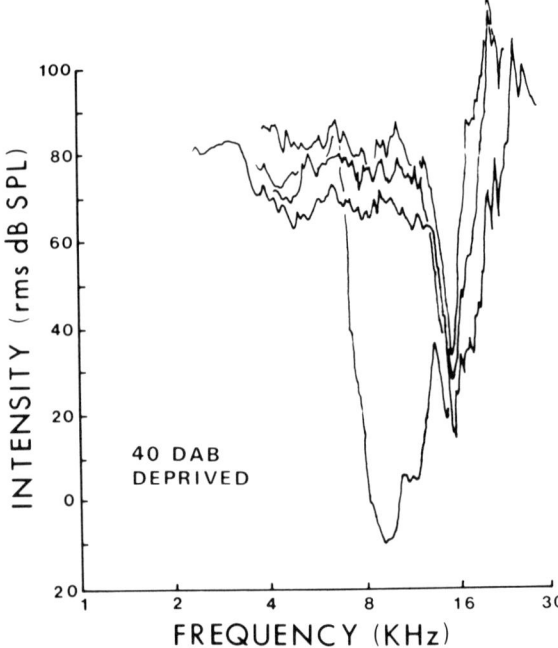

Fig. 4. Tuning curves from a rat partially deprived of hearing by a conductive block from 10 DAB to the time of recording at 40 DAB. Curves chosen to demonstrate the rapid drop in sensitivity for units with high CFs.

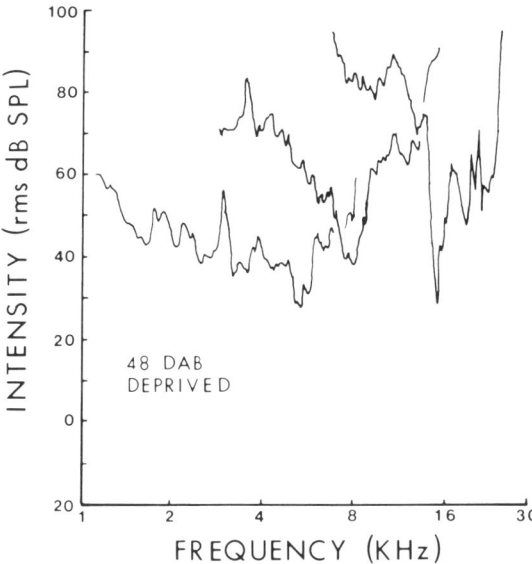

Fig. 5. Tuning curves for another deprived rat. Unit recording at 48 DAB revealed that many curves were characterized by high minimum threshold and poor selectivity for frequencies.

the rapid appearance of sharp tuning in units with high CFs during normal development. At 33 DAB the curve shown is approaching a typical adult curve (dashed line) except for the lack of a tail in the low frequencies and somewhat broader tuning. Units with lower CFs, illustrated for one at 24 DAB, have a significant decrease in minimum threshold. As suggested by these curves, sensitivity in the high frequencies continues to lag in development. As the adult curve demonstrates, sharp tuning with very steep slopes on the side of the curve for high frequencies, very low minimum thresholds, and a pronounced tail in the low frequencies approximately 40 dB up from the tip, characterize the responses of adult, normally experienced animals.

There are some initial observations on tuning curves from animals that had early auditory deprivations. Figures 4 and 5 present curves from 2 animals deprived of sound from 10 DAB. Curves from the subject at 40 DAB illustrate the striking progressive loss of sensitivity in going from approximately 10 kHz upward. While the curves may retain selectivity of frequencies at higher frequencies, their peak thresholds are elevated, and they have a more symmetric shape than adult curves. Some units with low CFs have excellent sensitivity, but their tuning is broad and reminiscent of immature curves. At 48 DAB, the other deprived subject had some units with sensitivity approaching normal, but most were well represented by the 3 curves in Figure 5. Units with low CFs had little tuning. Midfrequency units had some selectivity to frequencies, but most were notice-

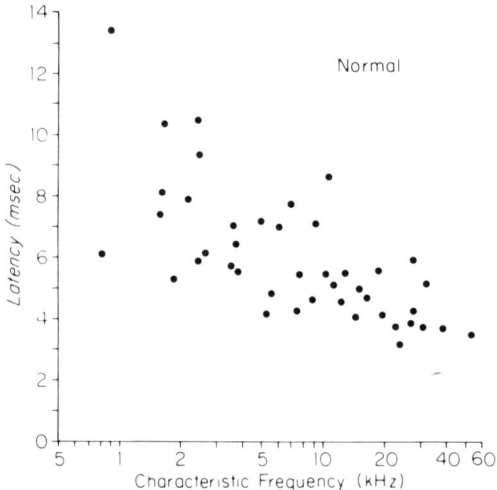

Fig. 6. Relationship of latency of onset of unit responses in a poststimulus histogram, to clicks 30 dB above threshold, for units at the inferior colliculus driven by normally experienced ears. The decrement in latency for the neural response represents differential delays in travel at the basilar membrane and probable central differences in transmission [20].

ably broadly tuned, symmetric, and insensitive. This electrophysiologic evidence clearly indicates a lack of resolution of frequencies, and lack of maximum sensitivity in unit responses at the cochlear nucleus due to 30–38 days of partial deprivation of sound.

The findings with tuning curves are in agreement with previous studies of units at the inferior colliculus. One such study investigated the effect of developmental deprivation on the latency and duration of unit responses [20]. The relationship of spike latencies, driven by clicks, at the colliculus to those produced by controls' ears normally experienced with sound is shown in Figure 6 as a function of each unit's CF. The latencies decline from about 10 msec for CFs near 1 kHz to 3–4 msec for those above 30 kHz. This finding reflects the traveling time along the basilar membrane as well as probable differential transmissional times in the brainstem's pathways.

Deprivation of sound for 3–5 months results in the latency shown in Figure 7. These latencies to clicks presented to deprived ears were comparable to latencies in controls except for the clearly separate group of units with CFs in high frequencies above 10 kHz. They had latencies that were 2–3 times the latencies of controls. Animals deprived for the same duration but starting at 60 DAB had a small increase in latencies at high frequencies, usually less than 1 msec. The early deprivation was very effective in disrupting normally rapid transmission in pathways for high frequencies in the auditory system of the brainstem. Deprivation after maturity was relatively ineffective.

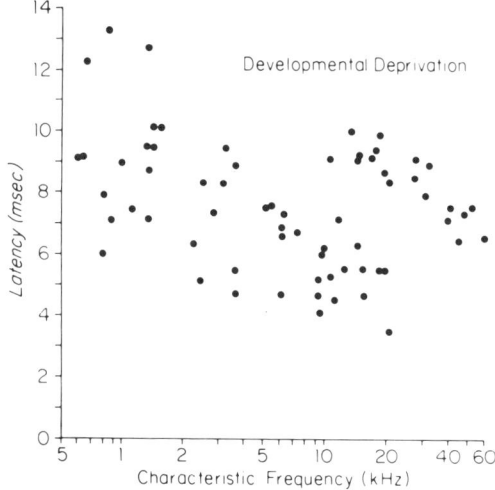

Fig. 7. Latencies for unit responses at the colliculus activated by an ear deprived of early input of sound. Units with CFs above 10 kHz had latencies 2–3 times those for comparable units for high frequencies in Fig. 6. Adult animals deprived for an equal period had a much smaller (≤1 msec) increment for units for high frequencies.

The pattern of unit response was also influenced by the developmental deprivation. The units for high frequencies that had long latencies, in deprived animals, spiked for only about 2 msec after the onset of the response, in contrast to durations of 3–4 msec for responses for other units. We interpreted the changes in latencies to arise from central sequelae of deprivation because the N_1 response of the auditory nerve was not delayed at the deprived ear relative to what normally would be expected.

The first study we made of the effect of deprivation of sound on central responses concerned binaural processing in the brainstem as reflected in unit responses at the colliculus [21, 22]. In this series of studies, we investigated the contrasting results of monaural versus binaural deprivation as well as the influence of starting the deprivation at different times after birth. It was an attempt to define developmental features of an important and quantifiable integrative process in the auditory system of the brainstem. The rat has a relatively predictable neural response at the colliculus for binaural stimulation by clicks at both ears.

As Figure 8 indicates, the primary influence of clicks to the opposite ear from the collicular recording site (contra) is facilitative, and the ipsilateral ear (ipsi) tends to suppress the responses evoked by contralateral stimulation. This binaural interactive process can be quantified by establishing the number of spikes a unit will produce in response to monaural stimulation of the opposite ear, and then presenting clicks to both ears with a chosen relationship of intensity, and observ-

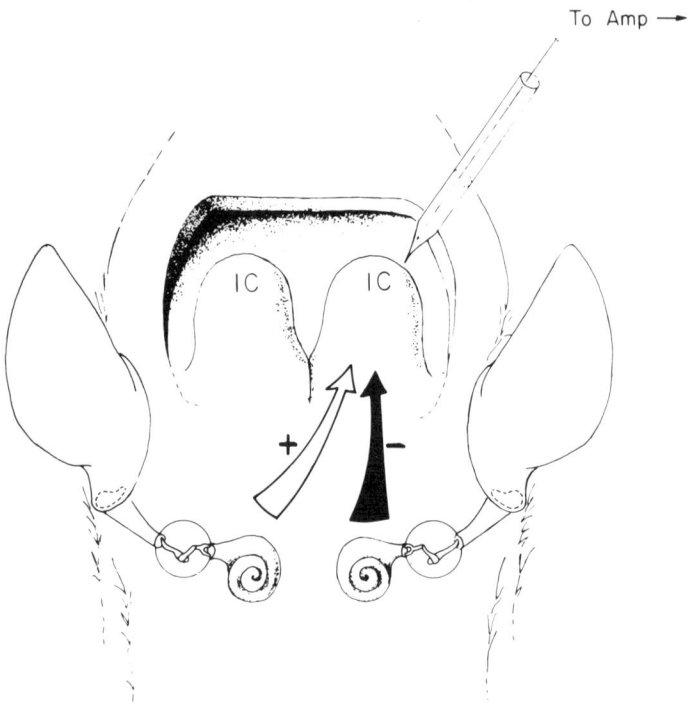

Fig. 8. Schematic representation of the predominant influences on unit firing at the inferior colliculus (IC) of the rat. Binaural interaction appears as a suppression of unit responses to clicks to the contralateral ear by more intense clicks at the ipsilateral ear.

ing the decrement in spikes counted. The decrement is referred to as ipsilateral suppression and is a convenient indicator of convergence and interaction of neural activity within the brainstem's auditory system. By varying contralateral and ipsilateral intensities of clicks inversely so as to model a source of sound moving around the head, it is possible to collect a profile of binaural interaction that is very stable across the population of neurons in the central nucleus of the inferior colliculus. This profile is characteristic of individual neurons in most cases. In the normally experienced animal, ipsilateral clicks suppress the response to contralateral clicks if the ipsilateral clicks are more intense, even by a few dB.

A comparison of binaural profiles for normal controls and subjects deprived of sound in one or both ears is shown in Figure 9. The response to monaural clicks from threshold to 40 dB above threshold was noted, and the change in the units' spiking with addition of ipsilateral clicks determined. Ipsilateral suppression of about 30% is present in the controls when a 30 dB difference in interaural intensity exists (contra = 5 dB, ipsi = 35 dB). Ipsilateral suppression exists

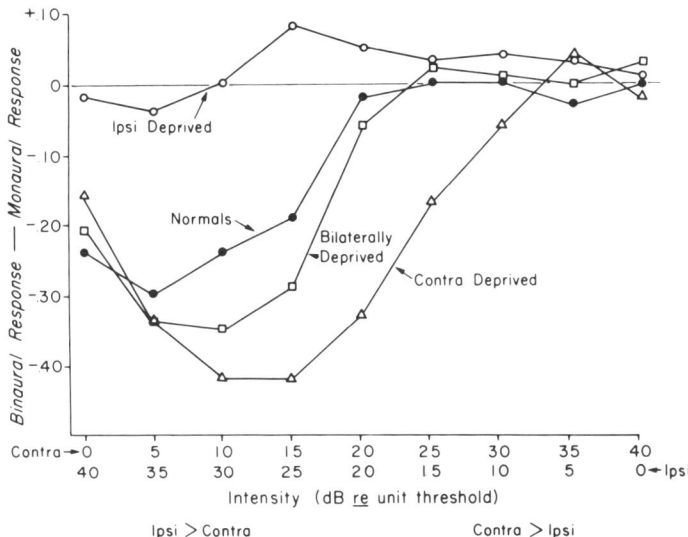

Fig. 9. Binaural interaction for populations of units in the colliculi of normally experienced rats and of rats monaurally or binaurally deprived from 10 DAB. The difference in spikes counted for monaurally (contralateral) and binaurally evoked responses are shown on the abscissa normalized relative to the monaural count. The binaural response is less than the monaural response due to ipsilateral suppression which is present in all instances except for suppression mediated through deprived ears.

only if the ipsilateral clicks are more intense so that a rather precisely indicated "midline" exists. This midline is a good measure of the balance of input from the 2 sides.

If both ears are deprived of normal input of sound from 10 DAB, the binaural profile after 3–5 months was remarkably similar to the profile for controls. Units driven by a deprived ear (contra deprived) received strong ipsilateral suppression through the undeprived ear on the same side, although the midline was shifted. We interpreted this shift of midline to be due to an attenuation of about 5–10 dB at the deprived ear due to some wax remaining on the tympanic membrane. This was supported by an equivalent attenuation in the cochlear microphonic at the deprived ear. In contrast, a deprived ear produced essentially no ipsilateral suppression of collicular activity even if it received clicks that were 40 dB more intense than clicks in the opposite, undeprived ear. The lack of stimulation during development thus eliminated the ability of clicks to produce ipsilateral suppression through the deprived ear, although the activation of the opposite colliculus through that ear was compromised much less.

If the external meatus was ligated at different times after birth, the lack of

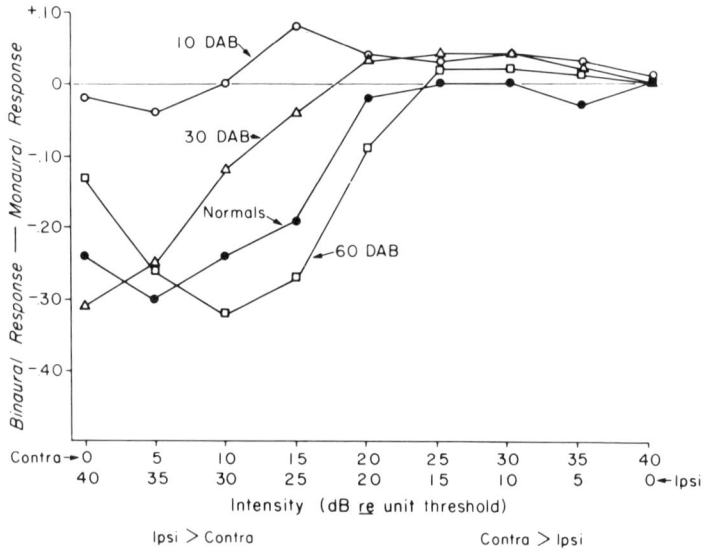

Fig. 10. Binaural interaction in rats monaurally deprived from 10, 30, or 60 DAB. All recording is from the colliculus on the same side as the deprived ear. (Normals included for comparison.)

ipsilateral suppression at the end of 3–5 months of deprivation depended on the time of ligation [21]. The progression of effects is seen in Figure 10. Ligation at 60 DAB had little impact on the binaural profile, but deprivation from 30 and 10 DAB increasingly eliminated ipsilateral suppression. This finding strongly suggests that a critical period applies to the maintenance or onset of binaural interaction in the brainstem. In order to determine whether this interaction was, indeed, prevented from developing or caused to disappear from lack of stimulation, we observed units in the colliculi of rats at 14–17 DAB. This population of units demonstrated binaural interaction with strong ipsilateral suppression and an accurate midline, in agreement with other findings in kittens [23]. Surprisingly, 20% of the units in young animals displayed ipsilateral suppression for the entire range of the binaural profile, an unusual finding in normal adults.

The conclusion is that binaural interaction is present in the rat soon after the onset of hearing, and adequate binaural stimulation is necessary to validate and maintain it, and possibly to optimize it. Asymmetric deprivation during a critical period from about 10–60 DAB will result in distortion of normal interaction, primarily through loss of ipsilateral suppression from the deprived ear. Figure 11 is an attempt to schematize the result of the binaural studies and the critical period for binaural plasticity inferred from them.

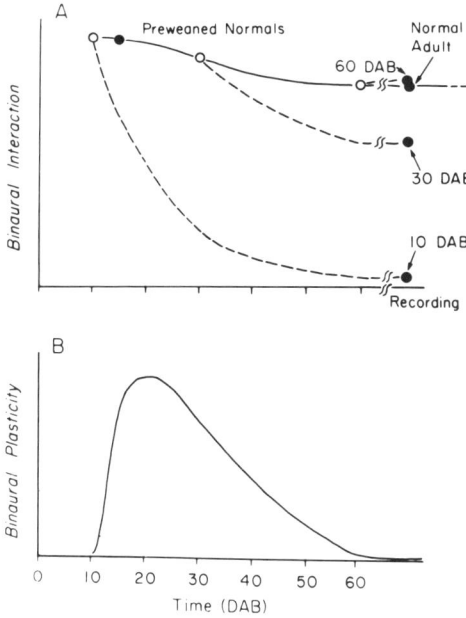

Fig. 11. A) Binaural interaction (total ipsilateral suppression) as a function of age. Filled circles represent actual observations. Open circles are inferred. Departure of binaural interaction from usual developmental magnitude (solid line) shown with dotted lines for 3 ligational times. B) Period of binaural plasticity inferred from data.

DISCUSSION

The changes encountered with these experiments caused by developmental deprivation of sound probably arise from plasticity at more than one site and affect numerous functions in the maturing auditory system. The distortion of tuning curves in the cochlear nucleus may reflect a lack of development in cochlear analysis. This becomes more plausible in light of current experimental support for cochlear processes, beyond the traveling wave, that enhance analysis of frequencies [24]. Such mechanisms might well require activation to attain adult levels of function. It is also known that efferent projections to the cochlea mature late in development and influence the sharpness of tuning and maximal sensitivity [12, 25]. Maturational and deprivational changes observed in the rat are especially apparent as changes in selectivity to frequencies and in minimum threshold.

Central susceptibility to lack of stimulation by sound is supported by a number of results. The very significant change in latency and pattern of responding neurons for high frequencies, in the colliculus, in contrast to no change in the N_1

latency, even after compensation for threshold shifts, is strong evidence for aberrant central transmission. The binaural results also imply selective deprivational changes in central pathways. Mechanisms mediating suppression of unit responses in the colliculus are more vulnerable than those responsible for driving activity. This is not easily reconciled with changes at the cochlear level alone. The small changes in thresholds for contralateral clicks seen in the binaural study can be due to numerous factors, the most plausible being that the wideband spectra of clicks should be little affected by reductions in the sensitive peaks of tuning curves. Differential transmission paths from the cochlear nuclei might also exist. Some indication is present for unique contributions from the dorsal and ventral projections of the cochlear nuclei to binaural processing [26].

These neurophysiologic observations strongly support the growing clinical concern about the viability of neural processing after early deprivation of sound. Important and intriguing questions obviously remain. Major concern, for example, must focus on the reversibility of the effects of deprivation. On the basis of current knowledge, neurophysiologic techniques can contribute heavily to resolving these questions.

ACKNOWLEDGMENTS

I would like to express appreciation to M. S. Silverman who contributed much to the experimental work, and to M. Garvey who helped in collection of data and preparation of the illustrations.

REFERENCES

1. Downs MP: The expanding imperatives of early identification. In Bess FH (ed): "Childhood Deafness." New York: Grune & Stratton, 1977, pp 95–106.
2. Downs MP: Hearing loss: Definition, epidemiology and prevention. Public Health Rev 4:225–280, 1975.
3. Eagles E: The survey. In "Proceedings of Conference on the Collection of Statistics of Severe Hearing Impairment and Deafness in the United States." Washington, DC: Public Health Service Publication No. 1227: 43, 44, 1964.
4. Kessner DM, Snow CK, Singer J: "Assessment of Medical Care in Children. Contrasts in Health Status," Vol 3. Washington, DC: National Academy of Sciences, 1973.
5. Kuhl PK, Miller JD: Speech perception by the chinchilla: Voiced-voiceless distinction in alveolar plosive consonants. Science 190:69–72, 1975.
6. Marler PR: Development and learning of recognition systems. In Bullock TH (ed): "Recognition of Complex Acoustic Signals." Berlin: Dahlem Konferenzen, 1977.
7. Spoendlin H: Retrograde degeneration of the cochlear nerve. Acta Otolaryngol 79:266–275, 1975.
8. Bosher SK, Warren RL: A study of the electrochemistry and osmotic relationships of the cochlear fluids in the neonatal rats at the time of the development of the endocochlear potential. J Physiol 212:739–761, 1971.

9. Crowley DE, Hepp-Raymond MC: Development of cochlear function in the ear of the infant rat. J Comp Physiol Psychol 62:427–432, 1966.
10. Hinojosa R: A note on development of Corti's organ. Acta Otolaryngol (Stockh) 84:238–251, 1977.
11. Wada T: Anatomical and physiological studies on the growth of the inner ear of the albino rat. Am Anat Mem 10:1923.
12. Kikuchi K, Hilding D: The development of the organ of Corti in the mouse. Acta Otolaryngol (Stockh) 60:207–222, 1965.
13. Pierce ET: Histogenesis of the dorsal and ventral cochlear nuclei in the mouse. An autoradiographic study. J Comp Neurol 131:27–54, 1967.
14. Shaner RF: The development of the nuclei and tracts related to the acoustic nerve in the pig. J Comp Neurol 60:5–19, 1934.
15. Milonyeni M: The late states of the development of the primary cochlear nuclei in mice. Brain Res 4:334–344, 1967.
16. Morest DK: The growth of synaptic endings in the mammalian brain: A study of the calyces of the trapezoid body. Anat Entwickl Gesch 127:201–220, 1968.
17. Moore DR, Aitkin LM: Rearing in an acoustically unusual environment – Effects on neural auditory responses. Neuroscience Lett 1:29–34, 1975.
18. Webster DB, Webster M: Neonatal sound deprivation affects brain stem auditory nuclei. Arch Otolaryngol 103:392–396, 1977.
19. Aitkin LM, Moore DR: Inferior colliculus. II. Development of tuning characteristics and tonotopic organization in central nucleus of the neonatal cat. J Neurophysiol 38:1208–1216, 1975.
20. Clopton BM, Silverman MS: Changes in latency and duration of neural responding following developmental auditory deprivation. Exp Brain Res 32:39–47, 1978.
21. Clopton BM, Silverman MS: Plasticity of binaural interaction. II. Critical period and changes in midline response. J Neurophysiol 40:1081–1089, 1977.
22. Silverman MS, Clopton BM: Plasticity of binaural interaction. I. Effect of early auditory deprivation. J Neurophysiol 40:1266–1274, 1977.
23. Aitkin LM, Reynolds A: Development of binaural responses in the kitten inferior colliculus. Neuroscience Lett 1:315–319, 1975.
24. Evans EF, Wilson JP: The frequency selectivity of the cochlea. In Moller AG (ed): "Basic Mechanisms in Hearing." New York: Academic Press, 1970, pp 519–551.
25. Wiederhold ML: Variations in the effects of electrical stimulation of the crossed olivocochlear bundle on cat single auditory-nerve fiber responses to tone bursts. J Acoust Soc Am 48:966–977, 1970.
26. Bengry MF, Silverman MS, Clopton BM: Effects of lesioning the dorsal and intermediate acoustic striae on binaural interaction at the inferior colliculus. Exp Brain Res 28:211–219, 1977.

DISCUSSION

Dr. Ben Clopton: There's a lot of evidence to suggest that there are severe neurologic changes with early auditory deprivation in humans.

Dr. Isabelle Rapin: I agree that very serious things happen if a child has a partial auditory deprivation early in life. Probably a hearing loss of 15 dB, even though it may be quite acceptable for adults, can be quite serious in children.

Dr. Robert Ruben: In a recent workshop that addressed this particular problem, nearly all thought that it could, yet it hasn't really been proven in a population of children. The thought was also expressed that perhaps a lot of this loss of learning could be made up afterwards. However, in a more public setting, I think I am constrained to say that it has not been proven.

Dr. Charles Berlin: I remember there was a consensus that there's a potential uniform effect on children's speech and language perception. But proving that the effect has occurred is another issue, it's an issue of evidence.

Dr. Ben Clopton: The major point I want to make is that there's a loss of learning experienced with hearing loss as small as 15 dB.

Dr. Charles Berlin: Tomorrow I'll be showing you a computer simulation of what a child would miss if he had a 20 dB hearing loss, and it predicts pretty much the kinds of problems that people have been reporting in the literature for years.

Dr. Ralph Wedgwood: I thought there was some fairly decent data on language development and hearing loss.

Dr. Isabelle Rapin: I have reviewed that literature and basically the studies fall into several categories. A number of studies done a long time ago seem to show an effect. The problem with those studies is that they did not separate sensorineural from conductive hearing loss, and that there were at least some moderately impaired children mixed in with the mildly impaired. Thus the data is difficult to evaluate.

Dr. Ralph Wedgwood: However, it doesn't change the idea that hearing loss affects speech.

Dr. Isabelle Rapin: Of course not. That we'd all accept. What we're talking about are effects of mild hearing loss. These studies were done in unusual populations such as in Baffin Island, and in Alaskan Eskimos, and in Australian aborigines. One felt a little uncomfortable when one had to go to these categories.

Dr. Harold Schuknecht: Dr. Berlin, do you have any interpretations of these observations relative to dysmorphogenesis?

Dr. Charles Berlin: The Websters, in our laboratory, have done a similar deprivation experiment but with a control that I think answers some of the objections that might be raised to surgically interfering with the ear. We've developed a technique for raising animals in silence that leads to the same morphologic slowness of development as surgical occlusion of the ear. The only common variable, therefore, is the lack of stimulation, which has the same effect whether it's from closing off the ear with atresia or raising the animal in silence. We did not know at that time that Dr. Clopton had done this experiment. It was our observation that the binaural interaction units failed to develop properly at the level of the trapezoid bodies and inferior colliculus.

We reasoned that there are units in the central nervous system that only react when impinged upon simultaneously from both sides. Rather than look for them individually, we thought we could get a gross picture of them in this fashion. First, we stimulated the left ear of the guinea pig, and then the right ear, and summed those data digitally. We were recording from brainstem from each of those major nuclei. This is the brainstem-evoked response. This prediction is what one would expect if you had two separate generators, one for each side of the head. Then we stimulated the ears binaurally, and found that we got exactly the correct prediction except in one area. When we digitally subtracted the true binaural stimulation from the predicted stimulation, we got a difference potential. This difference potential is ubiquitous in binaurally normal animals. Humans have this binaural interaction if they're normal, and the few abnormals we have studied who have had a history of chronic deprivation but normal audiograms at the time of testing do not show that potential.

Dr. Robert Ruben: We should know more about the effects on the CNS from deprivation of inner ear function during development. Livi-Montachalini extirpated the chick otocyst at about 1½ to 3 days. It's a long, very fascinating human story of the experimental conditions under which this was done. She was playing the Anne Frank game in a little Italian farmhouse during World War II. Instead of eating the eggs, what does a good embryologist do? She experimented with them, and found with relatively few eggs and very crude processing that there were real distortions in the auditory nuclei of the chick.

Dr. David Lim: I haven't seen the data myself, but there are some evidences that in the Pallid mouse, which doesn't have otoconia of smaller cells in the vestibular nuclei, the effect of the deprivation of the vestibular system to the CNS is much more complex and grave.

Dr. Charles Berlin: We were able to raise animals in perceptual silence by knowing what their basic audiogram was. The Websters raised two groups of animals, a deprived group in silence and an operated group, and then a control group of normals. In the initial studies, looking at the length of the globular cells and the length of the medial nucleus of the cells of the trapezoid, those were the significant differences that were found. The original study only evaluated cell length in the dorsocochlear nucleus: globular cells, small spherical cells, large spherical cells, and so forth. And these were the only two significantly different cell groups. However, subsequent studies that were completed studied the volume of the cells and found that virtually every cell except those in the dorsocochlear nucleus was significantly reduced in volume. The volume of the cells seems to have changed. The projections to the trapezoid body and the lateral and medial superior are binaural units for the most part and that's what led us to the experiment of studying the two ears and trying to see if we could evaluate the effect of that deprivation.

Dr. Robert Ruben: So far we have looked at sensitivity and binaural interaction. Do you have any ideas if we may find a greater difference when we look at an expected pattern of auditory perception instead of looking at our highly redundant cues of pure tones?

Dr. Ben Clopton: Yes. For example, as in the visual system, rather than depriving the system of input, you can warp it or put it in a special environment.

We presented a very special pattern to rats early in development. The patterns consisted of tone sweeps that went up and we found that we could, in effect, bias cells in the colliculus toward the pattern to which they had been exposed. You soon realize that our ignorance about auditory processing in very complex patterns is really great.

Dr. Charles Berlin: Were you aware that there's an asymmetry of the cochlear level for (rising vs falling) tones?

Dr. Richard Bobbin: It's sort of unrelated, but do you have any evidence that the effects you see are middle ear or infracochlear? For instance, have you measured primary fibers?

Dr. Joseph Nadol: Since the maximal change in threshold sensitivities seems to be about 10 kHz, how do you think this might affect the encoding of speech?

Dr. Ben Clopton: Well, I presume that basically the cochlea encodes the temporal pattern of speech, so we can speculate that not only do we get energy through those very sensitive tips of the inner ear, but we also get the cadence of speech the way it forms. If the high frequency cells are gone, the activation of the cochlea in essence doesn't get through the same way.

Dr. Ruediger Thalmann: Rats have extremely high frequency "speech." If you transpose this to the human, it's conceivable that one would have lower frequencies being affected, and that would affect speech. One cannot take rats' speech and compare it to human speech.

Dr. Ralph Wedgwood: By auditory deprivation, what happens if you do the opposite, raise the background noise level during the critical period, as happens in most large cities?

Dr. Charles Berlin: That experiment has been done in rodents and it often engenders various kinds of seizures. In other animal groups, it's supposed to make them insensitive to vocal communications.

Microtia — Clinical Observations

Jon M. Aase, MD

The most common developmental abnormality of the external ear is microtia. This term has been used as a description for a wide variety of auricular malformations whose common feature is small size. When a large number of individuals with microtia are studied, the observed abnormalities span a remarkable spectrum, ranging from diminutive ears with essentially normal configuration to complete absence of the pinna and auditory canal. The gradations in this spectrum blend into one another, so that no clear anatomic demarcations are seen between the so-called Type I, Type II, and Type III microtias (Figs. 1–3). These classifications, while useful to the plastic surgeons, are entirely arbitrary and are based largely on an estimate of ear tissue available for plastic repair. As a general rule the severity of malformation of the external ear provides only a rough guideline for predicting the likelihood and extent of malformation in the middle and inner ear. For example, in microtic ears with atresia of the auditory canal, severe to profound hearing loss is common, but in many such instances the ossicular chain and inner ear have been found to be intact [1]. In such cases, surgical reconstruction of the ear canal can result in virtually normal hearing.

In order to appreciate the sometimes subtle developmental abnormalities in the microtic ear, a clinician needs at least a nodding acquaintance with the architecture of the normal pinna. Unfortunately, but understandably, the auricular landmarks and their rather abstruse nomenclature are eminently forgettable after completion of the gross anatomy course. For review, the major topographic features shown in Figure 4 are the helix, the antihelix with its Y-shaped cruces, the tragus, the antitragus, and the lobule. The root of the helix dives into the concha and blends with its floor.

Perhaps the most minimal degree of structural abnormality of the auricle is abnormal formation of the superior crus of the antihelix (Fig. 5), which sometimes results in failure of support of the upper curve of the helix, producing a so-called lop-ear (Fig. 6). Jaffe [2] has pointed out that this abnormality is often

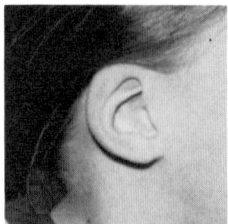

Fig. 1. Microtia Type I.

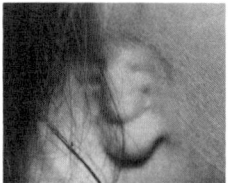

Fig. 3. Microtia Type III.

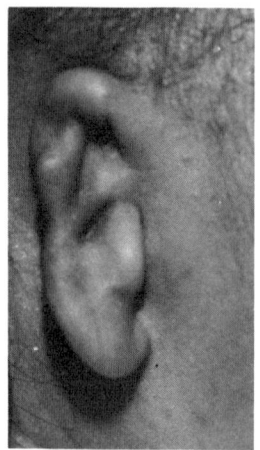

Fig. 2. Microtia Type II.

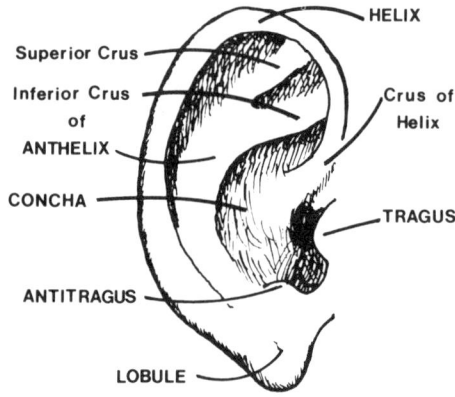

Fig. 4. Normal anatomy of the pinna.

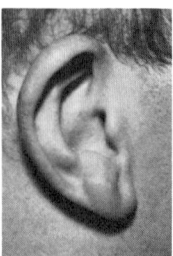

Fig. 5. Absence of superior crus of the anthelix.

the only external clue to the presence of hearing deficit caused by occult malformations of the middle ear, and he calls upon clinicians to consult this oracle when examining young children.

Another subtle alteration of ear architecture, while not strictly falling in the category of microtia, does serve as a useful diagnostic aid for children with the fetal alcohol syndrome. The abnormality consists of a marked prominence of the crus of the helix, forming a diagonal bar across the concha, parallel to and as high as the anthelix (Fig. 7). This "railroad track" configuration is quite rare in normal ears, but has appeared in approximately 30% of children we have seen with the fetal alcohol syndrome. In addition, some affected children do show more gross ear malformations and aberrant ear placement.

A most unusual variant of microtia is one in which the helix gives the appearance of having burrowed under the skin of the temporal scalp (Fig. 8). The pinna is held snugly under the fold of scalp skin, but is not adherent to it. This abnormality has been named *cryptotia* [3]. It is usually bilaterally symmetric, occurs much more frequently in males, and seldom seems to be associated with hearing loss. The pathogenesis of this bizarre malformation is unknown.

Most microtic ears are somewhat low-set, reflecting probable failure of complete migration of developing tissues from their more caudal and ventral position in early embryonic life. The clinical criteria for "low-set" ears are rather nebulous, being based upon landmarks in the face, some of which may themselves be altered in an associated pattern of developmental anomaly. Perhaps the most clinically useful topographic markers are these: a line drawn from the lateral corner of the orbit, perpendicular to the plane of the face, should intersect the helical root (otobasion superius) (Fig. 9A). Alternatively, portrait artists use an imaginary

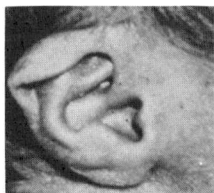

Fig. 6. Lop-ear secondary to absent superior crus.

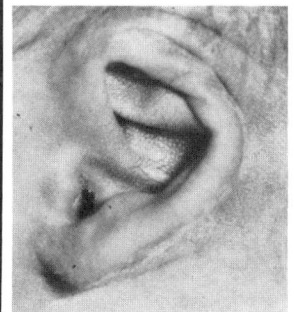

Fig. 8. Cryptotia.

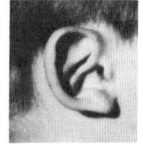

Fig. 7. "Railroad track" ear in fetal alcohol syndrome.

horizontal line from the eyebrow to locate the upper edge of the helix, and a parallel line from the base of the columella to fix the lower helical insertion (otobasion inferious) (Fig. 9B).

Many syndrome diagnoses are associated with greater or lesser degrees of microtia. In Down syndrome, for example, the ears are characterized as "small, square, and thickened" (Fig. 10). Actual measurement of ears in children with Down syndrome (Fig. 11) shows that length of the pinna does indeed fall well below the average at all ages [4]. In other syndromes, involvement of the external ear seems to be one manifestation of a more generalized developmental failure involving the face, head, and neck. Classic examples are Treacher Collins syndrome (Fig. 12), oculoauriculovertebral dysplasia, and Apert syndrome. Other reasonably well-defined syndromes which include microtia as a feature are: Bixler syndrome [5], in which hypertelorism, cleft lip/palate, and mild syndactyly are features; Beals syndrome [6] of contractural arachnodactyly; branchio-oto-renal syndrome [7]; thalidomide syndrome; the Rubinstein-Taybi syndrome; and several others with microtia as an occasional finding. However, before we succumb to eponymphomania, let us return to the topic of microtia as an isolated manifestation.

In several large studies [8–12], the incidence of isolated microtia has been reported to be from 5–19 per 100,000 live births. There seem to be clear racial differences in occurrence of this malformation, with the highest figures reported from Japan. In a study which Dr. Tegtmeier and I undertook in New Mexico [13], we found the prevalence of microtia in our 3 predominant racial subgroups to be as shown in Table 1. Jaffe [14] had pointed out the extraordinary frequency of microtia in the Navajo as early as 1968, and our figures, gathered from a state-wide population base, confirmed his impression.

In our study, as in others based on large populations, there were striking differences in distribution by sex, as well as a predilection for involvement of the right ear [10–16] (Tables 2 and 3). With regard to laterality of the defective ear, our own study revealed that 11% of "unilaterally affected" individuals had a functionally significant loss of hearing acuity on the contralateral side where the ear architecture was judged to be normal. This suggests that we are unable to detect

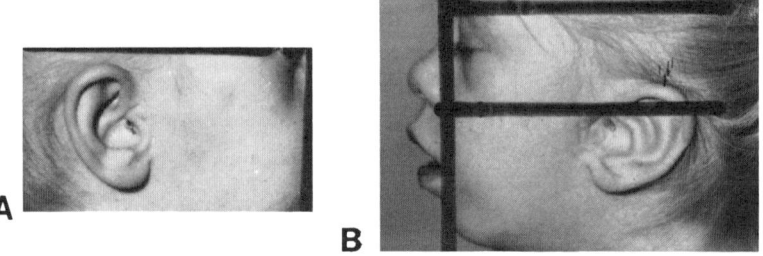

Fig. 9. Low-set ear measured A) from lateral canthus and B) by "artists' criteria."

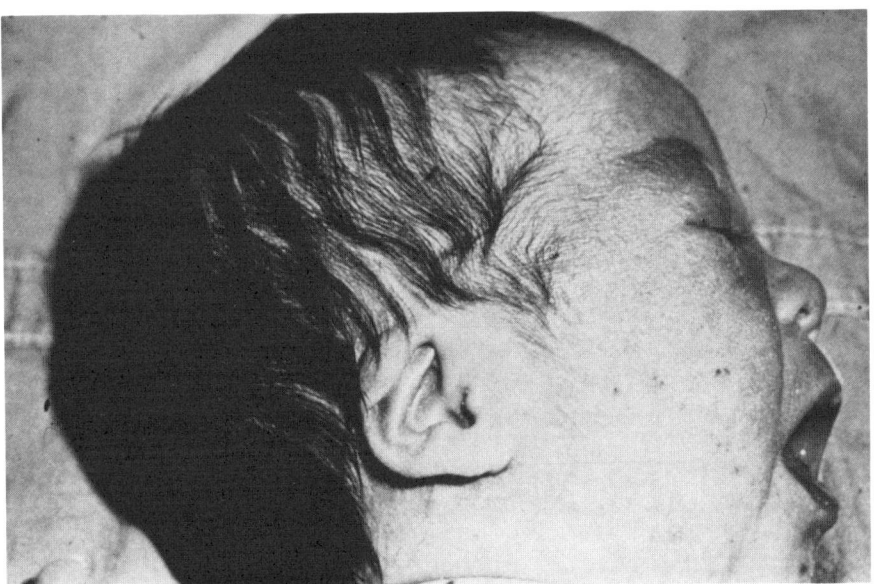

Fig. 10. Small, malformed ear in Down syndrome.

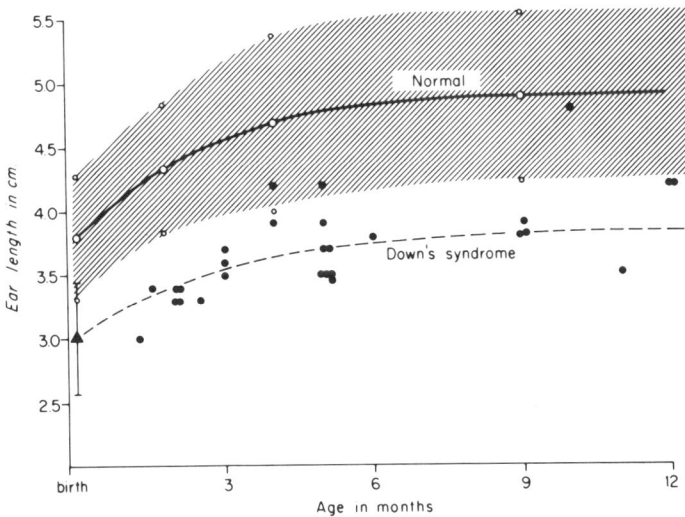

Fig. 11. Comparison of ear lengths of normal infants with those of infants with Down syndrome. (From Aase JM, Wilson AC, Smith DW: Small ears in Down's syndrome: A helpful diagnostic aid. J Pediatr 82:845–847, 1973, with permission.)

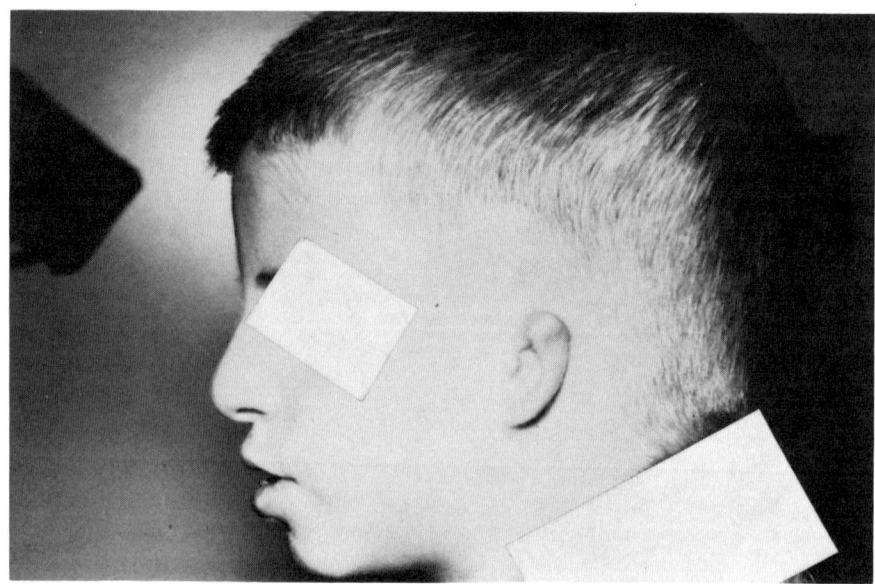

Fig. 12. Microtia in Treacher Collins syndrome.

TABLE 1. Prevalence of Microtia by Race

	Per 100,000 Population
American Indian	53.8
Spanish-American	11.1
Anglo	6.3
All New Mexico patients	13.4

TABLE 2. Sex Distribution of Microtia

	Male	Female
Conway and Wagner (1965) [10]	193	119
Grabb (1965) [11]	63	39
Patanguy (1969) [15]	50	23
Gill (1971) [12]	52	18
Harada and Ishii (1972) [1]	34	15
Fukuda (1974) [16]	629	262
Aase and Tegtmeier (1976) [13]	63	38
Totals	1,084	514
	68%	32%

TABLE 3. Laterality of Microtia

	Right	Left	Bilateral
Grabb (1965) [11]	51	39	12
Patanguy (1969) [15]	33	28	12
Gill (1971) [12]	25	26	18
Harada and Ishii (1972) [1]	47	18	8
Fukuda (1974) [16]	503	315	73
Aase and Tegtmeier (1976) [13]	67	27	4
Totals	726	453	127
	55%	35%	10%

even subtle structural abnormalities in some ears where occult disruption of the hearing mechanism has occurred. In addition, this observation emphasizes the necessity for audiologic testing in other family members with normal auricles, in whom hearing loss may be the only expression of the disorder.

Recurrence rates are low: in our study, only 4 of 116 affected individuals had affected first-degree relatives. The empiric recurrence risk rate for unaffected parents was 4.3%. Other studies have shown comparable figures, providing evidence for a multifactorial mode of inheritance for this abnormality [9, 11, 12, 17]. There are, however, reports of a few families in which isolated microtia seems to be transmitted in both autosomal dominant and recessive modes [18, 19] (J. Derstine, personal communication, 1976).

The actual degree of clinical involvement, both in our series and in others, has encompassed a broad spectrum, as mentioned earlier. The presence of preauricular tags and pits, and especially the occurrence of various degrees of hemifacial microsomia in some patients certainly support the concept of an embryonic field defect as the pathogenesis for this disorder. That is, structures which are physically adjacent during embryonic time seem to share a relatively similar degree of clinical involvement, despite their origin from different embryologic tissues.

While the basic etiology of this "field defect" remains to be elucidated in man, a strong hypothesis has emerged from Poswillo's elegant experiments in rats and macaque monkeys [20]. By administration of thalidomide or triazene at appropriate developmental stages, he was able to show hemorrhage and hematoma formation in the exact region of the embryonic auricle. Depending on the extent of bleeding, there was more or less disruption and eventual hypoplasia of adjacent structures such as the ramus of the mandible, zygoma, ossicles, and temporal bone — mimicking closely the findings in hemifacial microsomia. At present, this or some similar mechanism would seem to provide the best explanation for the broad spectrum of manifestations of microtia in man.

In summary, microtia in its many forms is the most common congenital anomaly of the external ear. Clinicians should be alerted to the importance of even minor aberrations of auricular architecture as a clue to possible hearing deficit. In addition, the contralateral ear, even if normal in appearance, must be tested for hearing acuity as well. Close relatives with normal ears should also be tested for occult hearing loss. Finally, in the absence of other affected family members, it seems justifiable to provide counseling with recurrence risk figures on the order of 3–8%, based upon the probable multifactorial pattern of occurrence.

REFERENCES

1. Harada O, Ishii H: The condition of the auditory ossicles in microtia. Plast Reconstr Surg 50:48–53, 1972.
2. Jaffe BF: Pinna anomalies associated with congenital conductive hearing loss. Pediatrics 57:332–341, 1976.
3. Kantu K, Aretsky PJ, Polisar IA: Cryptotia. Laryngoscope 82:161–165, 1972.
4. Aase JM, Wilson AC, Smith DW: Small ears in Down's syndrome: A helpful diagnostic aid. J Pediatr 82:845–847, 1973.
5. Bixler D, Christian JC, Gorlin RJ: Hypertelorism, microtia, and facial clefting. Am J Dis Child 118:495–500, 1969.
6. Beals RK, Hecht F: Delineation of another heritable disorder of connective tissue. J Bone Joint Surg [Am] 53:987, 1971.
7. Melnick M: Branchio-oto-renal dysplasia and branchio-oto dysplasia: Two distinct autosomal dominant disorders. Clin Genet 13:425–442, 1978.
8. Holmes EM: The microtic ear. Arch Otolaryngol 49:243–264, 1949.
9. Ohmori S: Congenital deformities of the auricle. Clin Plast Surg 1:3–25, 1974.
10. Conway H, Wagner K: Congenital anomalies of the head and neck. Plast Reconstr Surg 36:71–79, 1965.
11. Grabb WC: The first and second branchial arch syndrome. Plast Reconstr Surg 36:485–508, 1965.
12. Gill NW: Congenital atresia of the ear. A review of the surgical findings in 83 cases. J Laryngol Otol 85:551–587, 1971.
13. Aase JM, Tegtmeier RE: Microtia in New Mexico: Evidence for multifactorial causation. In Bergsma D, Lowry RB (eds): "Numerical Taxonomy of Birth Defects and Polygenic Disorders." New York: Alan R Liss for The National Foundation–March of Dimes, BD:OAS XIII(3A):113–116, 1977.
14. Jaffe BF: The incidence of ear diseases in the Navajo Indians. Laryngoscope 79:2126–2134, 1969.
15. Pitanguy I: Dysplasia auricularis. Trans 4th Int Congr Plast Surg, Excerpta Medica, Amsterdam, 1969, pp 660–666.
16. Fukuda O: The microtic ear: Survey of 180 cases in 10 years. Plast Reconstr Surg 53:458–463, 1974.
17. Karmody CS, Feingold M: Autosomal dominant first and second branchial arch syndrome: A new inherited syndrome? In Bergsma D (ed): "Malformation Syndromes." Miami: Symposia Specialists for The National Foundation-March of Dimes, BD:OAS X(7):31–40, 1974.
18. Ellwood L, Winter S, Dar H: Familial microtia with meatal atresia in two sibships. J Med Genet 5:289–291, 1968.
19. Konigsmark BW, Nager GT, Haskins HL: Recessive microtia, meatal atresia, and hearing loss. Arch Otolaryngol 96:105–109, 1972.
20. Poswillo DE: The pathogenesis of the first and second branchial arch syndrome. Oral Surg 35:302–328, 1973.

DISCUSSION

Dr. Jon Aase: In answer to a question, cryptotia is a condition in which the ear is partly hidden by a fold of skin on the temporal side, that is to say, the cryptic part is actually the outer helix.

Dr. LaVonne Bergstrom: Do you have any comparison between Navajo and Oriental peoples with microtia?

Dr. Jon Aase: The best study was carried out in Japan because of the number of people with the disorder. The rates are higher than in other populations including Australia and other essentially Caucasoid groups. But the Navajo figure is yet above that by a factor of two, so that I think we're looking at an anomaly that may be related to the Mongoloid background of the American Indian.

Dr. Robert Gorlin: One has an almost direct parallel with clefting. Among the Navajo it's about 1:150; among the Ojibwe or Chippewa in Minnesota about 1:250; in the Sioux, approximately 1:250; among the Japanese it's about 1:350. Among whites, the best data we have is Scandinavian: it's about 1:600. In blacks, clefting occurs about 1:3,000.

Dr. Jon Aase: Yes, a perfect example of the kind of continuum that I think we're talking about here. In my years in Alaska, I collected a lot of data on local American Indian and Eskimo populations. I truly expected that their rates [of microtia] would be intermediate between the Navajo rates and those in Japan. They weren't. They were low. I don't know what this means. There is very clear genetic relationship between some of the Athabaskan tribes in Alaska and the Navajo, but the Navajo still lead the list, as far as this particular abnormality goes.

Ear Muscles and Ear Form *

David W. Smith, MD and Hirotada Takashima, MD

The form of the external cartilaginous auricle tends to be specific by species [1]. Only recently, the mechanism for forming the auricles has been found to be clearly related to the sites of attachment and function of the auricular muscles. The cat is said to have 30 ear muscles and their function is readily evident as the cat's auricle swivels up to 90 degrees in response to sound stimuli. The human usually has 3 external auricular muscles and 6 intrinsic ones. Though the function of human ear muscles is seldom noticeable, Seiler [2] demonstrated by electromyographic techniques that they are responsive to sound stimuli.

Moss [3] first implicated these muscles in the positioning and forming of folds (plicae) of the cartilaginous auricle. Recent studies of Chiu et al [4] have demonstrated that early postnatal denervation of the auricle in rats results in a simple form of the auricle, without its usual folds (plicae). Clinically, Smith and Takashima [5] have shown that a protruding auricle is usually the consequence of a defect in the posterior auricular muscle. Here we report that lop ear relates to a defect of the superior auricular muscle, and comment on the clinical relevance of various defects in form of the external auricle.

METHODS AND RESULTS

Dissection of the superior auricular muscle was conducted on normal human fetuses obtained through the courtesy of Dr. Thomas H. Shepard of the University of Washington. The muscle fans out from the superior cartilaginous auricle to the temporal region. It appears to help hold the top of the auricle toward the head and also appears to affect the relative vertical positioning of the auricle on the head. Not uncommonly, fetuses with anencephaly have abnormally formed auricles, protruding ears, lop ears, or both lop and protruding ears. The external auricles

---

*Supported by HEW Project 913, NIH grant HD 05961, and USPHS grant GM 15253.

TABLE 1. Relationship of Ear Muscles to Ear Form

Muscle	Normal relation to form	Deficiency may cause
Posterior auricular	Pulls auricle back toward head	Protruding auricle
Superior auricular	Pulls auricle up toward head	Lop auricle, may appear 'low set'
Anterior auricular	Pulls superior auricle forward	? Slanted auricle
Intrinsic ear muscles	Responsible for ear folds	? From aberrant ear folds, to simple auricle

of anencephalic infants, obtained through the courtesy of Drs. Ronald J. Lemire and Benjamin C. Moffett of the University of Washington, were dissected by one of us (HT). Among 9 anencephalics, 2 had only protruding ears, one had only lop ears, 3 had lop and protruding ears, and 3 had normal auricles. Assessment of the auricular muscles revealed marked hypoplasia to absence of the posterior auricular muscle of the protruding ears (as previously noted [5]); marked hypoplasia to absence of the superior auricular muscle in instances with lop ear; and deficiency to absence of both muscles when there was the combination of both protruding and lop ears.

DISCUSSION

The relation of the auricular muscles to the form of the external cartilaginous auricle may be implied by observing the more specific function of each of the auricular muscles. We have had the good fortune to examine a person who can demonstrate the function of these muscles. Mr. Alan Hughes, of the University of Johannesburg Department of Anatomy, has the remarkable ability to selectively utilize each of the auricular muscles. The relationship of each muscle to the cartilaginous form of his auricles was dramatically evident. Further evidence of the relation of ear muscles to ear form is provided by study of the abnormalities of ear form which are the consequence of defects in development and/or function of particular ear muscles. Table 1 summarizes the relationship between defects of particular ear muscles and abnormalities of ear form. Figure 1 depicts the specific relationship between protruding and/or lop ear and the posterior and/or superior auricular muscles. These latter examples are the only ones which have been studied in humans. Hypotheses about the relationship between defects of the anterior auricular muscle and ear form, and between problems of intrinsic ear muscles and ear form have yet to be resolved.

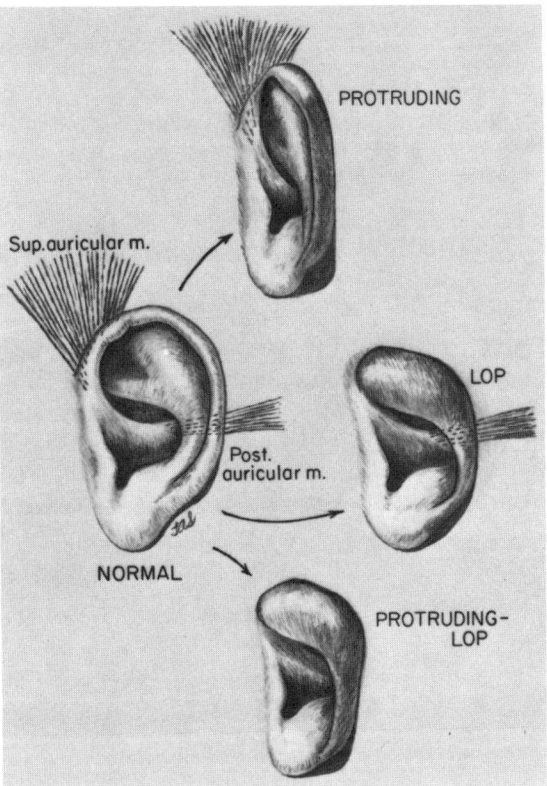

Fig. 1. Posterior and superior ear muscles in the normal, in the lop, and in the protruding plus lop ear. (Illustration by Thomas A. Stebbins, Director, Health Sciences Illustration, University of Washington.)

Thus, aberrant form of the external ear is usually a sign of a neuromuscular problem. The significance is analogous to that of ptosis of the eyelid, and as with eyelid ptosis, the sign does not clearly indicate whether the basic problem is neural or muscular. These are nonspecific signs which may be present in a number of different disorders.

REFERENCES

1. Boas J: "Ohrknorpel und äusseres Ohr der Saugetiere." Copenhagen: Nielsen and Lydike, 1912.
2. Seiler R: Die Muskeln des äusseren Ohres und ihre Funktion bei Menschen, Schimpansen und Makaken. Gegenbaurs Morphol Jahrb 120:78, 1974.

3. Moss ML: New studies of cranial growth. In Bergsma D (ed): "Morphogenesis and Malformation of Face and Brain." New York: Alan R Liss for the National Foundation–March of Dimes, BD:OAS XI(7):283–295, 1975.
4. Chiu DT, Crikelair GF, Moss ML: Epigenetic regulation of rodent auricular shape of position. Plast Reconstr Surg. 63(3):411–17, 1979.
5. Smith DW, Takashima H: Protruding auricle, a neuromuscular sign. Lancet 1:747, 1978.

DISCUSSION

Dr. Robert Gorlin: So the protruding ear is nonspecific?

Dr. David Smith: One can find, as with ptosis of the eyelid, families in which the protruding auricle runs as a simple dominant trait. One can find this anomaly with fetal alcohol syndrome, with the fetal hydantoin syndrome, with various environmental agents, and with chromosomal abnormalities such as Down syndrome syndrome (we found 55% had protruding auricles). The ear muscles are felt to be innervated from the VIIth nerve, and so if you have Moebius syndrome, it's not uncommon to have a protruding auricle as one feature.

The Etiology of External Ear Malformations and Its Relation to Abnormalities of the Middle Ear, Inner Ear, and Other Organ Systems

Michael Melnick, DDS, PhD

This investigation* of malformations of the external ear is part of a larger ongoing study of congenitally malformed children [1] who were born to mothers registered in the NINCDS Collaborative Perinatal Project (NCPP), a cooperative effort between the National Institute of Neurological and Communicative Disorders and Stroke and 12 medical centers throughout the United States. The objective of the Collaborative Project was to observe, record, and study events which affect mothers before and during pregnancy and to relate them to the outcome of pregnancy [2]. More than 50,000 pregnant women were followed from the first months of their pregnancy through labor and delivery and the children born to these mothers were followed to 8 years of age. The collection of information, medical examinations and laboratory tests were done in a uniform manner and according to preestablished protocol. The population in the project is about 45% white, 47% black, and the remaining 8% a variety of other ethnic groups, mostly Puerto Rican.

GENERAL CHARACTERISTICS

There were 600 children ascertained with malformations of the external ear or branchial cleft or both. This is an incidence of 0.0113 (600/53,257). Of these, there were 591 persons with at least one malformed ear, an incidence of 0.0111, and 12 persons with at least one branchial cleft malformation, an incidence of 0.0002. These 600 persons had a total of 626 malformations of the external ear

---

*This paper represents a synopsis of a larger work on malformations of the external ear. For the interested reader, a more extensive account of the data and analyses may be found in Melnick M, Myrianthopoulos NC: "External Ear Malformations: Epidemiology, Genetics, and Natural History." New York: Alan R. Liss, Inc., for The National Foundation–March of Dimes, BD:OAS XV(9), 1979.

or branchial cleft or both, and are listed in Table 1 along with their frequencies in the population. Note that bilateral cases of any given type of malformation were counted as one for these calculations of incidence. Of those persons affected, 78% of the cases were diagnosed during the neonatal period, 16% at 4 months of age, and the remaining 6% by 1 year.

As detailed in Table 2, 42 of the 600 persons presented with dysmorphic syndromes of both known and unknown etiology. We have been able to place 25 of these cases conclusively in recognized nosologic designations. The remaining 17 had findings either too nonspecific to be categorized, or completely unknown to us. These syndromes have been listed in Table 2 according to the suggested

TABLE 1. Distribution of All External Ear and Branchial Cleft Malformations

Malformation	Number	Rate per 10,000*
Preauricular sinus	446	83.74
Preauricular tags	91	17.09
Microtia	16	3.00
Other malformed pinna**	61	11.45
Branchial cleft sinus	12	2.25

*Based on a total NCPP population size of 53,257. Bilateral cases of any given malformation were counted as one for purposes of incidence calculations.
**Includes all other cases of malformed pinna. With the exception of microtia, the diagnostic labels and/or descriptions of the anomalies were not sufficiently clear to be certain of the precise nosologic category.

TABLE 2. Syndromic External Ear Malformation Cases in the NCPP Population

A) Known Genesis Syndromes
   1) Pedigree syndromes
      a) Branchio-oto-dysplasia (autosomal dominant) with bilateral preauricular sinuses, bilateral branchial cleft sinuses and bilateral severe mixed hearing loss.
      b) Smith-Lemli-Opitz syndrome (autosomal recessive) with left preauricular sinus.
   2) Chromosomal syndromes
      a) Trisomy 21 (9 cases) with microear and other pinna dysplasias.
      b) Trisomy 18 (2 cases), one with bilateral dysplastic pinnas and one with hypoplastic lobes.
   3) Environmentally-induced syndromes
      a) Rubella syndrome (2 cases), one with a right preauricular sinus and the other with bilateral dysplastic pinnas.
      b) Toxoplasmosis syndrome with left preauricular sinus.
      c) Amniotic band syndrome (2 cases), one with bilateral severe pinna dysplasia, the other with right preauricular sinus; both cases had bilateral cleft lip and palate and congenital amniotic bands and amputations of the digits.
      d) Fetal diabetes mellitus syndrome with right microtia; absence of coccyx; posterior displacement of upper limbs; macerated and stillborn.

(continued next page)

Malformations of the External Ear / 305

TABLE 2. (Continued)

B) Unknown Genesis Syndromes
  1) Recurrent pattern syndromes
     a) Abdominal muscle deficiency syndrome with right preauricular sinus.
     b) 1st and 2nd branchial arch syndrome (2 cases), one with right preauricular sinus, the other with bilateral preauricular tags.
     c) Holoprosencephaly with bilateral microtia and normal chromosomes.
     d) Prader-Willi syndrome with bilateral lop ears.
  2) Provisionally-unique pattern syndrome
     a) Case 1: right preauricular sinus; bilateral isolated cleft palate; multiple hemangiomas of the face; synophrys; brachydactyly of fingers and toes; clinodactyly of 5th fingers bilaterally; abnormal separation of big toes; failure to thrive as an infant; spastic diplegia; bilateral conductive hearing loss (30–40 dB); ?Klippel-Trenaunay-Weber syndrome or Sturge-Weber syndrome?
     b) Case 2: bilateral lop ears; hemangiomas of the nasal bridge, nape of neck, and sacrum; antimongoloid obliquity of the eyes; bilateral iris colobomas; bilateral cataracts; microphthalmia; downturned corners of the mouth; coarctation of aorta; atrial septal defect; ventricular septal defect; accessory spleen; polycystic kidneys; bicornuate uterus; hypertonia. Patient died at 10 days of age; ?Klippel-Trenauny-Weber syndrome or Sturge-Weber syndrome?
     c) Case 3: left preauricular sinus; macrocephaly; downturned corners of the mouth; severe hypoplasia of left frontal bone; bilateral inguinal hernias; bilateral cryptorchidism; retarded locomotor development.
     d) Case 4: bilateral preauricular sinuses; right conductive hearing loss; Arnold-Chiari malformation; meningomyelocele (L3-5); microphthalmia (left > right); lumbar lordosis.
     e) Case 5: bilateral lop ears with left preauricular sinus; mitral and aortic atresia; hypoplastic left atrium, ventricle, and aortic arch; patent ductus arteriosus; patent foramen ovale; accessory spleen; acute gastric ulcers; microscrotum; bilateral cryptorchidism.
     f) Case 6: bilateral preauricular sinuses; exophthalmos; hypertelorism; web neck; spina bifida occulta (S-1); wide-spaced nipples; increased carrying angle; omphalocele; bilateral inguinal hernias; hypoplastic labia majora; cardiac arrhythmia; normal hairline; karyotype 46,XX (no banding).
     g) Case 7: right preauricular sinus; microcephaly; bilateral exotropia; left VII nerve paresis; pectus carinatum; psychomotor retardation.
     h) Case 8: left preauricular tag; hydrocephalus; ventricular septal defect; patent ductus arteriosus; patent foramen ovale; aortic arch dysmorphia; hypoplastic labia majora.
     i) Case 9: bilateral microears; trigonocephaly; cerebellar dysfunction; antimongoloid obliquity to the eyes with left eyelid ptosis; left VII nerve palsy; short neck; low hairline; bilateral cryptorchidism; normal IQ, speech and hearing. ? 9p– or r(9)?
     j) Case 10: bilateral poorly differentiated, protruding ears with small external auditory canals; incomplete fusion of median and lateral nasal processes just under nares with normal vermilion border; mongoloid obliquity to the eyes; left hand postminimus; bilateral clinodactyly of the 2nd and 5th digits; normal IQ, speech and hearing.
     k) Case 11: bilateral cryptotia; isolated cleft palate; epicanthal folds; small orbits; short, webbed neck; pulmonary hypoplasia; agenesis of left diaphragm; congenital

(continued next page)

TABLE 2 (Continued)

heart disease (unspecified); stenosis of ureters (hydroureters) and bilateral hydronephrosis; brachydactyly of 5th fingers with fusiform middle phalanges; right hammer toe; pes valgus; died at 44 minutes.
l) Case 12: bilateral dysplastic pinnas; epicanthal folds; hypertelorism; microdontia; pyloric stenosis; bilateral 5th finger brachydactyly; mental retardation.
m) Case 13: bilateral microtia with meatal atresia; large pigmented nevus above right eye; spindle-shaped hyperextensible fingers; hypoplastic thumb nails; bilateral calcaneovalgus; congenital phimosis.
n) Case 14: bilateral microtia; mongoloid obliquity to the eyes; micrognathia; flattened, crooked nose; webbed neck; gastric hypoplasia; pulmonary hypoplasia; digital dislocations of the left hand; left knee dislocation; bilateral talipes equinovarus; died at 11 hours; history of oligohydramnios $2°$ to chronic leakage.
o) Case 15: bilateral microears; plagiocephaly; right palpebral fissure > left; left VII nerve paresis; mental retardation; sensorineural hearing loss.
p) Case 16: bilateral microtia; isolated cleft palate; hypoplastic kidneys.
q) Case 17: right microtia; ventricular septal defect; absence of right thumb; 3 accessory spleens; single dysplastic kidney; absence of rectum and imperforate anus; absent urethra; tail remnant; stillborn.

C) Deformation
Potter syndrome (1 case) with bilateral large, flattened auricles and no extrarenal malformations.

classification of M. M. Cohen [3] and have been eliminated from most further analyses. Excluding syndromes, there were 549 persons (0.0103) with at least one aural malformation and 11 persons (0.0002) with at least one branchial cleft malformation. There was a total of 558 persons affected with 583 nonsyndromic malformations of the external ear or branchial cleft or both. These are listed in Table 3 along with their frequencies in the population. Again, both bilateral and unilateral cases of a given type of malformation were counted as one.

Etiologic Relationships

Since previously published cases of malformation of the external ear and/or branchial cleft (see References 4–8 for nonsyndromic examples and References 9 and 10 for syndromic examples) have shown combinations of the various types in the same person or in different members of the same family, chi-square analyses were used to determine 1) if in fact these different malformations tended to occur together more often than by chance in the same person, and 2) if they do tend to cluster, are they the result of single hits by multiple causes or multiple hits by single causes. Because there was no a priori knowledge of the etiologies of the nonsyndromic and most of the syndromic cases or of their complete pleiotropic manifestations, all 600 persons were considered together for these analyses.

TABLE 3. Distribution of All External Ear and Branchial Cleft Malformations Excluding Syndrome Cases

Malformation	Number	Rate per 10,000*
Preauricular sinus	431	80.93
Preauricular tags	89	16.71
Microtia	9	1.69
Other malformed pinna**	43	8.07
Branchial cleft sinus	11	2.07

*Based on a total NCPP population size of 53,257. Bilateral cases of any given malformation were counted as one for purposes of incidence calculations.
**Includes all other cases of malformed pinna. With the exception of microtia, the diagnostic labels and/or descriptions of the anomalies were not sufficiently clear to be certain of the precise nosologic category.

Table 4 lists the frequency of malformation "X" in cases with malformation "Y" and compares these frequencies with those of the general population without "Y." In nearly all comparisons, the probability of such clustering being random is less than 0.005.

The Poisson distribution tests the tendency of observed events to cluster. If the observations being scored occur independently and thus are the results of single hits by multiple causes, then their distribution should agree with that predicted by the Poisson. Analysis of the entire population studied (53,257) using standard computational methods [11] is presented in Table 5. It is apparent that multiple types of anomalies in a single individual are more likely associated with multiple hits by a single cause and thus, any given malformation of the type studied here is not necessarily etiologically distinct from any other of this type. Based on these analyses as well as the studies on animals by Poswillo [12] and on numerous clinical reports in the literature, all malformations in this study appear to share common, indistinguishable etiologies and thus are grouped together for all further analyses.

Familial vs Isolated Cases

On the basis of family history, the malformed probands can be divided into 2 groups, familial and isolated. *Familial* is defined in this study as the presence of any affected first-degree or second-degree relative(s). An affected first-degree or second-degree relative is one with any malformation of the external ear or branchial cleft or both, regardless of whether it is identical to that in the proband or not. Data on third-degree relatives were mostly unavailable and thus could not be included in the definition. All cases not familial are termed *isolated* in this study. Such cases are either *sporadic,* which include new mutations, phenocopies,

TABLE 4. Distribution of Malformation "X" in Cases With Malformation "Y"*

"Y"	"X"	Frequency (X/Y)	Multiple of the "without 'Y' population" frequency	χ^{2}**
Preauricular sinus (446)	Preauricular tag (7)	0.0157	9.87	43.64
	Microtia (1)	0.0022	7.89	1.01 (NS)
	Other malformed pinna (10)	0.0247	23.22	159.70
	Branchial cleft sinus (2)	0.0045	23.68	19.66
Preauricular tag (91)	Preauricular sinus (7)	0.0769	9.32	43.64
	Microtia (1)	0.0110	38.95	8.19
	Other malformed pinna (4)	0.0440	41.00	110.95
	Branchial cleft sinus (1)	0.0110	53.11	11.23
Microtia (16)	Preauricular sinus (1)	0.0625	7.48	1.01 (NS)
	Preauricular tag (1)	0.0625	36.97	8.19
Other malformed pinna (61)	Preauricular sinus (10)	0.1803	20.00	159.70
	Preauricular tag (4)	0.0656	40.09	110.95
Branchial cleft sinus (12)	Preauricular sinus (2)	0.1667	19.99	19.66
	Preauricular tag (1)	0.0833	49.30	11.23

*1) Numbers in parentheses are numbers of cases. 2) 2 × 2 contingency chi-square tables were constructed based on the incidence of the malformations in the general population as listed in Table 1; eg 7/446 were compared to 84/52,811 in the first line of the table. Note that the general population was defined in this example as all those without a preauricular sinus.

**All values less than P = 0.005 with the exception of the preauricular sinus–microtia combination which was not significant (NS).

TABLE 5. Observed and Expected Distribution of External Ear and/or Branchial Cleft Malformations

Number of anomaly types/proband[a]	Total number Observed[b]	Expected[c]	Deviation from expected[d]
0	52,657	52,637.5	+
1	574	615.9	−
2	26	3.6	+

[a]A proband with preauricular sinus and a preauricular tag, whether on the same side or not, was considered to have 2 anomaly types, while a proband with bilateral preauricular sinuses was considered to have 1 anomaly type.
[b]Total number in NCPP study = 53,257. Total number of considered malformations = 626. Mean number of considered malformations per NCPP study child = 0.0118. Total number of NCPP study children with considered malformations = 600.
[c]Calculated from Poisson distribution (pp 86–87 [11]).
[d]Goodness of fit χ^2 = 142.24 ($P < 0.005$).

TABLE 6. Distribution of Nonsyndromic Malformations: Familial vs Isolated

Malformation	Familial*	Isolated*
Preauricular sinus	27 (6.26)	404 (93.74)
Preauricular tags	6 (6.74)	83 (93.26)
Microtia	0 (0.00)	9 (100.00)
Other malformed pinna	7 (16.28)	36 (83.72)
Branchial cleft sinus	0 (0.00)	11 (100.00)
Total number	40 (6.86)	543 (93.14)
Percent of total NCPP study population (53,257)	0.08	1.01

*Numbers in parentheses are the frequencies in percent of familial and isolated in each malformation category.

chromosomal anomalies, and such; or *chance isolated,* ie, those which are due to segregation at the same locus as the familial case but for one reason or another (penetrance?) represent the only case in the family. The distribution of all cases of malformation according to the designations "familial" or "isolated" and the distribution according to type of malformation can be seen in Table 6. The proportion of isolated cases was greater than 80% in all categories of malformation.

Laterality

The analysis of laterality of malformation is presented in Table 7. It appears that the tendency to be bilateral or unilateral may be dependent on the type of case, familial or isolated ($\chi^2 = 3.78$, $P \approx 0.05$). The frequency of bilateral cases is considerably higher among familial cases (0.46) and, conversely, the frequency of unilateral cases is higher among isolated cases (0.71). The unilateral distribution, whether right or left, was independent of type of case (familial or isolated). However, there was a significant predilection for the right side ($\chi_1^2 = 40.32$; $P < 0.005$) if one takes the null hypothesis to be an equal distribution to both sides.

Additional Malformations in the Nonsyndromic Cases

Although we have already eliminated syndromes (2 or more malformations in addition to the one being studied) from the analyses, there exists a group of patients in whom a single additional malformation, major or minor, can be seen. Such events may represent a chance occurrence or a real association in which the occurrence of the two malformations happens with greater frequency than can reasonably be expected by chance alone. The pros and cons of whether these statistically significant associations can be classified as syndromes in their own right will not be discussed. Table 8 shows that the frequency of a single additional malformation in the nonsyndromic cases of aural malformation was significantly greater ($\chi_1^2 = 103.51$; $P < 0.005$) than the frequency of cases of malformation in the remaining NCPP population with no malformations of the ear. On closer inspection we can see that this frequency was significantly higher in the isolated cases but not so in the familial cases. For this reason the association of a particular malformation with a malformation of the external ear or branchial cleft or both is considered separately for familial and isolated probands.

In an attempt to avoid spurious associations, only those malformations which occurred 2 or more times in the probands' population were considered for analysis. For isolated probands, 22 such frequencies of malformation were analyzed, of which 11 were significant at the 5% level or less. On the basis of chance alone we would have expected only one to be significant. The significantly associ-

TABLE 7. Laterality of Malformations in Nonsyndromic Cases

	Bilateral	Unilateral	=	Right	+	Left	+	Unspecified
Familial	16	19		11		7		1
Isolated	150	373		202		166		5
$2 \times 2\ \chi^2$		3.78*			0.08			
Combined	166	392		213		173		6

*$P \approx 0.05$.

TABLE 8. The Frequency of a Single Additional Malformation in the Nonsyndromic Cases

Case type	Malformation type*			Combined vs combined (case type vs NCPP)
	Major	Minor	Combined	
Familial	2/35 (0.06)	6/35 (0.17)	8/35 (0.23)	$\chi^2 = 0.98$
Isolated	75/523 (0.14)	91/523 (0.17)	166/523 (0.32)	$\chi^2 = 104.05**$
Combined	77/558 (0.14)	97/558 (0.17)	174/558 (0.31)	$\chi^2 = 103.51**$
Remaining NCPP population	—	—	8,114/52,699 (0.15)	—

*The numerator is the number of malformed, the denominator is the total number of cases for each case type and the number in parentheses is the frequency which may be converted to percent by multiplying by 100.
**$P < 0.005$.

ated malformations are listed in Table 9. In addition, there were a number of malformations which could not be analyzed because of a lack of NCPP population frequencies. These included 2 cases of neonatal teeth, 2 of ankyloglossia, 2 of eyelid ptosis, and 4 of severe myopia.

Among the familial cases there was only one malformation which occurred more than once: stenosis of the lacrimal duct (2 cases). The frequency of this malformation with the aural malformation was significantly higher than it was among the remaining, aurally normal, NCPP population ($\chi_1^2 = 47.73; P < 0.005$). This contrasts with the isolated cases in which there were also 2 cases but the frequency was not significantly different from that among the remaining NCPP population without aural malformation ($\chi_1^2 = 1.09; P > 0.1$).

Sex Ratios

The male/female sex ratio was 1.06 for familial probands, 1.11 for isolated probands, and 1.11 overall. None of these ratios was significantly different from the 1.04 ratio found in the overall NCPP population and other large populations studied.

TABLE 9. Congenital Malformations at Age 1 Year With Frequencies Significantly Greater (P < 0.05) in Isolated Nonsyndromic Cases Than in Remaining NCPP Population at Age 1 Year

Malformation*	Rate per 10,000		$2 \times 2 \chi^2$
	Proband group	NCPP group	
Major			
1. Craniosynostosis (4)	76.5	4.6	38.22
2. Kyphoscoliosis (3)	57.4	6.8	11.83
3. Pectus carinatum (2)	38.2	2.5	12.54
4. Congenital heart disease (12)	229.4	74.1	14.63
5. Inguinal hernia (13)	248.5	133.3	4.35
6. Dysmorphic ureters (2)**	38.2	0.9	30.10
Minor			
1. Digital dysmorphia, mild (4)***	76.5	9.9	16.00
2. Strawberry/port-wine hemangioma (21)	401.5	225.9	6.42
3. Pigmented nevus (8)	153.0	45.3	10.77
4. Café-au-lait spots (31)	592.7	70.0	182.92
5. Vitiligo (2)	38.2	0.0	112.69

*There were 523 nonsyndromic isolated proband cases and the number in parentheses indicates how many of these had a particular malformation.
**Includes atretic and/or double ureters.
***Includes such anomalies as mildly hypoplastic distal phalanges, notched distal phalanges, etc.

Race

The frequency of malformations of the external ear and/or branchial cleft was more than 4 times greater in blacks than in whites, and this was highly significant (Table 10). It should be noted that the race of the proband was independent of whether the proband was a familial or isolated case ($\chi_2^2 = 0.146$; $P > 0.9$). Table 11 shows that the differences between the races are accounted for by the highly significant excess of preauricular sinuses among blacks. It should be noted, however, that the frequency of cases in which a proband had two or more different types of malformations of the external ear and/or branchial cleft is about 4% in both whites (4/101) and blacks (19/432) and thus, the phenomenon of a given cause being associated with more than one type of aural malformation in a single individual is evident in both races.

Institution

Table 12 shows that the overall frequency of persons with malformations was highly dependent on the institution studied ($\chi_{11}^2 = 793.19$; $P < 0.005$). In addition, the frequency of familial or isolated malformations was also highly dependent on institution, the χ_{11}^2 being 35.43 ($P < 0.005$) and 790.01 ($P < 0.005$), respectively. However, the proportion of familial to isolated cases was not quite as variable among institutions ($\chi_{11}^2 = 25.00$; $P < 0.01$). The incidence of familial cases tended to follow in magnitude the overall incidence of cases of malformation of the ear, hospital by hospital.

Racial and Institutional Variability

Upon inspection of Table 12, one finds that there is considerable variation among hospitals in racial composition of patients' population ($\chi_{11}^2 = 29,147.73$; $P < 0.005$), in addition to a significant variation among hospitals in frequency of malformations ($\chi_{11}^2 = 793.19$; $P < 0.005$). The problem arises whether this racial variation in frequencies of malformation is the same in all hospitals. That is, we had to determine whether there is interaction between race and institution. To do this we employed first an angular transformation of the binomial proportions and then applied an analysis of variance [13]. The results of this analysis are presented in Table 13.

As expected, the overall racial differences were highly significant ($\chi_1^2 = 47.04$; $P < 0.005$). This was even more apparent ($\chi_1^2 = 133.25$; $P < 0.005$) when racial variation was considered after eliminating the institutional differences. Similarly institutional variation, after eliminating racial differences, was also highly significant ($\chi_{10}^2 = 297.31$; $P < 0.005$). However, the interaction χ^2 was not significant, indicating that the racial variation in frequency of malformation was independent of the institutional variation. Nevertheless, although the racial variation was quite real, there remained considerable institutional differences after racial

TABLE 10. Racial Distribution of the Nonsyndromic Cases*

Case type**	Race**			Total
	Black	White	Other	
Familial				
Malformed	27 (0.11)	6 (0.03)	2 (0.05)	35
Remainder	25,099	24,147	3,976	53,222
$2 \times 2 \chi^2$	11.36***	0.14		53,257
Isolated				
Malformed	405 (1.61)	95 (0.39)	23 (0.58)	523
Remainder	24,721	24,058	3,955	52,734
$2 \times 2 \chi^2$	180.86***	2.37		53,257
Combined				
Malformed	432 (1.72)	101 (0.42)	25 (0.63)	558
Remainder	24,694	24,052	3,953	52,699
$2 \times 2 \chi^2$	193.66***	2.93		53,257

*Numbers in parentheses are malformed frequencies in percent.
**Racial type and case type (familial, etc) were independent of one another ($\chi_2^2 = 0.146$, $P > 0.9$).
***$P < 0.005$.

Malformations of the External Ear / 315

TABLE 11. Distribution of Nonsyndromic Malformations by Race and Phenotype

Malformation	Whites		Blacks	
	Number	Rate/10,000*	Number	Rate/10,000*
Preauricular sinus	43	17.80	374	148.85***
Preauricular tag	33	13.66	48	19.10 (NS)
Microtia	4	1.66	5	1.99 (NS)
Other malformed pinna**	20	8.28	18	7.16 (NS)
Branchial cleft sinus	5	2.07	6	2.39 (NS)

*Based on a total NCPP white population of 24,153 and NCPP black population of 25,126. Bilateral cases of any given malformation were counted as one for purposes of incidence calculations.
**Includes all other cases of malformed pinna. With the exception of microtia, the diagnostic labels and/or descriptions of the anomalies were not sufficiently clear to be certain of the precise nosologic category.
***Significantly greater than the incidence in whites ($\chi_1^2 = 250.48$, $P < 0.005$).
NS = no significant difference between the races.

variation was eliminated. A more precise visualization of this institutional heterogeneity can be obtained by dividing the mean institutional χ^2 by the mean interaction χ^2. In this case, this variance ratio ($F_{10,10} = 17.94$) is highly significant ($P < 0.001$).

GENETICS

It has already been demonstrated that there are highly significant racial differences in the incidence of malformations of the external ear and/or branchial cleft. These differences may reflect important genetic differences between blacks and whites. For this reason, it was decided to analyze the racial groups separately.

There were 2 family histories obtained in this study, one prior to the birth of the child studied, and one at that child's 7th year's pediatric examination. This provided an update of information on the family, particularly for those sibs born after the proband. In addition, it often contained information about other relatives (usually first or second degree or both) who had a particular minor aural malformation that was not recorded on the first family history. Apparently, the birth of a child with a particular external aural malformation prompted the mothers to investigate their families and communicate this information to the history-taker at the 7-year-old's exam. This often included new information on the proband's father, sibs, and grandparents. Nevertheless, information on second-degree relatives other than grandparents was generally sketchy.

TABLE 12. Distribution of Nonsyndromic Malformed Persons by Institution

	Hospital*												Total
	05	10	15	31	37	45	50	55	60	66	71	82	
Malformed-Familial (F)	6	0	4	2	1	4	0	4	7	0	1	6	35
Malformed-Isolated (I)	57	3	60	35	17	38	12	25	26	58	14	178	523
Total Malformed (M)	63	3	64	37	18	42	12	29	33	58	15	184	558
Total Normal (N)	11,540	2,322	2,458	2,055	3,996	3,225	3,080	4,298	3,175	9,484	3,932	3,271	52,836**
M/M + N × 100	0.54	0.13	2.54	1.77	0.45	1.29	0.39	0.67	1.03	0.61	0.38	5.33	1.05
F/M + N × 100	0.05	0.00	0.16	0.10	0.03	0.12	0.00	0.09	0.22	0.00	0.03	0.18	0.07
I/M + N × 100	0.49	0.13	2.38	1.67	0.42	1.17	0.39	0.58	0.81	0.61	0.35	5.16	0.98
F/M × 100	9.52	0.00	6.25	5.40	5.56	9.52	0.00	13.79	21.21	0.00	6.67	3.26	6.27
I/M × 100	90.48	100.00	93.75	94.60	94.44	90.48	100.00	86.21	78.79	100.00	93.33	96.74	93.73
Number of:													
Whites	10,282	2,244	0	617	879	814	2,934	258	2,274	855	3,027	21	24,205
Blacks	1,135	55	2,522	857	3,128	2,447	18	1,508	859	8,363	858	3,434	25,184
Others	186	26	0	618	7	6	140	2,561	75	324	62	0	4,005

*05: Boston Lying-in Hospital and Children's Hospital; 10: Children's Hospital of Buffalo; 15: Charity Hospital, New Orleans; 31: Columbia University; 37: Johns Hopkins Hospital; 45: Medical College of Virginia; 50: University of Minnesota; 55: New York Medical College; 60: University of Oregon; 66: Children's Hospital of Philadelphia; 71: Brown University, Providence; 82: University of Tennessee.
**Includes 137 individuals of unknown sex [1].

TABLE 13. Racial and Institutional Variability

	Hospital													Total
	05	10	15	31	37	45	50	55	60	66	71	82		
Whites														
Affected	46	3	0	4	0	2	12	1	19	2	11	1		101
Total	10,282	2,244	0	617	879	814	2,934	258	2,274	855	3,027	21		24,205
Blacks														
Affected	16	0	64	27	18	40	0	10	14	56	4	183		432
Total	1,135	55	2,522	857	3,128	2,447	18	1,508	859	8,363	858	3,434		25,184

Analysis of χ^2*

	Degrees of freedom	χ^2
Race	1	47.04**
Institution	10	297.31**
Interaction	10	16.57 NS
Total***	21	447.13**

*Since there were no whites in the population of Hospital 15, this hospital was not considered in the analysis.
**$P < 0.005$; NS = not significant.
***Note that the various components of χ^2 do not add up to the total because the proportions are based on different numbers [13].

Multifactorial/Threshold Inheritance

Since there were relatively few familial cases (approximately 6% in both blacks and whites), it was apparent that these malformations were not likely to be inherited in a simple Mendelian fashion, at least not in the population as a whole. Rather than entertain elaborate etiologic explanations, it was felt appropriate to investigate initially the suitability of the classic multifactorial/threshold model which includes polygenic inheritance as one of its features. Examination of the frequency of these malformations in the first-degree relatives of probands demonstrated a 3.3-fold increase in the incidence among white first-degree relatives and virtually no increase among black first-degree relatives. Utilizing the most conservative predictions, $p^{0.6}$ in whites and $p^{0.8}$ in blacks [14] for calculating the respective expected incidences of a polygenically determined trait in the first-degree relatives of white and black probands, the observed number of affected first-degree relatives in both races differed significantly from the expected; the χ^2 in whites was 6.49 ($P < 0.025$) and in blacks 23.12 ($P < 0.005$).

Again employing predictions from the model, the severity of the defect should be proportional to the number of genetic and/or environmental liability factors present in the affected individual. Theoretically, the relatives of more severely affected probands should be at greater risk to express the phenotype. This was not true for either whites ($\chi_1^2 = 0.19$; $P > 0.5$) or blacks ($\chi_1^2 = 0.018$; $P > 0.5$). Furthermore, holding constant by regression the number of children born after the proband, only 0.06% in blacks and virtually 0.00% in whites of the total variation in the number of children affected after the proband could be accounted for by the variation of the number affected up to and including the proband. Neither of the partial correlations associated with this prediction from the model was significantly different from 0. Even when the number of children born after the proband was allowed to vary freely, the number of children affected up to and including the proband could only account for 0.05% of the variation in risk to black sibs born subsequent to the proband and virtually 0.00% of this same variation in whites. Finally, there was no consanguinity in any of the families studied.

Heritability (h^2) estimates were calculated for each race from the population and observed first-degree data. For whites, h^2 (in percent) was 29.59 ± 11.02 and for blacks 0.16 ± 5.93. It should be noted that since these estimates are in large measure based on sib data, the values for both races are probably inflated unless one is willing to assume that the dominant component of the genetic variance is equal to 0, an assumption which is most likely untenable in the case of sibs. For this reason these estimates may be a closer approximation to a measure of the relative genetic determination of the malformations, ie a measure of that portion of the total phenotypic variance which is genetic and not just the additive component of that genetic variance. Unfortunately, there was not sufficient data on parents/offspring or data reliable enough on second-degree relatives to make better estimates of the heritability. In any case, it would appear that the degree of environmental determination in both races is considerable, strikingly so in blacks. In summary, then, the classic multifactorial/threshold model which includes polygenic inheritance was not a satisfactory explanation of these data.

Segregation Analysis

The frequency of familial probands among all probands was 6% in both races. The fact that the pedigrees of about half of the familial probands demonstrated vertical transmission through 2 and 3 generations made it reasonable to regard at least these probands as likely monogenic cases and to estimate the proportions of sporadic and familial cases among the total population of isolated cases as well as the segregation frequency of the familial cases. Segregation analysis, by race, of all cases [15] was accomplished by the SEGRAN method [16] which provides maximum likelihood estimates of ϕ (segregation probability), X (proportion of sporadic cases), and π (ascertainment probability). *For blacks,* iteration on all Normal by Normal (N X N) matings (N = 413) yielded as best estimates $\phi = 0.096 \pm 0.036$, $X = 0.804 \pm 0.062$, and $\pi = 0.750 \pm 0.104$. Iteration on all Affected by Normal (A X N) matings (N = 10) yielded as best estimates $\phi = 0.132 \pm 0.082$, $X = 0$, $\pi = 1.0$. *For whites,* iteration on all N X N matings gave best estimates of $\phi = 0.101 \pm 0.079$, $X = 0.828 \pm 0.118$, and $\pi = 0.358 \pm 0.231$. Unfortunately there were only 3 A X N matings. A calculation by the Weinberg Proband Method [17] estimated $\phi = 0.14$, consistent with the results in blacks.

Apparently there may be a substantial number of isolated cases in both races which are chance isolated and not sporadic. Regarding the cases presumed to be hereditary, with these data we cannot distinguish between a common recessive trait with about 40% penetrance, a rare dominant trait with about 20% penetrance, or genetic heterogeneity. Of particular note are the high estimates of the proportion of sporadic cases in both races. This would again suggest that there are major environmental determinants of external aural malformations.

ENVIRONMENTAL VARIABLES

Since one of the major objectives of this study was to test broad hypotheses about environmental effects by examining a large number of variables of unknown significance, a prospective-retrospective study was considered quite suitable, that is, retrospective analysis of prospectively collected data. Selection of an appropriate control group is undoubtedly one of the major methodologic problems encountered in the design of such retrospective analyses. Since the basic assumption underlying a retrospective analysis is that the selected control group is representative of all persons without the disorder, selection bias must be avoided at all cost. The ideal procedure would have been to review and abstract the complete NCPP records of all 44,969 non-malformed children. Obviously, the time and cost of such an undertaking made this impractical. It was decided that 400 non-malformed children would be randomly selected from the non-malformed NCPP population.

The number of controls chosen from each of the 12 centers was apportioned according to the percentage that that hospital contributed to the total NCPP population, with the aid of tables of 5-digit random numbers [18, 19]. For each hospital the choice of table was determined randomly by the toss of a coin. The racial distribution of this control group was 44.5% white, 48% black, and 7.5% other, a distribution almost identical to the total NCPP population. The distribution by sex of the children in the control group was 52% male and 48% female, again nearly identical to the 51% to 49% found in the total NCPP population.

Birth Order

In a multiple regression analysis with normal or isolated malformed ears as the dependent variable, and race, maternal age, paternal age, parity and the total number of sibs in each sibship as the independent variables, neither parity, maternal age, paternal age, nor total sibs was significantly correlated with being malformed. As expected, though, the independent variables were highly correlated with each other. Parity was not correlated with race, nor were the other independent variables correlated with race.

Socioeconomic Status

The socioeconomic status in the NCPP population was evaluated by Myriantho-poulos and French [20] using the technique recently developed by the U.S. Bureau of the Census. This combines scores for education, occupation, and family income to derive a composite numerical profile termed the socioeconomic index (SEI). The index ranges from a low of 0 to a high of 99. These SEI scores represent the socioeconomic status of the child's family at the time of antepartum registration.

The mean SEI and standard error were calculated separately for blacks and whites. The mean score for black isolated cases (34.36 ± 0.85) was significantly lower (t_{584} = 3.5326, P < 0.001) than the mean score for black normal controls (39.82 ± 1.32). However, the mean score for white isolated cases (54.73 ± 2.45) was *not* significantly different (t_{263} = 0.5394, P > 0.5) from the mean score for white normal controls (56.31 ± 1.66). Interestingly, the socioeconomic index of black familial cases (40.93 ± 2.88) was close to that of black normal controls. The difference between black familial cases and black isolated cases was close to the 5% level of significance (t_{421} = 1.94, P < 0.06). The number of white familial cases was too few (6) to make such a comparison.

Potential Teratogens

The finding of a lower socioeconomic status in a group of affected persons as opposed to controls suggests, in the case of congenital malformations of unknown etiology, the importance of environmental factors, particularly those that are related to nutrition and chronic infectious and noninfectious diseases. With this in mind, a large number of environmental factors were investigated with disappointing but not unexpected results (Tables 14–18). Since it is well recognized that large sample sizes are needed to detect a teratogenic effect, it was statistically inefficient to analyze by race. Instead, we sought to maximize the data by combining racial frequencies. With the exception of KUB infection and vaginitis (Table 15), there were no statistically significant risk ratios. It should be noted, however, that the 95% confidence limits were considerably wide for many of these parameters and thus it is not totally possible to rule out a teratogenic effect for at least those in which the risk ratio was well above 1, such as chronic lung disease and pyelonephritis (Table 14), Rh incompatibility (Table 17), a number of antibiotics, and barbiturates (Table 18). Nevertheless, if such an effect is present, the data suggest that it is not likely to be a strong one, and a much larger sample size would be needed to detect it. Since this is not likely to be available in the near future, animal studies might be profitable for some of the parameters just mentioned.

TABLE 14. Chronic Diseases During Pregnancy

Disease	Isolated probands (total = 525)	Normal controls (total = 400)	Relative risk**	95% Confidence limits
Diabetes mellitus[a]	7 (0.0133)*	8 (0.0200)	0.66	0.25–1.80
Hyperthyroidism	4 (0.0076)	4 (0.0100)	0.76	0.20–2.83
Hypothyroidism	4 (0.0076)	8 (0.0200)	0.38	0.13–1.26
"Epilepsy"[b]	1 (0.0019)	1 (0.0025)	0.76	0.08–7.35
Lung disease[c]	20 (0.0381)	8 (0.0200)	1.94	0.83–4.21
Organic heart disease[d]	10 (0.0190)	10 (0.0250)	0.76	0.32–1.80
Hypertension	53 (0.1009)	44 (0.1103)	0.91	0.59–1.38
Phlebitis	1 (0.0019)	2 (0.0050)	0.38	0.06–3.47
GI disorders[e]	5 (0.0095)	8 (0.0200)	0.47	0.17–1.44
Glomerulonephritis	1 (0.0019)	0 (0.0000)	undefined	–
Pyelonephritis	5 (0.0095)	2 (0.0050)	1.91	0.38–7.55
Sickle cell anemia	1 (0.0019)	1 (0.0025)	0.76	0.08–7.35
Nutritional anemia	169 (0.3219)	108 (0.2700)	1.28	0.94–1.74

*Frequency of the disorder in each study group is in parentheses.
**No significant differences between study groups.
[a]Nongestational diabetes mellitus only.
[b]Noneclamptic convulsive disorders.
[c]Asthma, chronic bronchitis, etc.
[d]Rheumatic heart disease, congenital heart disease and hypertensive heart disease.
[e]Peptic ulcer, appendicitis, cholecystitis and cholelithiasis.

TABLE 15. Infectious Diseases During First Trimester of Pregnancy

Disease	Isolated proband (total = 525)	Normal controls (total = 400)	Relative risk	95% Confidence limits
Influenza	20 (0.0381)*	21 (0.0525)	0.71	0.38–1.33
URI (nonspecific)	135 (0.2571)	128 (0.3200)	0.74**	0.55–0.98
Intestinal parasites	1 (0.0019)	2 (0.0050)	0.38	0.06–3.47
KUB (nonspecific)	113 (0.2152)	54 (0.1350)	1.76***	1.23–2.49
Syphilis	13 (0.0248)	12 (0.0300)	0.82	0.37–5.97
Gonorrhea	3 (0.0057)	0 (0.0000)	undefined	—
Vaginitis[a]	137 (0.2609)	82 (0.2050)	1.37**	1.00–1.86

*Frequency of the disorder in each study group in parentheses.
**$P < 0.05$.
***$P < 0.005$.
[a]Monilial, trichomonal, and nonspecific.

TABLE 16. Maternal Vaccinations During First Trimester of Pregnancy

Vaccine	Isolated probands (total = 525)	Normal controls (total = 400)	Relative risk**	95% Confidence limits
Polio (Sabin)	28 (0.0533)*	27 (0.0675)	0.78	0.45–1.34
Polio (Salk)	42 (0.0800)	46 (0.1150)	0.67	0.43–1.04
Influenza	7 (0.0133)	6 (0.0150)	0.89	0.31–2.53
Tetanus	4 (0.0076)	3 (0.0075)	1.02	0.24–3.99
Diphtheria	1 (0.0019)	1 (0.0025)	0.76	0.08–7.35
Smallpox	1 (0.0019)	0 (0.0000)	undefined	—
Measles (live)	1 (0.0019)	0 (0.0000)	undefined	—
Rabies	1 (0.0019)	0 (0.0000)	undefined	—

*Frequency of the disorder in each study group in parentheses.
**No significant differences between study groups.

Let us return briefly to the significantly increased risk to children whose mothers had either a nonspecific KUB infection or vaginitis (Table 15). Analyzed by race, the risk to children whose mothers had a nonspecific KUB infection was only significant for blacks. Again analyzed separately by race, the risk to children whose mothers had vaginitis during the first trimester was *not* statistically significant for either whites or blacks, although the estimated relative risk was nearly 1½ times higher in blacks than in whites. Concerning the increased risk to children whose mothers had first trimester KUB infections, the meaning remains obscure to us. Since this was found only in blacks, it may be related to the significantly lowered socioeconomic status. For this reason, as well as chance alone, this finding may be spurious. On the other hand, this finding could be real and possibly related to the effects of hyperthermia, medication, the infectious agent per se, or all three. Finally, it should be noted that a failure to identify clearly

TABLE 17. Other Complications of Pregnancy

Disorder	Isolated probands (total = 525)	Normal controls (total = 400)	Relative risk**	95% Confidence limits
Hyperemesis gravidarum	2 (0.0038)*	3 (0.0075)	0.51	0.11–2.76
Vaginal bleeding (1st trimester)	80 (0.1524)	52 (0.1300)	1.20	0.88–1.63
Polyhydramnios	3 (0.0057)	7 (0.0175)	0.32	0.10–1.26
Placenta previa	2 (0.0038)	3 (0.0075)	0.51	0.11–2.76
Abruptio placentas	1 (0.0019)	3 (0.0075)	0.25	0.05–2.21
ABO incompatibility[a]	91 (0.1904)	68 (0.1954)	0.97	0.68–1.37
Rh incompatibility[b]	33 (0.0690)	20 (0.0580)	1.21	0.68–2.11

*Frequency of the disorder in each study group in parentheses.
**No significant differences between study groups.
[a]ABO incompatibility data available for 478 isolated probands and 348 normal controls – frequencies based on these totals.
[b]Rh incompatibility data available for 478 isolated probands and 345 normal controls – frequencies based on these totals.

TABLE 18. Drug Use During the First Trimester of Pregnancy

Drug	Isolated proband (total = 525)	Normal controls (total = 400)	Relative risk**	95% Confidence limits
Diuretics	2 (0.0038)*	6 (0.0150)	0.25	0.07–1.25
Antihistamines	18 (0.0343)	19 (0.0475)	0.71	0.37–1.37
Barbiturates	18 (0.0343)	11 (0.0275)	1.26	0.58–2.61
Tranquilizers	15 (0.0286)	13 (0.0325)	0.88	0.41–1.83
Penicillin	48 (0.0914)	25 (0.0625)	1.51	0.91–2.46
Tetracycline	4 (0.0076)	2 (0.0050)	1.53	0.29–6.49
Streptomycin	1 (0.0019)	1 (0.0025)	0.76	0.08–7.35
Chloramphenicol	2 (0.0038)	1 (0.0025)	1.53	0.17–9.67
Sulfonamides	2 (0.0038)	1 (0.0025)	1.53	0.17–9.67
Antifungal agents	1 (0.0019)	3 (0.0075)	0.25	0.05–2.21
Insulin	4 (0.0076)	5 (0.0125)	0.61	0.18–2.17
Thyroxin	4 (0.0076)	7 (0.0175)	0.43	0.14–1.47
Estrogen	6 (0.0114)	9 (0.0225)	0.50	0.19–1.41
Progesterone	11 (0.0209)	10 (0.0250)	0.83	0.36–1.94
Pressor agents	13 (0.0248)	11 (0.0275)	0.90	0.40–1.97
Salicylates	158 (0.3009)	112 (0.2800)	1.11	0.83–1.47

*Frequency of the disorder in each study group in parentheses.
**No significant differences between study groups.

environmental risk factors may be due in part to our inability to eliminate the chance isolated (presumed genetic) cases from the total isolated case sample. Nevertheless, until such time as we can identify, positively, such chance isolated cases, we are forced to either accept this epidemiologic pollution or not do the analysis at all.

NATURAL HISTORY

Relatively little is known about the natural history of those children who have nonsyndromic isolated or familial malformations of the external ear and/or branchial cleft. There are some indications that congenital hearing loss is likely to be an important factor [21, 22]. Furthermore, Hanson et al [23] pointed out that prenatal growth deficiency is the most consistent single feature of major known teratogens yet recognized in man, being expressed as abnormal skeletal and psychomotor development. This factor may be of particular importance with regard to the sporadic cases in this study. In order to evaluate all these possibilities, a number of variables were investigated including low birthweight, intelligence (IQ), hearing loss, abnormal speech production in the absence of deafness, mental retardation, and anomalies of speech mechanism.

Birthweight and Isolated Malformations of the External Ear

In order to examine the possible effects of a less than optimum (teratogenic) environment in utero on the somatic and physiologic development of infants with isolated cases of malformations of the external ear and/or branchial cleft, a number of factors were considered: birthweight, Apgar score, and gestational age. Obviously some of these variables are likely to be correlated with each other and perhaps with race. Thus, it was decided that the most appropriate analysis was a multiple regression analysis with normal or malformed as the dependent variable, and race, Apgar score, birthweight, and gestational age as the independent variables. Birthweight, when the other independent variables were held constant, was not significantly correlated with malformation; similarly, neither was gestational age nor Apgar score. These data, then, betray no indication that prenatal growth deficiency expressed as low birthweight is a significant factor in children with isolated malformation of the external ear and/or branchial cleft.

Intelligence (IQ)

IQ was measured at age 4 years with the abbreviated version of the Stanford-Binet Intelligence Scale (Form L-M) and at age 7 years with the Wechsler Intelligence Scale for Children (WISC). It has previously been shown that the best predictors of IQ at 4 years in the NCPP population of blacks and whites are socioeconomic status and the Bayley motor and mental scores at 8 months of age [24]. Thus, since it is known that in the NCPP population blacks have considerably lower socioeconomic index scores than whites (see above and [20]), blacks and whites are considered separately. The frequency of mental retardation (IQ ≤ 69) in white isolated cases (3%) was not significantly different from that in the white control population (4%); the same was true of blacks (4% vs 7%, respectively). Since the number of familial cases was small, further stratification into black/white racial groups was not possible. Nevertheless, the frequency of mental retarda-

TABLE 19. IQ at Age 7 Years and Isolated External Ear Malformations

	Mean ± SE			
Race	Isolated cases	Normal controls	DF	t Value
White	100.01 ± 1.87	102.24 ± 1.20	227	1.02 (NS)
Black	90.97 ± 1.86	89.42 ± 0.94	533	0.58 (NS)

DF = degrees of freedom.
NS = not significant.

tion in the total of black and white familial cases (3%) was not significantly different from that in the combined black and white control population (5%).

Viewing IQ at age 7 years, it can be seen that the mean IQ of white isolated cases was not significantly different from the white control group; the same was true for blacks (Table 19). The mean IQ at age 7 years for black familial cases (91.04 ± 2.54) was also not significantly different (t_{393} = 0.59) from the black control group and the same was true of whites (mean for cases = 108.75 ± 13.58; t_{159} = 0.83), although the number of white familial cases (4) with IQ scores at 7 years was very small. These data suggest that the etiologic agents associated with familial and isolated malformations of the external ear and/or branchial cleft have no detectable effect on the mental development of affected infants, black or white.

Hearing

Audiologic screening by various methods was performed on the NCPP study children on numerous occasions. Detailed audiologic testing, including pure-tone audiometry, was carried out at ages 3 and 8. A loss of greater than 15 dB was considered abnormal. Among the isolated cases, adequate pure-tone audiometry at 8 years was completed for 77 of 95 whites and 369 of 405 blacks. Among controls, the same data were available for 172 of 178 whites and 186 of 192 blacks. For familial cases, 28 of 33 were so tested. Comparisons between affected and control groups are given in Table 20. The frequency of abnormal hearing loss of all kinds was significantly greater ($P < 0.05$) in isolated white cases than in white controls. This was not the case for blacks although the frequency in the black cases (10%) was twice that found in the black controls. For the combined (ie, black and white) familial cases, the frequency of abnormal hearing loss (7%) is almost identical with that found in the combined white/black control group (χ^2 = 0.09).

In order to characterize the laterality and nature of the hearing loss in the malformed cases, as well as the ipsilaterality or contralaterality to the malformed ear, an attempt was made to list the hearing loss by side in one of 3 broad

TABLE 20. Hearing Loss and Isolated External Ear Malformations

	Isolated cases		Normal controls
White			
Hearing loss	14		14
Normal	63		158
$2 \times 2 \chi^2$		4.42*	
Black			
Hearing loss	38		10
Normal	331		176
$2 \times 2 \chi^2$		3.19	
Combined			
Hearing loss	52		24
Normal	394		334
$2 \times 2 \chi^2$		5.13*	

*Significant, $P < 0.05$.

categories: conductive, sensorineural, and mixed. Those cases in which only air-conduction audiometry was done were classified as "type unknown." The 2 familial cases with hearing loss both had bilateral conductive impairment. One case had bilateral preauricular sinuses and the other, bilateral anomalies of the helix and anthelix. Of the 52 isolated cases with hearing loss, 11 were "type unknown." Of the remainder, 29 (71%) had conductive hearing loss, 8 (19%) sensorineural hearing loss, and 4 (10%) mixed hearing loss. Viewed another way, a conductive component was present in 81% of the cases with hearing loss, and a sensorineural component was present in 29%. There were 20 cases (38%) in which there was a hearing loss contralateral to the ear with the malformation, 8 of these 20 (40%) having no hearing loss on the ipsilateral side.

All these data are presented in Table 21. There are 4 points of great interest here: 1) the surprising number of unilateral external aural malformations with unilateral (mostly ipsilateral) sensorineural hearing loss; 2) the finding that all 4 cases of mixed hearing loss are bilateral regardless of the unilaterality of the malformations of the external ear; 3) the finding that only 1 of the 2 cases of "hemifacial microsomia" had a hearing loss and that was bilateral sensorineural; and 4) the finding that of the 11 cases of nonsyndromic branchial cleft sinuses, there were no instances of a hearing loss. These data would strongly suggest considerable dysmorphic asymmetry of the external, middle, and inner ear structures for each individual patient as well as great phenotypic variability among those patients who demonstrated a hearing loss.

TABLE 21. Isolated Cases, Hearing Loss, and Relative Laterality

Whites		Blacks	
External ear malformation	Hearing loss	External ear malformation	Hearing loss
L-PAS	L-S	B-PAS	B-TU
B-PAS	B-C	L-PAS	L-S
R-PAS	B-TU	L-PAS	B-C
R-PAT	B-S	B-PAS	B-TU
R-PAT	B-C	R-PAS	L-TU
L-PAT, R-DP	R-C	L-PAS	L-C
R-PAT, R-DP	R-S	R-PAS	R-C
R-DP	B-TU	B-PAS	B-C
B-DP	L-C	B-DP, L-PAS	L-C
R-MIC	R-TU	L-PAS	B-S
R-MIC	R-C	R-PAS	R-S
R-MIC	R-C	B-PAS	L-C
B-DP	B-C	B-PAS	R-C
HM	B-S	B-PAS	B-TU
		R-PAS	L-TU
		L-PAS	B-M
		R-PAS	B-C
		B-PAS	L-C
		R-PAS	L-C
		R-PAS	R-C
		B-PAS	B-M
		R-PAS	L-C
		L-PAS	B-C
		L-PAS	R-C
		R-PAS	L-C
		R-PAS	L-C
		R-PAS	B-M
		L-PAS	L-C
		R-MIC	R-C
		B-MIC	B-C
		R-MIC	R-C
		L-PAT	L-C
		B-PAT	R-TU
		L-PAT, R-PAS	B-TU
		L-PAT	L-TU
		R-PAT	L-S
		R-PAS	B-M
		L-PAS	L-C

L = left; R = right; B = bilateral; PAS = preauricular sinus; PAT = preauricular tag; MIC = microtia; DP = other pinna malformations; C = conductive hearing loss; S = sensorineural hearing loss; M = mixed hearing loss; TU = unknown type of hearing loss (bone conduction studies not done).

Speech Production

Evaluation of the mechanisms of speech and of the production of speech was performed in detail at ages 3 and 8 years. Among the isolated cases, sufficient data were available for 77 of 95 whites and 384 of 405 blacks. Among controls, the same studies were completed for 172 of 178 whites and 189 of 192 blacks. For familial cases, 32 of 33 were so tested. Comparisons between affected and control groups are given in Table 22.

It is important to remember that the anomalies in speech considered here are only those of production of speech in the absence of hearing loss, mental retardation, and pathologic mechanisms of speech. The frequency of such anomalies in production of speech (disarticulation) in white isolated cases was significantly greater ($P < 0.05$) than that in the white controls. This was very much different in blacks, where the frequency for isolated cases was not significantly different from that in controls ($P > 0.1$). Regarding familial cases, the frequencies of abnormal articulation of speech (15%) were not significantly different from those found in the combined white/black control group ($\chi_1^2 = 0.99; P > 0.1$).

CONCLUSIONS

In the past, 2 abnormalities have been associated frequently with malformations of the external ear: conductive hearing loss associated with anomalies of the middle ear, and malformation of the urinary tract. As Jaffe [22] pointed out, however, malformations of the external ear are far more commonly associated with anomalies of the middle ear (conductive hearing loss) than with anomalies of the urinary tract. This clinical observation by Jaffe [22] has been substantiated

TABLE 22. Speech Articulation and Isolated External Ear Malformations

	Isolated cases		Normal controls
White			
Abnormal	11		10
Normal	66		162
$2 \times 2 \chi^2$		3.91*	
Black			
Abnormal	45		18
Normal	339		171
$2 \times 2 \chi^2$		0.42	
Combined			
Abnormal	56		28
Normal	405		333
$2 \times 2 \chi^2$		3.79**	

*Significant, $P < 0.05$.
**$P \approx 0.05$.

by the NCPP data, at least as it relates to dysfunctional anomalies of the urinary tract. The frequency of a hearing loss with a conductive component, among the isolated probands in the NCPP population, was about 6% while the frequency of dysfunctional anomalies of the urinary tract (dysmorphic ureters) was about 0.4%. This, however, does not minimize the importance of the latter finding.

Regarding the hearing loss, there were a number of surprising findings. First, the frequency of hearing loss in familial, presumed monogenic, cases of malformations of the external ear was *not* significantly different from that in the normal control population. The opposite was found in the isolated cases. Second, more than one-third of the isolated cases with hearing loss had a loss contralateral to the ear with the malformation, 40% of these having no hearing loss on the ipsilateral side. Third, nearly one-third of the isolated cases with hearing loss had a sensorineural component.

Another interesting finding in the NCPP population with isolated external aural malformations is the significantly increased incidence of anomalous pigmentation of the skin (nevi, café-au-lait spots, and vitiligo) and anomalies in production of speech (disarticulation). In light of these findings, along with that of the surprising frequency of sensorineural hearing loss, it is tempting to speculate that at least some of the isolated cases may represent an earlier, more basic defect in the neuroectoderm prior to or at the time of development of the neural crest. Finally, assuming that there are etiologic differences between the isolated and familial cases of malformation of the external ear, it is instructive to highlight any relationship which may exist between supposed etiology and epidemiologic, morphologic, and natural historic characteristics. As shown in Table 23, there are many interesting differences and, although the reasoning is somewhat tautologic, one is forced to concede that there is very likely an etiologic difference be-

TABLE 23. Summary: Familial vs Isolated Cases

Characteristic	Familial	Isolated
Laterality	More likely bilateral	More likely unilateral
Other major malformations (frequency)	6%	14%
Lacrimal duct stenosis (frequency)	6%	0.4%
Skin pigmentation anomalies	Frequency the same as general population	Frequency significantly greater than general population
Congenital malformations in sibs (frequency)	0.8%	2.3%
Hearing loss	Frequency the same as normal controls	Frequency significantly greater than controls
Dysarthria	Frequency the same as normal controls	Frequency significantly greater than controls

tween familial and isolated cases. Similarly, throughout, we have stressed differences between the races for a number of parameters and this may also be indicative of frequent differences in etiologic triggers for blacks and whites concerning malformation of the external ear.

REFERENCES

1. Myrianthopoulos NC, Chung CS: "Congenital Malformations in Singletons: Epidemiologic Survey." Bergsma D (ed). Miami: Symposia Specialists for The National Foundation—March of Dimes, BD:OAS X(11):1–58, 1974.
2. Niswander KR, Gordon M: "The Women and Their Pregnancies." Bethesda: National Institutes of Health, 1972.
3. Cohen MM: On the nature of syndrome delineation. Acta Genet Med Gemellol (Roma) 26:103–119, 1977.
4. Ruttin E: Zur Frage der Fistula auris congenita und der Aurikularanhänge. Wien Med Wochenschr 77:1019–1020, 1927.
5. Muckle TJ: Hereditary branchial defects in Hampshire family. Br Med J 1:1297–1299, 1961.
6. Hunter AGW: Inheritance of branchial sinuses and preauricular fistulae. Teratology 9:225–228, 1974.
7. Edmonds HW, Keeler CE: Natural "ear-ring" holes. Inherited sinuses of the ear lobes. J Hered 31:507–510, 1940.
8. Rogers BO: Microtic, lop, cup and protruding ears: Four directly inheritable deformities? Plast Reconstr Surg 41:208–231, 1968.
9. Grabb WC: The first and second branchial arch syndrome. Plast Reconstr Surg 36:485–508, 1965.
10. Melnick M, Hodes ME, Nance WE, Yune H, Sweeney A: Branchio-oto-renal dysplasia and branchio-oto-dysplasia: Two distinct autosomal dominant disorders. Clin Genet 13:425–442, 1978.
11. Sokal RR, Rohlf FJ: "Biometry." San Francisco: WH Freeman and Co, 1969, pp 86–87.
12. Poswillo D: The pathogenesis of the first and second branchial arch syndrome. Oral Surg 35:302–328, 1973.
13. Rao CR: "Advanced Statistical Methods in Biometric Research." New York: John Wiley and Sons, 1952, pp 210–214.
14. Czeizel A, Tusnady G: A family study on cleft lip with or without cleft palate and posterior cleft palate in Hungary. Hum Hered 22:405–416, 1972.
15. Melnick M: Recurrence risks for nonsyndromic external ear malformations. In Epstein CJ, Curry CJR, Packman S, Sherman S, Hall BD (eds): "Risk, Communication and Decision Making in Genetic Counseling." Alan R Liss for The National Foundation – March of Dimes, BD:OAS XV(5C):155–161, 1979.
16. Morton NE: Genetic tests under incomplete ascertainment. Am J Hum Genet 11:1–16, 1959.
17. Crow JF: Problems in ascertainment in the analysis of family data. In Neel JV, Shaw MW, Schull WJ (eds): "Epidemiology and Genetics of Chronic Diseases." Washington DC: HEW, 1965, pp 23–41.
18. Guenther WC: "Concepts of Probability." New York: McGraw-Hill, 1968, pp 355–360.
19. Rohlf FJ, Sokal RR: "Statistical Tables." San Francisco: WH Freeman and Co, 1969, pp 152–156.

20. Myrianthopoulos NC, French KS: An application of the U.S. Bureau of the Census socioeconomic index to a large, diversified patient population. Soc Sci Med 2:283–299, 1968.
21. Harada O, Ishii H: The condition of the auditory ossicles in microtia. Plast Reconstr Surg 50:48–53, 1972.
22. Jaffe BF: Pinna anomalies associated with congenital conductive hearing loss. Pediatrics 57:332–341, 1976.
23. Hanson JW, Myrianthopoulos NC, Harvey MAS, Smith DW: Risks to the offspring of women treated with hydantoin anticonvulsant, with emphasis on the fetal hydantoin syndrome. J Pediatr 89:662–668, 1976.
24. Broman SH, Nicholas PL, Kennedy WA: "Preschool IQ. Prenatal and Early Developmental Correlates." Hillsdale, NJ: Lawrence Erlbaum Associates, 1975.

Intervention in Mild-to-Moderate Conductive and Sensorineural Hearing Losses

Charles I. Berlin, PhD

There are a few definitive published studies which deal with the effects of conductive hearing loss on the speech and language communication of children. In my own professional development, using normative data on perception of speech, I found it difficult to believe that hearing losses on the order of 15–30 dB could materially affect communication and, therefore, doubted the value of early intervention. Evidence is mounting that mine was an overly conservative opinion and deserves reevaluation. The research of Webster and Webster [1], Clopton and Silverman [2, 3], and many others suggested that conductive hearing loss, auditory deprivation, or both, lead to an underdevelopment of central auditory structures in the brainstem. To date, we still do not know the behavioral consequences of such deprivation in humans. I will only touch here on some of the literature on conductive hearing loss and its presumed effects on humans, and describe a technique we have developed which may measure these effects physiologically in vivo.

THEORETIC ISSUES

Children who have chronic otitis media generally suffer from malaise and chronic absence from school, as well as fluctuating conductive hearing loss. It is difficult to separate the effects of the first two variables from the effects of the hearing loss alone. Needleman and Menyuk [4] have recently shown that children having otitis media between birth and 18 months, whose episodes have continued for 2 years thereafter, are significantly retarded in articulation of isolated words, articulation of connected speech, and reproduction of word-endings that have to do with tense and case (ie go[es], John['s], cat['s], etc). Recently, we predicted such a finding by computer simulation [5]. We generated, by computer, signals of speech and subjected them to a 20 dB attenuation and correction for human hearing sensitivity, and then examined the resultant oscillographic tracings. This examination showed a loss of faint morphologic markers, such as plural endings and fricatives in a final position. We concluded that a child with a conductive hearing loss in both ears might be subject to the following reduction in information from the acoustic signal: 1) morphologic markers might be lost or sporadically misunderstood; 2) in a related fashion, very short words or segments which are spoken quickly in connected speech will lose considerable loudness because of the critical relationship between intensity, duration, and loudness; and 3) inflections or markers carrying subtle nuances such as questioning and related intonational contouring can, at the very best, be expected to come through inconsistently.

There is less than overwhelming evidence that conductive hearing loss actually causes such misperceptions or has any long-term effect on behavior; what we have demonstrated was that conductive hearing losses could cause misperceptions under certain conditions. In order to determine whether intervention is either necessary or possible, and when and if to introduce the intervention, we need answers to questions such as the following:

a) Are there any distinct aspects of language or development of speech or of both which can be earmarked as arising from mild deprivation?

b) What other variables (such as parental attention or solicitousness, intelligence, socioeconomic class, and so on) are related to chronic, untreated aural problems which may contribute to development of language?

c) Do other diseases, or malaise in general, have similar effects on development of language in the presence of chronic otitis or other fluctuating hearing losses?

d) How long must we wait before it is too late to intervene appropriately in a child's development of speech and language? (Adapted from Menyuk [6].)

Unfortunately, there are no definitive answers to these questions, yet.

How Early Do Speech and Language Develop?

In recent years, it has become almost axiomatic that awareness of speech and neural organization for perception begin virtually at birth. There is, of course, the ubiquitous evidence that the brain is morphologically asymmetric, even in the fetus. This asymmetry, along with behavioral orientation and responsiveness of young infants to speech sounds is taken as evidence for a predisposition of the human infant towards the processing of human speech material. Does congenital deafness affect this morphologic asymmetry and the ability of the nervous system to process speech material? Unfortunately, there are few documented brains and brainstems of congenitally deaf people available and none, to my knowledge, study the asymmetry of the temporal lobe. Many temporal bones, and far fewer brains and brainstems, are available from deaf patients but, in the presence of peripheral deafness, it is impossible to study central organization for perception of speech.

Therefore, until or unless some form of by-passing stimulation becomes available, we have no way of assessing the effect of "intervention" on patients with total peripheral sensorineural loss. For the rest of this discussion, then, we can speak effectively of only 2 types of patients: patients with conductive loss, or those with incomplete sensorineural losses.

Effects in Conductive Loss

Kokko [7] and Bluestone et al [8] have both reported audiometric data from ears subsequently proven to have effusions at surgery. Kokko's series of 161 ears had a mean air-conduction pure-tone average (at 500, 1,000, and 2,000 Hz) of 27.6 dB, with a standard deviation of 12.8 dB. The mean air/bone gap was 24.6 dB. Bluestone et al report similar results: mean pure-tone average for 58 ears was 26.0 dB, with a standard deviation of 9.9 dB. The composite audiogram from Kokko's data is shown in Figure 1. The loss is predominantly flat, although there is a definite peak in threshold sensitivity at 2,000 Hz. This may represent a crossover point between separate mass and stiffness components of the loss.

To predict the effect a loss such as this will have on perception of speech, we can turn to available data on powers of speech. Fletcher [9] has presented, in graphic form, the typical frequencies and relative amplitudes for the common sounds of speech in English. If we plot these on a graph of intensity (SPL) versus

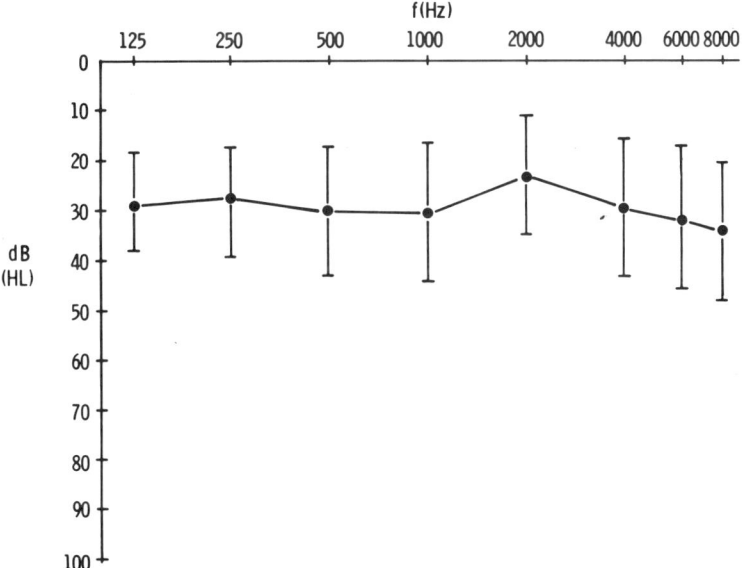

Fig. 1. Average hearing loss of 161 ears with conductive losses due to middle ear effusion. (Adapted from Kokko [7].)

frequency, assuming the vowels will have an average intensity of 65–70 dB SPL (sound pressure level), and then plot on the same graph the composite audiogram for Kokko's patients with middle ear effusions (after conversion from HL to SPL), we can see the areas of expected interference (Fig. 2). Note, however, that no corrections for loudness versus duration are available from those data. If only 6 dB of "loudness shift" is introduced, the projected effects can be quite serious.

It appears that the upper and lower ends of the spectrum of speech are most vulnerable, with the formant peaks in the middle regions (500–3,000 Hz) being 5–15 dB above the line representing the mean loss plus 1 SD. However, some patients (about 1/6) will have losses greater than this, and should have severe problems in communication. Further, this graph assumes an average speech-power of 65–70 dB. This refers primarily to the vowels; the consonantal energy will often be considerably less. Furthermore, in actual situations in school, poor signal-to-noise ratios may abound. The actual degree of interference with speech experienced by children with effusions of the middle ear in relevant environments is, so far as we know, a matter of conjecture. However, one would predict, based on the comparison made above, that at least a significant proportion of these children are unable to hear many sounds of speech in normal listening situations.

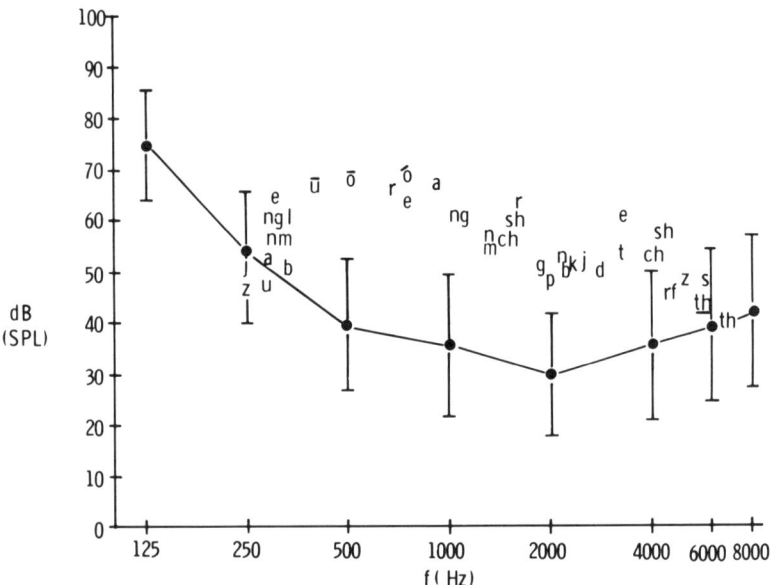

Fig. 2. Hearing loss from Kokko data [7] superimposed upon average spectral peak positions of speech sounds [9].

Intervention in Hearing Losses / 337

Mini-Experiment I From Dobie and Berlin [5]

Since we could find nothing in the literature actually predicting what sort of difficulties children with otitis might have in perception of speech, we decided to simulate a few seconds of speech from a standardized test of auditory comprehension. 1) A 10-second recording was made from the Durrell Reading Analysis test at the lowest grade level. The test is as follows:

   a) Muff is a little yellow kitten.
   b) She drinks milk.
   c) She sleeps on a chair.
   d) She does not like to get wet.
   e) What color was the kitten?
   f) What does she drink?
   g) Where does she sleep?
   h) Why doesn't Muff like to go out on rainy days?

2) This utterance was recorded through "correcting filters" which shaped the signal as if it were processed through an ear at about the 40-phon level (a scale correction). 3) The selection was digitized in our Interdata 8/32 computer and displayed oscillographically. 4) It was then attenuated by 20 dB and displayed again underneath the unattenuated oscillographs. The oscillographs were then read independently by a number of readers to segment, mark, and locate, as best we could, the onsets of the various phonetic utterances.

Inspection of this synthesis of a 20 dB hearing loss reveals the following. A potential loss of transitional information, especially plural endings and related fricatives in final positions, was highly likely. Vocalic information appeared to be preserved, as was temporal information (syllable length); however, very brief utterances or information at high frequencies could be either distorted or degraded if signal-to-noise conditions were less than satisfactory. Thus, as we noted earlier, the child with otitis media might be subject to the following reductions in information from the acoustic signal. 1) Morphologic markers might be lost or sporadically misunderstood. For example, "Where are Jack's gloves to be placed?" might be perceived as "Where Jack glove be place?" 2) In a related fashion, very short words which are elided often in connected speech (see *"are"* and *"to"* above) will lose considerable loudness because of the critical relationship between intensity, duration, and loudness. 3) Inflections or markers carrying subtle nuances such as questioning and related intonational contouring can, at the very best, be expected to come through inconsistently.

A three-dimensional plot of part of the tested utterance reveals one surprising feature: the acoustic input can be quite inconsistent despite a rather fixed hearing loss. Note that the components in the three-dimensional plot have such variability that a 20 dB loss relative to an arbitrary signal-to-noise level may not always obliterate a given segment of information. Thus, markers for the beginning and ending of words and ideas may be inconsistently noted.

Assessing Physiologic Effects of Conductive Hearing Loss

Since there is some evidence that conductive hearing loss does affect brainstem nuclei, especially at the level of binaural interaction, we have developed a technique for assessing neural interaction at the presumed level of underdevelopment [10]. A system for measuring the response evoked from the brainstem (BSER) is used with a number of salient modifications: 1) The electrodes, for example, are put in the midline with a hot electrode on the vertex, the ground electrode at the nasion, and the referent electrode at the nuchal region at the base of the skull. 2) Click-evoked BSERs are obtained first from the left ear alone, then the right ear alone. 3) The digitized results from left and right ears are added to each other by computer. 4) This resultant sum of the left and right ears is stored in the computer for later use. 5) A brainstem-evoked response to binaural stimulation is acquired, and this result is subtracted from the previously stored sum of the 2 ears. 6) A resultant "difference potential" is obtained in normal subjects, indicating a depolarization of binaurally stimulated neural elements. To date, our experiments show this binaural interaction is ubiquitous in guinea pigs as well as normal human subjects. Results also show that by systematically varying time-of-arrival of the clicks, or relative intensity of the clicks, we still show binaural interaction within certain limits of stimulation.

Armed with this technique for potentially identifying subjects with underdeveloped brainstem nuclei, we hope to study children with chronic conductive hearing losses, adults with long-standing conductive losses surgically cured, children with atresias who may have temporary remission of their hearing loss and, of course, children with the diagnosis of "auditory-perceptual disabilities" (APDs) for the presence or absence of this potential for binaural interaction. Incidentally, this "difference potential" is observed also in the so-called "middle components" and may lend itself to studies of the functional organization of the binaural lateralization system in humans. It is too early to tell whether there are always behavioral consequences of deprivation, true linguistic consequences, or other communicative interference of fluctuating conductive loss. However, if we can "label the children" who show the effects of maldevelopment of the brainstem, we can then look for more and closer relationships between the presence of such deficiencies and possible development of behavioral aberrations.

The Efficacy of Intervention, Even in Adulthood, in a Unique Form of Sensorineural Loss

The most common forms of sensorineural loss are those in which high-frequency sensitivity is poorer than low-frequency sensitivity. The literature abounds with routines for management and intervention for such patients. However, some years ago, we uncovered a unique form of hearing loss among the so-called "deaf" in which hearing through the frequencies for speech was severely impaired, but considerable residual hearing (in fact, almost normal hearing) was remaining in areas above the traditional audiogram [11]. The remainder of this discussion will outline how we discovered such a hearing loss, and the effect of an unusual type of "translation hearing aid" on the communicational skills of the only 2 people in the world who now have this type of aid.

The first patient came to our attention a number of years ago and had been diagnosed as having an "hysterical hearing loss." Superficially, the diagnosis was reasonable, based on the following observations: 1) She produced a voluntary audiogram between 91 and 116 dB sound pressure level (SPL) in the frequencies for speech, yet detected speech unaided at about 50 to 60 dB overall SPL. She did not hear as well under earphones. 2) She was unable to use the telephone despite her ability to detect speech at relatively low intensities. 3) She found conventional hearing aids unacceptable. 4) She had a remarkably precise articulation rate and prosody, even though she had the hypernasality and poor control of pitch characteristic of a "deaf" voice. She had been treated elsewhere for 10 years with outpatient psychiatric and psychologic care before being evaluated by tympanometry, reflexes, and electrocochleography at the Kresge Hearing Research Laboratory of the South. These revealed a peripheral physiologic loss but also indicated the possibility of nearly normal hearing in the extremely high frequencies. This was later confirmed by voluntary audiometry using a specially developed high-frequency audiometric system, and this explained her difficulty in hearing speech through traditionally limited transducers.

A special 2-channel translation hearing aid was built (by Henry Halperin, M.D., John K. Cullen, Jr., Ph.D., and the staff of the Kresge Hearing Research Laboratory). One channel modulates a very high-frequency carrier, producing essentially the sum of low-frequency signals for speech plus the high-frequency carrier [12]. The other channel is unmodulated straight through amplification to a unique hearing aid/transducer that is sensitive out to 20 kHz (Knowles BP-1712). Both patients report unusual changes in their own speech after the use of the aid, and changes in their awareness of sound around them. With the permission of one of the subjects, who lost her hearing at age 4, I would like to quote from portions of her diary which reflect on the successful attempt we appear to have made on late intervention in this unusual form of sensorineural loss. Since she is post-lingually deaf, the patient is able to describe her experiences eloquently and give us insight as to what it is like to experience this unusual form of intervention.

> July 1, I was fitted with the translating hearing aid and the sounds seemed to come at me all at once. Voices sounded like 'jabberwocky' because they sounded so different. I opened a door and let it slam. I expected the slam would be loud, as it would have been with other hearing aids, but it wasn't — a surprise! My husband and I took a walk down Bourbon Street and I listened to the sounds of the lively New Orleans jazz band. The music was really jumping, it was loud, but not blaring. The rush of traffic made

me a little jumpy but not disconcertingly so. When we returned to the hotel, Ron practices some sentences on me and I was surprised that I could pick up fragments of what he said without watching him. Possibly for the first time in my adult life, I could hear his voice, while the water was running in the bathroom. I wore my hearing aid later in the evening as we walked around the French Quarter and I could hear the tap of my shoes against the pavement — it sounded just like that, a tap! A sharp clopping of the horse-drawn carriages on the street sounded the same. I am at a loss for descriptive adjectives for these sounds because I have never heard quite this way.

Back in New York City, Ron and I walked over to the Plaza Hotel for dessert and coffee at the Palm Court. The music at the Palm Court left me 'thunderstruck' as the violins began to play. I felt the richness of the music would lift me from my chair. What incredibly lovely haunting sounds the violins were making! My husband was struck by the radiance in my face which, for me, was associated not only with the total absorption of the music but also in some way with the hearing aid. For two hours I sat totally mesmerized by the music. It was a lovely experience — a very lovely thing. Altogether, this was a very heady and fulfilling day with my new hearing aid.

Tonight something surprising occurred. The television was turned on. Usually the sound precedes the picture and I miss the prologue to the news because the anchor man isn't on yet. Tonight I heard, 'Good evening, CBS news.' I thought I was kidding myself. I hurried to Ron. Did he just say 'Good evening, CBS news?' and Ron said 'yes.' A small victory to be savored — I've never been able to catch that before!

[One month after the hearing aid has been used.] I am becoming sensitive to environmental sounds. I am listening to the tap, tapping of my shoes against the pavement. Without the hearing aid it sounds as if I am just scraping the surface. I listen to the voices of children playing outside underneath my bedroom window. They are happy voices — high laughing voices — they begin to sing. Their mouths move like sleepy fish. It was difficult to understand at first but their voices were so sweet. It was sad that I had never heard those children before. I am even able to understand more and more on the telephone.

[This woman owns and rides a horse named Tozha. She talks about an experience she had with him.]

It is my habit after a ride to brush Tozha down and treat him to a bag of carrots. How he loves his carrots! I listened to him as he crunched on his treat and for me the clarity of this sound was one of the most arresting I could ever hope to hear. After dinner, I listened to 'Exodus' on the stereo. I did not realize how the change in sounds would betray my exceptional sensitivity to the music. So stirring was the music that I began to cry, tears that almost degenerated into hysteria. The beauty of the sounds I was hearing was almost torture — I simply could not get enough of it. I had rarely experienced the swells, changes in color and character of music that was now developing into an elaborate network of sound for me. I must have played these records for hours and the last thing I remember was listening to 'And the Angels Sing' before I fell asleep.

It's three weeks since I have had the hearing aid. Vocal sounds are so many and varied. Howls, growls, chucklings, crying, roaring, screams, slurping, burping, kissing, laughing. While I heard these sounds before, years ago, I hear them now with finer distinctions so that the emotions accompanied with such sounds become more and more meaningful. Unfortunately, I am encountering [occasional failure] of the translator and it's playing hell with my ability to pay attention to unrecognizable noises . . . there is some intolerable buzz from the telephone attachment while talking to Mama on the phone. The translator occasionally seems to disappear only to emerge with lower intensity. Persistent light tapping on the aid will generally bring it on again but this is worrisome since it is creating an erosion of my desire to wear the aid even though I do love it. *I wish this thing would work consistently.*

There was in fact a "cold solder joint" in the translator circuit which has since been repaired. Note, however, her dependence on the aid and her sensitivity to the translator portion of the device. She continues to keep her journal and, essentially, reveals that she is now virtually completely competent over the telephone. She is able to take directions, proper names, spelling letters, and telephone numbers and addresses over the telephone from her mother as well as from me. Reinspection of her audiogram reveals that no such intelligibility is possible unaided, and with ordinary hearing aids she is essentially "masked out" in the high-frequency regions she uses to hear.

One of our patients with this type of loss has evidence of a genetic etiology. Causative factors are unclear in the other.

The Absence of Recordable BSER to Supra-Threshold Signals

We studied the latter patient's BSER to 60 dB SL 13 kHz signals, and were surprised to find no measurable synchronous discharge. Despite excellent electrodal impedance, checking all triggers, asking the patient to describe the signal (it was quite loud to her), and repeating all measures 4 times, we still were unable to elicit a synchronous BSER discharge although we obtained a small AP-like discharge at the beginning of the analysis. Does this mean the BSER she generates has very few synchronously discharging units? Does she have enough functioning units in the brainstem to respond to the signals with great enough magnitude for our technique? Has she suffered some maldevelopment of the brainstem? Do normal people show a BSER to 13 kHz signals or are there too few synchronously discharging neurons in all of us to generate the waveform?

It is too early to tell the answers to these, but the questions themselves are provocative. We have briefly touched on the putative effects of deprivation after conductive loss and how we might measure these effects despite normal audiograms. We have also discussed an unusual form of sensorineural loss which, despite residual audiometric hearing and good results with a translating aid, shows little central physiologic response to sound. Have such patients suffered too much deprivation already to synchronously discharge many central units?

REFERENCES

1. Webster DB, Webster M: Neonatal sound deprivation affects brainstem auditory nuclei. Arch Otolaryngol 103:392–396, 1977.
2. Silverman MS, Clopton BM: Plasticity of binaural interaction. I. Effect of early deprivation. J Neurophysiol 40:1266–1274, 1977.
3. Clopton BM, Silverman MS: Plasticity of binaural interaction. II. Critical period and changes in midline response. J Neurophysiol 40:1275–1280, 1977.
4. Needleman H, Menyuk P: Effects of hearing loss from recurrent otitis media and speech and language development. In Jaffe B (ed): "Hearing Loss in Children." Baltimore: University Park Press, 1977, pp 642–649.
5. Dobie RA, Berlin CI: Influence of otitis media on hearing and development. Ann Otol Rhinol Laryngol 88 (Suppl 60):48–53, 1979.
6. Menyuk P: Design factors in the assessment of language development in children with otitis media. Ibid.
7. Kokko E: Chronic secretory otitis media in children. A clinical study. Acta Otolaryngol (Stockh) 327(Suppl):1–44, 1974.
8. Bluestone CD, Beery QC, Paradise JL: Audiometry and tympanometry in relation to middle ear effusions in children. Laryngoscope 83:594–604, 1973.
9. Fletcher H: "Speech and Hearing in Communication." Princeton, NJ: Van Nostrand, 1953.
10. Dobie RA, Berlin CI: Binaural interaction in brainstem evoked responses. Arch Otolaryngol 105:391–396, 1979.
11. Berlin CI, Wexler KF, Jerger JF, Halperin HR, Smith S: Superior ultraaudiometric hearing: A new type of hearing loss which correlates highly with unusually good speech in the "profoundly deaf." Otorhinolaryngology 86:111–116, 1978.
12. Halperin HR, Cullen JK Jr, Berlin CI, Killion MC: Translating hearing aid for "deaf" patients with nearly normal ultra-audiometric hearing. Paper presented at the 94th Meeting of the Acoustical Society of America, December 13, 1977, Miami, Florida.

DISCUSSION

Dr. Harold Schuknecht: There's not a temporal bone in existence that has been studied for the basin-shaped pattern, which as you know is a relatively common type of congenital hearing loss, bilaterally symmetric usually. I've looked and I've been waiting to get one, but we don't have any. One would assume that the sensorineural deafnesses would correspond fairly well to your threshold pattern, so there should be good neuronal and hair cell population in the basal turn up to the 8 kHz area. But what was the discrimination score?

Dr. Charles Berlin: Zero. These people have no discrimination without this hearing aid. With the hearing aid, they have extremely good discrimination.

Dr. Harold Schuknecht: The milder basin-shaped type audio patients show excellent discrimination.

Dr. Charles Berlin: Remarkably good discrimination. I might add that I cannot get any physiologic synchrony from a patient like that, doing extratympanic cochleograms with BSER, even at 60 or 70 dB sensation level; I can't measure synchronous neural discharge.

Dr. Heinrich Spoendlin: You said you have no electrocochleographic response.

Dr. Charles Berlin: Extratympanically.

Dr. Heinrich Spoendlin: But not even when you place it with these high frequencies?

Dr. Charles Berlin: Let me review the situation. I did get an extratympanic 12 kHz response. But it is so artifact-fraught that I couldn't call it a true response. You can appreciate this.

Dr. Heinrich Spoendlin: Theoretically, you shouldn't get a response. And how is the intensity difference limen in the area, let's say of about 10,000? Because in normal hearing the intensity is very important.

Dr. Charles Berlin: There was a 2 dB difference limen on these patients. This patient has no apical turns, no other hair cells, and therefore she's released from a lot of interference. But this patient has an exceptional difference limen.

Dr. Heinrich Spoendlin: I'm not so sure whether we can think that this patient has only the hook, or in low spots in the basal turn level, because if she has such a good discrimination score, she must have quite a considerable neuronal population there. It appears more likely that a whole frequency range has shifted, maybe from injury to the cochlea.

Dr. Charles Berlin: The middle ear is quite normal. We can elicit reflexes in this patient, so we don't see any evidence of resonal shift.

Dr. Ruediger Thalmann: I don't understand how she speaks at all with that high-pitched voice, before you translate it.

Dr. Charles Berlin: Well, she obviously didn't read the books. Remember, the second lady who's doing so well with the hearing aid was adventitiously deaf, she had 4 years of normal hearing, so she had more than enough time to learn. Her speech does not sound normal, she has a strange high voice. Incidentally, when they put the hearing aid on, the voice drops. Her speech stays a little clipped.

Dr. LaVonne Bergstrom: You have one adventitiously deaf and some congenitally deaf individuals who have high-pitched, precise speech, who have zero discrimination in the ordinary speech range. It is interesting because after the loss is restored, their voices go down.

Dr. Charles Berlin: I think they've had progressive loss. In "discrimination scores," you have noncontextual clues. When you test these people and use contextual clues, discrimination is much better than zero because they have cues from prosody and from the linguistic code, and they do quite well inferring or inducing what's been said, if they have other kinds of cues, synthetic cues.

Dr. LaVonne Bergstrom: But the input then, that a young child gets — the only contextual kinds of things he has until he acquires verbal language are things he sees, actions going on around him, smiles and such — nonverbal cues. He still has to acquire things that go into verbal context. I think you're right, the hearing must be better earlier, because people don't speak in that range.

Dr. Charles Berlin: Dr. Schuknecht says that all his patients have exceptionally good discrimination. Maybe it started out this way, then their hearing went down and they had some sort of loss. Also, when these patients have colds or allergies which introduce a mass effect into the middle ear, they call and tell me the hearing aid is broken because they've lost hearing.

Dr. Robert Ruben: You show dishpan and U-shaped audiograms. Have you asked the question of what they are actually perceiving below, say, 2 kHz or whether they can identify a tone, and what's the difference limen in use of frequency.

Dr. Charles Berlin: We've done low-frequency and high-frequency psychophysics on only one of the two good patients, so far: I can tell you the one who's doing so well on the hearing aid has a better difference limen for intensity frequency and a narrower masking function at 13K than she has at 4K, and at 2K she can't do anything in psychophysics. She's a marvelous example of what causes periodicity pitch and she has 100 cycles periodicity pitch, by modulating the 13K tone 100 times a second. That's a theoretic issue, as to where pitch arrives on the basilar membrane.

Dr. Robert Ruben: So at least with this sample of one, they are not really perceiving the same type of auditory input below 2 kHz; what we may be looking at then is that they are really perceiving the harmonics or the subharmonics in this case.

Dr. Charles Berlin: That's possible. There's certainly an enormous amount of spectral energy of speech well above 3,000 Hz. We were taught that the speech frequencies are 300 to 3,000, but that isn't so. Analysis of the speech code says that the vowels and some of the consonants have their peak discriminants between 300 and 3,000, not their peak energy, and I could show you slides that show 40 dB more energy at 9,000 cycles than at 1,000 cycles for the final "s" in a word like bus.

Dr. Heinrich Spoendlin: What is the outer frequency limit at which these patients could hear? Is it higher than normal? And what is the highest mark on the audiogram?

Dr. Charles Berlin: We were able to study out to 20,000 cycles, and then these patients begin to drop off. The highest mark on the audiogram is 14,000.

Dr. Heinrich Spoendlin: What is the dynamic range in this part? In normal ears, one would have almost no dynamic range here.

Dr. Charles Berlin: For the transducers we use, the dynamic range is about 75 dB. I stopped plotting the audiogram because the zero hearing level for normal started to drop, and it would have looked as if hearing was getting better. The technique of doing high-frequency audiometry is very frustrating. We're talking about additional spectral content to speech that for most of us is unintelligible.

Dr. David Smith: And this precludes what they can hear in the environment?

Dr. Charles Berlin: Yes. These patients used to complain that when you turn TV on, they would hear the rasper of the TV, the 15,000 cycles; their parents wondered what they complained about. Also, they would hear the ultrasonic alarms in department stores, where they have ultrasonic and scanning alarms around 16 to 18 kHz. Patients would say they had a ringing in their ears and given the deaf audiogram they were not believed.

Concluding Remarks of Chairmen Ruben, Schuknecht, and Gorlin

Dr. Robert Ruben: Two and a half days ago we began this meeting with a discussion of the symbiotic relationship between pursuing knowledge for its own sake and the constraints for those in clinical medicine to effect prevention, cure, and care. During the last 72 hours we have seen this operative. There are very real deficits in our basic science. This was evident from lack of discussion of the molecular biology of hearing, for example. This pertains to what Dr. Deol has done with mutant mice and ultimately to what Drs. Schuknecht, Nadol, and Bergstrom have shown clinically. This is an area in which we have to increase our effort. The most effective thing we could do for intervention would be to attract more individuals who can begin to pursue some of the many avenues for advancements which even this short conference has revealed. Science should be carried out for science's sake. Those of us who have the privilege of working in clinical medicine must be able to understand, utilize, and effect the advances made by our basic-science colleagues.
up with.

Dr. Harold Schuknecht: I have been very interested and excited during this meeting, seeing all of the work that is going on in a number of areas. Obviously, it has to continue, especially that work concerning embryology and pathology. But we need more temporal bones. We need gathering of good data from population studies, and from individual cases. We need to correlate the human morphologic changes with those seen in animals, and I would hope that genetic counseling would become a more effective means of preventing some of these problems in the future. Surgically, we have a long way to go. It is the most difficult of all types of surgery — it is more difficult than tumor surgery, the results are generally mediocre, and, unless performed by an experienced surgeon, the procedures almost always fail. Thus, I would make a plea that surgery for congenital anomalies of the external and middle ear be performed only by very experienced surgeons and those who have the probability of seeing more than one or two cases during their professional careers. At the moment, this is not well understood by otologists and I think that in many cases harm is being done. I believe that the other clinicians will agree with me in that respect.

Dr. Robert Gorlin: On behalf of both The National Foundation and myself, I want to thank all of you for coming here, spending the time, sharing your knowledge with us, and, we hope, ultimately with the world. I suppose it is because people aren't perfect that we have these meetings, and maybe for not being perfect we're each a little better. I suppose that maybe Mariana says it best in *Measure for Measure*: "Some say best men are molded out of faults, and for the most, become much more the better, for being a little bad."

Index

Acetylcholine, 100
Adenylate cyclase, 85, 92, 95, 97
Afferent transmitters, 107–8
Aging, 121–22, 136
Alport syndrome, 48–50
Aminoglycoside antibiotics, 93–94
Amniotes, 154
Amphibia, 148, 154
Aneuploidy, 55–57
Animal models, 111–38, 273
Antibiotics, 93–94
Architecture, ear, 289–97
Aspirin, 241
ATP, 86, 87, 89, 91, 95, 97, 98, 101
Auditory deprivation, 271–88, 333
    333–45; see also Deafness
Auditory transduction, 83–85
Auricles, 299–302
Autism, 146

Bing-Siebenmann anomaly, 76, 81
Birth defects, 202–30
Bone dysplasia, 183–97
Bony labyrinth, 47, 260; see also
    Labyrinth; Mondini dysplasia
Branchial arch, 202

Caloric test, 136, 143–44
Carbonic anhydrase, 129
Central nervous system, 2, 3, 145,
    287
Cerebrospinal fluid, 93
Chorioallantoic grafts, 168–70
Chromosomal abnormalities, 55–
    57, 201–2, 220
Clefting, 297, 315, 324, 326

Cochlea, 245, 252, 254, 255
  anomalies, 73, 76, 78
  and aspirin, 241
  development of, 240
  nuclei of, 138, 145, 217, 273–
    75, 278, 283–84
Cochlear duct, 83–101, 121, 124–
    25
Cochlear microphonic, 83, 94, 97–
    98
Cochleosaccular degeneration, 124
Cochleosaccular dysgenesis, 55, 127;
    see also Scheibe dysplasia
Conductive hearing loss, 138, 217,
    227, 233–35, 326, 328
  genetic syndromes in, 182–202,
    207–9
  mild, 333–38
  nonprogressive, 199–202
  progressive 183–98
Congenital hearing loss, 2, 3, 75,
    217–19, 234
Connective tissue abnormalities,
    198, 199
Craniofacial defects, 218–19, 223
Crista, 247, 249, 250, 251, 253
Crouzon syndrome, 200–201
Cryptotia, 291, 297
Crystal deficiency, 131
Cupulolithiasis, 121, 124
Cyclic AMP, 98
Cyclic GMP, 98–100

Dancer gene, 247–49
Deafness
  causes of, 1–3

350 / Index

and central nervous system, 2–3
cure of, 1
development of, 2
profound prelingual, 263–69
see also Auditory deprivation;
Conductive hearing loss;
Congenital hearing loss;
Sensorineural hearing loss
Digit malformation, 223
Disease, 211–23
Diuretics, 95
Down syndrome, 292
Dreher gene, 247, 259–60
Drugs,
and otoconia, 126
ototoxic, 93–95, 122–24
see also Teratogens
Dysplasia, 48, 61–71, 183–97

Ear form, 299–302
Ear muscles, 299–302
Electronystagmogram, 143
Embryonic induction, 172–74
Endolymph, 116–17, 119, 121, 125
Endolymphatic duct and sac, 246, 247, 250–52, 259
experiments on, 17–19, 40–41
variations in, 47
and vestibular anomalies, 73
Endolymphatic potential, 83–85, 89, 91–92, 95–96, 101
Energy reserve, 87, 101
Environment, 126–27, 319–23
Enzyme deficiency, 181
Epithelio-mesenchymal interactions, 29–31, 42
Ethacrynic acid, 95, 97, 101, 122
Explantation procedures, 167
External ear, 299–302
evolution of, 148–53
malformations, and relation to other abnormalities, 303–30
morphogenesis of, 147–76

see also Microtia; Microtia/atresia
Extirpation procedures, 166–67
Eyelid ptosis, 301, 302

Fate-mapping, 20–27
Fetal alcohol syndrome, 291, 302
Fetal hydantoin syndrome, 302
Fidget gene, 249, 260
Fish, 150
Friedreich ataxia, 81–82
Furosemid, 95

γ-Aminobutyric acid, 100
Genetics and
conductive hearing loss, 182–202, 207–9
congenital hearing loss, 217–19, 240
external ear, 171–72, 315–19
inner ear malformation, 243–57, 259–61
middle ear, 171–72, 181, 212
otoconia malformation, 127–35
profound prelingual deafness, 263 263–69
Glutamate, 107–8
Gravity receptors. See Otoconia

Head and neck examination, 221–23, 224, 227
Hearing test, 224–25, 325–26
Histidinemia gene, 250–51, 256, 257
Hurler syndrome, 198–99, 208–9
Hydrops, 125
Hypopigmentation gene, 254–56; see also Pigmentation
Hypothyroidism, 243, 255–57

Infection, 124, 126–27
Inner ear
abnormalities, 303–30
anomalies, 73–82
biochemistry of, 83–101
damage, 93–100

dysmorphogenesis, 47–71
dysplasia, 48; *see also* specific syndromes
malformation, 243–57, 259–61
ontogenic aspects of development of, 5–42
and toxic drugs, 93–95
Intelligence, 324–25
Intervention, 333–45
Ischemia, 87, 89–91, 101

Kidney, 94, 97, 221, 223
Kinky gene, 252
Klippel-Feil syndrome, 53
Kreisler gene, 243–45, 259

Labyrinth, 75–81, 251; *see also* Bony labyrinth; Membranous labyrinth
Language, 271, 272, 286, 333–45; *see also* Speech
Lateral duct, 249, 253
L-azetidine-2-carboxylic acid, 36–40
Limb malformations, 223
Lop-ears, 289–91, 299–300
Low-set ears, 291

Macula, 145, 245, 250, 251
Malformations. *See* Birth defects; specific malformations
Mammals
 inner ear of, 5–42
 middle ear of, 148, 153, 158
Manganese, 127–29, 133, 144, 145, 254; *see also* Trace elements
Membrane rupture, 125
Membranous labyrinth, 47–48, 260; *see also* Labyrinth; Mondini dysplasia
Mesenchyme
 condensation of, 251

 ventral, 35–36
 whole, 31–35
 see also Epithelio-mesenchymal interactions
Mesoderm, 200
Michel anomaly, 76, 81
Microtia, 289–97
Microtia/atresia, 221, 224, 289
Middle ear
 abnormalities, 303–30
 anatomy of, 154–60
 anomalies, 211–16
 evolution of, 148–52
 malformations, 181, 217–35, 240–41
 morphogenesis of, 147–76
 muscles in, 239–40
 pathoembryology of, 181–204
Mondini-Alexander anomaly, 76, 81
Mondini dysplasia, 61, 67–71
Mouse
 inner ear malformations, 243–56, 259
 tilted-head, 130
Mucopolysaccharidoses, 198–99
Mutant genes, 243–57, 259–61
Mutant phenotypes, 171–72

Neomycin, 94, 122, 124
Nerves, middle ear, 211
Neural crest, 160–66, 171, 175, 209, 329
Neural induction, 27–29, 42
Neural tube, 244–47, 249–51
Neurophysiology, hearing, 271–88
Neurotransmission, 100
Neurotrophic interactions, 6–16, 60–61
Nijmegen waltzer gene, 252–53
Noise damage, 97–100

Ontogeny, inner ear, 5–42
Organ of Corti, 83–101, 107, 247,

250–52, 254–56, 259–60
Organ systems, 303–30
Ossicle, 202–3, 211, 218, 224–25, 227, 239
Otic labyrinth, 251; see also Labyrinth
Otic vesicle, 244–46
Otitis media, 124, 227, 271, 333, 337
Otoconia
  absence of, 144
  and aging, 121–22
  and central nervous system, 145
  and cochleosaccular dysgenesis, 127
  and drugs, 122–24, 126
  and environmental factors, 126–27
  fate of, 119–21
  genetic factors, 127–35
  and hydrops, 125
  and infection, 124, 126–27
  loss of, 121
  and macula, 145
  and membrane rupture, 125
  malformation, 111, 236–38
  and mechanical trauma, 125
  morphogenesis of, 111, 116–19, 138
  morphology, 112–16
  and pallid agenesis, 127–30
  and sensory degeneration, 124–25
  terminology about, 112
  and trace elements, 126
  and vascular insufficiency, 125
  and weightlessness, 127
Otoliths, 254
Ototoxic drugs, 93–95, 122–24

Pallid agenesis, 127–35
Pallid gene, 254, 260
P-creatine, 85, 86, 97
Perilymph, 93, 100, 107–8, 125
Phospholipids, 94

Pigmentation, 127–30, 144, 145, 254–56, 329
Pinna, 223, 224, 291, 292
Polyphosphoinositides, 94
Polytomography, 224–27; see also Tomography
Protruding ears, 299–302
Ptosis, eyelid, 301, 302

Racial differences and
  ear malformation, 313–15, 318, 325, 328, 330
  microtia, 292, 297
Railroad track ears, 291
Regional defects, 200
Reptiles, 148, 153
Retina, 98, 99
Retinitis pigmentosa, 51–54
Rotating gene, 253
Rubella, 57–61, 221

Saccule, 245, 250–52, 254–55;
Scheibe anomaly, 61–67, 76, 81;
  see also Cochleosaccular dysgenesis
Semicircular canals, 73
Semicircular ducts, 254–53
Sensorineural deafness, 146, 224, 232, 233, 272, 326, 329
  mild, 333, 335, 338–41
Sensory degeneration, 124–25
Sex differences and
  ear malformation, 312, 320
  microtia, 292
Shaker-with-syndactylism gene, 251
Sightless gene, 245–46, 259
Socioeconomic status, 320
Speech, 328–29; see also Language
Stapedial anomalies, 211–12
Stapedius muscle, 240
Statoconial deficiency syndrome, 136, 137
Statoconial membrane, 112, 115, 116 116, 119, 121, 124, 125, 129, 130

Stria vascularis, 83–101, 119, 255
Sudden infant death syndrome, 129
Surgery, 225, 226, 230–235

Tectorial membranes, 256, 260
Teratogens, 57–61
    and external ear malformation, 321–23, 324
    microtia, 295
    middle ear anomalies, 219–20, 240
    middle and external ear morphogenesis, 170–71, 175
Tetrapod
    evolution of, 148–53
    and middle ear development, 154–60
Thalidomide, 57, 200, 223
Thyroid, 255–57
Tilted-head mouse, 130
Tissue interactions, 172–74
Trisomy 18, 57, 211
Trisomy 13, 55, 73–75, 212
Tomography, 146; see also Polytomography
Toxicity, 93–95, 122–24
Trace elements, 126, 138; see also specific elements

Trauma, 125
Treacher Collins syndrome, 200–201, 209, 211–12, 227
Twirler gene, 252
Tympanic cavity, 211–12

Urinary tract malformation, 328–29
Usher syndrome, 51–54, 82
Utricle, 245, 249–51

Vascular insufficiency, 125
Vestibular
    abnormalities, 142–45, 247–48, 252, 259
    anomalies, 73, 78, 227, 235
    endolymph, 101

Waltzer-type gene, 249–50, 260
Weightlessness, 127

Xenopus laevis lateral line, 107–8
X-rays, 225–27, 233

Zigzag gene, 253
Zinc, 129, 133, 144, *See also* Trace elements

BOOKS PUBLISHED BY ALAN R. LISS, INC. FOR THE MARCH OF DIMES BIRTH DEFECTS FOUNDATION

BIRTH DEFECTS: ORIGINAL ARTICLE SERIES

1975 — Volume XI

No. 7 **Morphogenesis and Malformation of Face and Brain,** Daniel Bergsma and Jan Langman, *Editors*

1976 — Volume XII

No. 1 **Cancer and Genetics,** Daniel Bergsma, R. Neil Schimke, Robert L. Summitt, and David J. Harris, *Editors*

No. 3 **The Eye and Inborn Errors of Metabolism,** Daniel Bergsma, Anthony J. Bron and Edward Cotlier, *Editors*

No. 4 **Developmental Disabilities: Psychologic and Social Implications,** Daniel Bergsma and Ann E. Pulver, *Editors*

No. 5 **Cytogenetics, Environment and Malformation Syndromes,** Daniel Bergsma and R. Neil Schimke, *Editors*

No. 6 **Growth Problems and Clinical Advances,** Daniel Bergsma and R. Neil Schimke, *Editors*

No. 8 **Iron Metabolism and Thalassemia,** Daniel Bergsma, Anthony Cerami, Charles M. Peterson, and Joseph H. Graziano, *Editors*

1977 — Volume XIII

No. 1 **Morphogenesis and Malformation of the Limb,** Daniel Bergsma and Widukind Lenz, *Editors*

No. 2 **Morphogenesis and Malformation of the Genital System,** Richard J. Blandau and Daniel Bergsma, *Editors*

No. 3 **Annual Review of Birth Defects, 1976,** Daniel Bergsma and R. Brian Lowry, *Editors*
Proceedings of the 1976 Vancouver Birth Defects Conference. Published in 4 volumes:
    3A **Numerical Taxonomy of Birth Defects** *and* **Polygenic Disorders**
    3B **New Syndromes**
    3C **Natural History of Specific Birth Defects**
    3D **Embryology and Pathogenesis** *and* **Prenatal Diagnosis**

No. 5 **Urinary System Malformations in Children,** Daniel Bergsma and John W. Duckett, *Editors*

No. 6 **Trends and Teaching in Clinical Genetics,** Daniel Bergsma, Frederick Hecht, Gerald H. Prescott, and Joan H. Marks, *Editors*

1978 — Volume XIV

No. 1 **Genetic Effects on Aging,** Daniel Bergsma and David E. Harrison, *Editors*

No. 2 **The Molecular Basis of Cell-Cell Interaction,** Richard A. Lerner and Daniel Bergsma, *Editors*

No. 3   **The Genetics of Hand Malformations,** by Samia A. Temtamy and Victor A. McKusick
No. 5   **Neurochemical and Immunologic Components in Schizophrenia,** Daniel Bergsma and Allan L. Goldstein, *Editors*
No. 6   **Annual Review of Birth Defects, 1977,** Robert L. Summitt and Daniel Bergsma, *Editors*
Proceedings of the 1977 Memphis Birth Defects Conference. Published in 3 volumes:
- 6A   **Cell Surface Factors, Immune Deficiencies, Twin Studies**
- 6B   **Recent Advances** *and* **New Syndromes**
- 6C   **Sex Differentiation** *and* **Chromosomal Abnormalities**

No. 7   **Morphogenesis and Malformation of the Cardiovascular System,** Glenn C. Rosenquist and Daniel Bergsma, *Editors*

1979 — Volume XV

No. 1   **Sex Chromosome Aneuploidy: Prospective Studies on Children,** Arthur Robinson, Herbert A. Lubs, and Daniel Bergsma, *Editors*
No. 2   **Genetic Counseling: Facts, Values, and Norms,** Alexander M. Capron, Marc Lappé, Robert F. Murray, Jr., Tabitha M. Powledge, Sumner B. Twiss, and Daniel Bergsma, *Editors*
No. 3   **Recent Advances in the Developmental Biology of Central Nervous System Malformation,** Ntinos C. Myrianthopoulos and Daniel Bergsma, *Editors*
No. 4   **Continuous Transcutaneous Blood Gas Monitoring,** A. Huch, R. Huch, and J. Lucey, *Editors*
No. 5   **Annual Review of Birth Defects, 1978,** Proceedings of the 1978 San Francisco Birth Defects Conference. Published in 3 volumes:
- 5A   **Diagnostic Approaches to the Malformed Fetus, Abortus, Stillborn, and Deceased Newborn,** Mitchell S. Golbus and Bryan D. Hall, *Editors*
- 5B   **Penetrance and Variability in Malformation Syndromes,** James J. O'Donnell and Bryan D. Hall, *Editors*
- 5C   **Risks, Communication, and Decision Making in Genetic Counseling,** Charles J. Epstein, Cynthia J.R. Curry, Seymour Packman, Sanford Sherman, and Bryan D. Hall, *Editors*

No. 6   **Dermatoglyphics — Fifty Years Later,** Wladimir Wertelecki and Chris C. Plato, *Editors*
No. 7   **Newborn Behavioral Organization: Nursing Research and Implications,** Gene Cranston Anderson and Beverly Raff, *Editors*
No. 8   **Developmental Aspects of Craniofacial Dysmorphology,** Michael Melnick and Ronald Jorgenson, *Editors*
No. 9   **External Ear Malformations: Epidemiology, Genetics, and Natural History,** by Michael Melnick and Ntinos C. Myrianthopoulos